MAKING MULTIPLE BABIES

Fertility, Reproduction and Sexuality

GENERAL EDITORS:
Soraya Tremayne, Founding Director, Fertility and Reproduction Studies Group and Research Associate, Institute of Social and Cultural Anthropology, University of Oxford.
Marcia C. Inhorn, William K. Lanman, Jr. Professor of Anthropology and International Affairs, Yale University.
Philip Kreager, Director, Fertility and Reproduction Studies Group, and Research Associate, Institute of Social and Cultural Anthropology and Institute of Human Sciences, University of Oxford

Understanding the complex and multifaceted issue of human reproduction has been, and remains, of great interest both to academics and practitioners. This series includes studies by specialists in the field of social, cultural, medical and biological anthropology, medical demography, psychology, and development studies. Current debates and issues of global relevance on the changing dynamics of fertility, human reproduction, and sexuality are addressed.

Recent volumes:

Volume 52
Making Multiple Babies: Anticipatory Regimes of Assisted Reproduction
Chia-Ling Wu

Volume 51
Sexual Self-Fashioning: Iranian Dutch Narratives of Sexuality and Belonging
Rahil Roodsaz

Volume 50
Inconceivable Iran: To Reproduce or Not to Reproduce?
Soraya Tremayne

Volume 49
Good Enough Mothers: Practicing Nurture and Motherhood in Chiapas, Mexico
J.M. López

Volume 48
How Is a Man Supposed to Be a Man? Male Childlessness – a Life Course Disrupted
Robin A. Hadley

Volume 47
Waithood: Gender, Education, and Global Delays in Marriage and Childbearing
Edited by Marcia C. Inhorn and Nancy J. Smith-Hefner

Volume 46
Abortion in Post-revolutionary Tunisia: Politics, Medicine and Morality
Irene Maffi

Volume 45
Navigating Miscarriage: Social, Medical and Conceptual Perspectives
Edited by Susie Kilshaw and Katie Borg

Volume 44
Privileges of Birth: Constellations of Care, Myth and Race in South Africa
Jennifer J.M. Rogerson

Volume 43
Access to Assisted Reproductive Technologies: The Case of France and Belgium
Edited by Jennifer Merchant

For a full volume listing, please see the series page on our website:
http://www.berghahnbooks.com/series/fertility-reproduction-and-sexuality

MAKING MULTIPLE BABIES

ANTICIPATORY REGIMES OF ASSISTED REPRODUCTION

Chia-Ling Wu

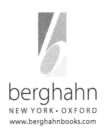

berghahn
NEW YORK · OXFORD
www.berghahnbooks.com

First published in 2023 by
Berghahn Books
www.berghahnbooks.com

Library of Congress Cataloging-in-Publication Data
Names: Wu, Chia-Ling, 1966- author.
Title: Making multiple babies : anticipatory regimes of assisted reproduction /
Chia-Ling Wu.
Description: [New York] : Berghahn Books, 2023. | Series: Fertility,
reproduction and sexuality ; volume 52 | Includes bibliographical
references and index.
Identifiers: LCCN 2022045290 (print) | LCCN 2022045291 (ebook) |
ISBN 9781800738522 (hardback) | ISBN 9781800738850 (open access
ebook)
Subjects: LCSH: Fertilization in vitro, Human. | Fertilization in vitro,
Human—Government policy. | Fertilization in vitro, Human—Moral and
ethical aspects. | Fertilization in vitro, Human—Social aspects.
Classification: LCC RG135 .W83 2023 (print) | LCC RG135 (ebook) |
DDC 618.1/780599—dc23/eng/20221122
LC record available at https://lccn.loc.gov/2022045290
LC ebook record available at https://lccn.loc.gov/2022045291

British Library Cataloguing in Publication Data
A catalogue record for this book is available from the British Library

ISBN 978-1-80073-852-2 hardback
ISBN 978-1-80073-885-0 open access ebook

https://doi.org/10.3167/9781800738522

This open access edition has been made available thanks to the support of the
National Taiwan University.

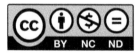

In loving memory of my father Hung-Pin Wu
and
To my mother Pi-Ying Yu

Contents

List of Illustrations   viii
Acknowledgments   xi
List of Abbreviations   xv

Introduction   1

Chapter 1. Multiple Embryo Transfer: Anticipating Success
           and Risk   23

Chapter 2. eSET: Anticipating New Success and
           Re-networking IVF   57

Chapter 3. When IVF Became a Nationalist Glory   88

Chapter 4. The Making of the World's Most Lenient
           Guideline   108

Chapter 5. Optimization within Disrupted Reproduction   129

Chapter 6. Women Encounter Fetal Reduction   153

Chapter 7. *An-Tai*: Active Maternal Body Work   172

Conclusion   187

References   196
Index   235

ILLUSTRATIONS

Figures

2.1. Anticipatory Governance of IVF: The Belgian Project.
   © Chia-Ling Wu   74

2.2. The JSOG Project. © Chia-Ling Wu   83

3.1. Dr. Masakuni Suzuki Showing the Photo of Japan's
   First IVF Baby at Tohoku University Hospital,
   October 1983. © Yomiuri News Photo Center
   (Yomiuri Shimbun)   93

3.2. The Celebratory Birthday Cake at the Discharge of
   "Baby Boy Chang," Taiwan's First IVF Baby, at Taipei
   Veterans Hospital, April 1985. Courtesy of Academia
   Historica.   94

3.3. Report on the Birth of Quadruplets at Chang-Gung
   Hospital in Taiwan, February 1988 Courtesy of Hope
   Information Technology Co. Ltd.   96

4.1. The Disconnected Patchworks of SET and the
   Dominance of MET in Taiwan, 2005–2020.
   © Chia-Ling Wu   125

Graphs

0.1. Twin Rate, Triplet + Rate, and Multiple Rate of Fresh
   Nondonor IVF and ICSI Transferred Cycles in 2011, in
   Selected Countries. © Chia-Ling Wu   6

0.2. Number of Women Giving Multiple Birth, the Multiple
   Birth Rate, and the Premature Birth Rate after IVF in
   Taiwan. © Chia-Ling Wu   17

2.1. NET by Selected Countries. © Chia-Ling Wu and Wei-
 Hong Chen　　82
2.2. Percentage of SET in All IVF Cycles for Selected
 Countries. © Chia-Ling Wu and Wei-Hong Chen　　84
3.1. The Distribution of NET by Selected Countries in 1998.
 © Chia-Ling Wu　　103
4.1. Taiwanese Government Statistics for 2002 Cited by
 Legislator Huang. © Chia-Ling Wu　　116
4.2. Percent (%) of Live Births by NET in Taiwan in 2003.
 © Chia-Ling Wu　　118
4.3. Trends of SET, Multiple Pregnancy, and Low
 Birthweight Babies in Taiwan, 1998–2019.
 © Chia-Ling Wu　　128
5.1. Changes in Year of First Marriage and Birth in Taiwan,
 1975–2020, Showing the Reproductive Trajectories of
 Four Interviewees. © Chia-Ling Wu　　131
5.2. Multiple Birth Rate of Live Birth Cycles with NET
 among Four Age Groups in Taiwan in 2019.
 © Chia-Ling Wu and Wei-Hong Chen　　140
6.1. Triplet (and Higher-Order) Births and the Triplet (and
 Higher-Order) Birth Rate per Thousand Deliveries in
 Taiwan, 1998–2019. © Chia-Ling Wu.　　158
7.1. Trends in Preterm Birth in Taiwan, 2004–2019.
 © Chia-Ling Wu　　175

Tables

1.1. Framing IVF Anticipation. © Chia-Ling Wu　　53
2.1. Guidelines on NET for Countries with and without
 Public Financing for IVF. © Chia-Ling Wu　　71
2.2. The Belgian Regulation on NET in IVF in 2003.
 © Chia-Ling Wu　　73
2.3. The JSOG Opinion on NET in IVF in 2008.
 © Chia-Ling Wu　　77
3.1. Anticipatory Governance of IVF in Japan and in
 Taiwan. © Chia-Ling Wu　　106
4.1. ASRM and TSRM Guidelines in 2004 and 2005.
 © Chia-Ling Wu　　113
4.2. TSRM Voluntary Guidelines in 2005, 2012, and
 2016. © Chia-Ling Wu　　119

4.3. ASRM 2017 Guideline on the Maximum Number of
     Embryos to Transfer. © Chia-Ling Wu   120
4.4. The Making of MET Regulation in Taiwan,
     1980s–2007. © Chia-Ling Wu.   127
5.1. Changes in Attitude toward Marriage and Parenthood
     in Taiwan, 1991–2015. © Chia-Ling Wu   143
5.2. Anticipation Trajectories with Different Optimizations
     within Disruptive Reproduction in Taiwan.
     © Chia-Ling Wu   149

ACKNOWLEDGMENTS

The conception of *Making Multiple Babies* took more than fifteen years, and the "anticipatory labor" I did to bring it to fruition was eased tremendously by the staunch support I received from members of many different communities. First of all, my heartful thanks go to all the women and their families, medical practitioners, research scientists, government officials, and activists who generously spent so much time and energy talking and working with me. Some of them kindly helped me conduct my fieldwork in various settings in Taiwan, Japan, and South Korea. For reasons of privacy, I cannot list individual names here. However, as I read pages and pages of interview transcription and fieldwork notes, all the struggles, reflection, tears, and smiles vividly emerge and remind me of the stern challenges people have gone through. Although this book cannot tell all the stories and solve all the puzzles, I hope it is at least a serious response to their difficult dilemmas and serves as a resource for some policy reforms.

My super-capable assistants have been my dream teammates on this long research journey. I am grateful for all the hard work done by Wei-Hong Chen, Hsin-Yi Hsieh, Yu-Hsiang Huang, Wen-Chyn Jwo, Yili Liao, Chun-Liang Liu, Nien-Yun Liu, Sam Robbins, Hinata Sakai, Denzel Chun-Kiu Tan, Yi-Fang Wang, Kuei-Yen Wu, and Chuan Yang. I learned so much from their insights on the topics of this book while carrying out the interviews, conducting the fieldwork, coding the news and policies, and making the figures and graphs. It was my privilege to work with these young talents. I am indebted to those who interpreted for me when I conducted the interviews in Japan: Wei-Rong Chang, Yu-Hsiang Huang, Yukiko Komiya, Jung-Yang Lin, Hinata Sakai, and Yuichi Tan. I was very lucky to have had Li-Ling Hsieh and Longta Wei kindly help me translate the Korean data and information. And I am particularly thankful to my full-time research assistant Wei-Hong Chen and

English-language copyeditor Victoria R. M. Scott, who have been
like caring midwives supporting me with their expertise and witty
encouragement both in refining the draft chapters and during the
final intensive stage of preparing the work for publication. As the
first readers of the manuscript, their insights and assurances were
very calming as the book grew in size.

Colleagues, students, and friends not only inspired but also nur-
tured me during the pregnancy of the book. I have been so fortu-
nate to receive so much wise and stimulating support from several
intellectual communities over for years. I would like to thank all
the staff, students, and colleagues at the Department of Sociology
at National Taiwan University, which is truly the most vibrant of
working environments; the community of science, technology, and
society (STS) in Taiwan as well as globally, whom I met through
working with the international journal *East Asian Science Technology
and Society*; the history of hygiene research group led by Angela Ki
Che Leung; the Global Asia Research Center, led by Pei-Chia Lan,
and the Women's and Gender Research Program at National Taiwan
University; and the community of feminist scholars and activists
from the Birth Reform Alliance in Taiwan. Some of the early findings of my study were presented at the various sociological, feminist, and STS conferences that I regularly attend. I thank all those
who commented on and engaged with the subject, who pushed me
to work further. Some portions of the book have appeared in the
journals *Social Science and Medicine*; *Taiwanese Sociology*; *East Asian
Science, Technology and Society*; and the *Taiwan Journal of Democracy*. I
thank all the editors and reviewers who contributed to making them
better. I also appreciate the participants at the various invited talks,
conferences, and workshops who gave me useful feedback.

Many wise doulas sustained me in making the delayed birth
of the book a learning and growing journey. At the stage of the
book proposal, I am indebted to Mei-Hua Chen, Adele Clarke,
Catelijin Coopmans, Yun Fan, Pei-Chia Lan, John Lie, Hsiang-lin
Sean Lei, Jen-der Lee, Stefan Timmermans, and Yen-Fen Tseng
for their constructive and spiritual guidance in helping *Making
Multiple Babies* reach embryonic book form. Many colleagues and
students provided me with useful research materials, answers to my
requests, and crucial comments and encouragement: Stine Willium
Adrian, Herng-dar Bih, Susan L. Burns, Shirai Chiaki, Dung-Sheng
Chen, Lingfang Cheng, Yawen Cheng, Yu-Ju Chien, Tasing Chiu,
Adele Clarke, John P. DiMoia, Chung-Yeh Deng, Chen-Lan Janet
Kuo, Jung Ok Ha, Ke-Hsien Huang, Yu-Hsun Huang, Yu-Ling

Huang, Ming-Sho Ho, Aya Homei, Minori Kokado, Jen-der Lee, Hsiang-lin Sean Lei, Holin Lin, Kuo-ming Lin, Wei-Ping Lin, Yi-Ping Lin, Hwa-Jen Liu, Jung-En John Liu, Osamu Ishihara, Eri Maeda, Karen M. McNamara, Izumi Nakayama, Wenmay Rei, Li-Wen Shih, Kuo-shien Su, Wen-Ching Sung, Fan-Tzu Tseng, Azumi Tsuge, Sharmila Rudrappa, Yukari Samba, Malissa Kay Shaw, Ayo Walhberg, Bettina Wahrig, Anne-Chie Wang, Jeffrey Weng, Andrea Whittaker, Hsiao-Wen Wong, Cherry Wu, Hideki Yui, and Shiao-min Yu. Several Japanese colleagues helped me conduct the fieldwork in Japan: *arigato gozaimashita* to Shirai Chiaki, Osamu Ishihara, Yukari Samba, and Azumi Tsuge. When we first met in 2005, the Korean scholar Jung Ok Ha asked me why Taiwan had the highest number of embryos transferred in IVF, prompting me to research this topic. I thank her for her inspiration and for helping me with the fieldwork conducted in Seoul. Also in Taiwan and Japan, the stimulating discussions that Yu-Ling Huang and I had whenever we did fieldwork together always made the research labor doubly rewarding. Deep appreciation, too, to those who commented on early draft chapters or on the whole manuscript, particularly Ting-She Chang, Shiau-Fang Chao, Wei-Hong Chen, Wei-Yun Chung, Chieh Hsu, Tsugn-Yi Michelle Huang, Chen-Lan Janet Kuo, Pei-Chia Lan, Hsiang-lin Sean Lei, Yen-Fen Tseng, and Chi-Mao Wang. I am also very lucky to work with Berghahn Books, which helped speed up publication of this long-overdue book project. I thank Marcia Inhorn and Soraya Tremayne, the editors of Berghahn's series on Fertility, Reproduction, and Sexuality, for their encouragement; editor Tom Bonnington for his helpful guidance; and the two anonymous reviewers for their most encouraging and constructive comments. It is most rewarding to have Kuo-Hsuan Ku, a paper-cutting artist from Taiwan, create the amazing artwork "The Dance of Life between Nature and Manipulation" for the cover image.

This long research project has been supported by grants from the Ministry of Science and Technology (102-2410-H-002-076-MY2, 104-2410-H-002-196-MY2, 106-2410-H-002-168-MY2) in Taiwan and by National Taiwan University. I am also grateful for the administrative and financial support extended by the College of Social Sciences and the Department of Sociology at National Taiwan University, especially the teaching load reduction program, which helped me better concentrate on writing this book, and the fundings to make open access of this book possible.

Finally, I would like to thank my family, friends, and hiking mates for all their support, love, care, and patience during the intensive writing days. My mentor Yen-Fen Tseng nurtures me on a daily basis with her food, fun, and wisdom. My beloved son Da-Rong and his cat Seventy always teach me how wonderful growth and adventure are. My brother Chia-Wei brings me endless laughter and eye-opening conversation. This book is dedicated to my late father, Hung-Pin Wu, and my mother, Pi-Yin Yu. Even before they had their first singleton, they began planting and tending a garden with love and devotion in anticipation of their little girl growing up happily and freely. I benefit from that flourishing garden even today.

Chia-Ling Wu
Department of Sociology, National Taiwan University

ABBREVIATIONS

ACOG	American College of Obstetrics and Gynecologists
AI	artificial intelligence
ART	assisted reproductive technology
ASRM	American Society for Reproductive Medicine
BESST	Birth Emphasizing a Successful Singleton at Term
BFS	British Fertility Society
CDC	Centers for Disease Control and Prevention (US)
Co-IVF	co–in vitro fertilization
CP	cerebral palsy
cp value	cost-performance ratio value
cSET	compulsory single-embryo transfer
CVS	chorionic villus sampling
DET	double embryo transfer
DI	donor insemination
EBM	evidence-based medicine
eDET	elective double-embryo transfer
EIM	European IVF-Monitoring (Programme/Consortium)
eSET	elective single-embryo transfer
ESHRE	European Society of Human Reproduction and Endocrinology
ET	embryo transfer

FINE   Fertility Information Network (Japan)

FINRRAGE   Feminist International Network for Resistance to
                Reproductive and Genetic Engineering

FSROC   Fertility Society of the Republic of China

GCPG   Genetic Counseling Professional Group

GIFT   gamete intrafallopian transfer

hCG   human chorionic gonadotrophin

HFE Act   Human Fertilisation and Embryology Act (1990, UK)

HFEA   Human Fertilisation and Embryology Authority (UK)

hMG   human menopausal gonadotrophin

ICMART   International Committee for Monitoring Assisted
                Reproductive Technologies

ICSI   intracytoplasmic sperm injection

IFFS   International Federation of Fertility Societies

iPS   induced pluripotent stem

ISLAT   Institute for Science, Law and Technology (Illinois
                Institute of Technology)

IUI   interuterine insemination

IVF   in vitro fertilization

IWGRAR   International Working Group for Registers on
                Assisted Reproduction (later transformed into
                ICMART)

JAOGMP   Japan Association of Obstetrics and Gynecology for
                Maternal Protection

JSOG   Japan Society of Obstetrics and Gynecology

KCl   potassium chloride

LH   luteinizing hormone

MET   multiple embryo transfer

MFPR   multifetal pregnancy reduction

MHB   Men Having Babies

NET	number of embryos transferred (or to transfer)
NGO	nongovernmental organization
NHI	National Health Insurance (Taiwan)
NHS	National Health Services (UK)
NICU	neonatal intensive care unit
NTU	National Taiwan University
OHSS	ovarian hyperstimulation syndrome
PBFT	Premature Baby Foundation of Taiwan
PCOS	polycystic ovary syndrome
PGS	preimplantation genetic screening
PGT-A	preimplantation genetic testing for aneuploidies
RCT	randomized clinical trials
ROC	Republic of China
ROPA	reception of oocytes from partners
SART	Society for Assisted Reproductive Technology
SET	single embryo transfer
SNU	Seoul National University
STD	socially transmitted disease
STS	science, technology, and society
TSRM	Taiwanese Society for Reproductive Medicine
TWL	Taiwan Women's Link
VLA	Voluntary Licensing Authority (UK)
WHO	World Health Organization
ZIFT	zygote intrafallopian transfer

INTRODUCTION

When the doctor congratulated Wen-Min on having success-fully conceived after a nine-year quest to do so, her first reaction was a pang of disappointment because the blood test indicated she was pregnant with *only* a singleton.[1] "I had made tremendous efforts for so long ... I responded to the doctor that I deserved to have twins," she told me in a café in Kaohsiung, Taiwan. Wen-Min regarded having twins as the ideal reward for her hard work. The list of her efforts to achieve pregnancy was indeed long: following traditional Chinese medicine, taking fertility drugs, trying nutrition supplements, exercising regularly, and even considering divorce so that her husband could have biological offspring with someone who did not have fertility problems. She remembered how tears had silently flowed down her cheeks during one painful procedure in the operation room, and how she had sworn that this would be her last attempt. And then she finally became pregnant.

With her seven-year-old triplets playing next to us, Wen-Min, a cheerful elementary school teaching assistant, resumed sharing the story of her reproductive journey with me. Yes, triplets! Neither a singleton nor twins. Although the blood test had shown a singleton pregnancy, at Wen-Min's next maternal checkup two fetal heartbeats had been detected, and when she was three months pregnant, the ultrasound images revealed three fetuses moving around. "I was shocked and speechless. The doctor did mention that taking fertility drugs for the insemination might increase the chance of twins, but I did not expect triplets." Wen-Min's emotional roller coaster continued. She was advised to undergo fetal reduction—the surgery to reduce one or two fetuses during pregnancy—but she decided not to do it after navigating through the complicated information and undergoing difficult moral struggle. Carrying triplets, she could hardly walk in the late stage of pregnancy and had to take sick leave from work to rest at home. The strategies to prevent preterm birth were not effective, so the triplets were born prematurely, staying in incubators for between twenty and forty days before going home. When I interviewed Wen-Min, her three boys were fooling around happily in the café, occasionally interrupting us to ask questions like, "What is fetal reduction?"

I first met Wen-Min at the annual gathering of triplet families in Tainan, Taiwan. These triplets were conceived in different ways—naturally, with the help of fertility drugs, or through multiple embryo transfer (MET) during in vitro fertilization (IVF). Their parents organized an annual get-together on the third Sunday in March, which they named the Day of Triplets. I served as a volunteer there several times, helping the parents arrange the outdoor picnic and games and activities for the kids. Being with so many lovely toddlers and children simply brightened me up. Wen-Min's three chubby little boys were so much fun to play with that I could not take my eyes off them. The annual group photo, full of smiles, was often published by the media the next day. Yet amid the joyful and noisy laughter, it was hard to ignore the fact that one or two kids were sitting in wheelchairs, and some were wearing glasses on their tiny faces. The gathering was also meant to support those families whose triplets had health problems, especially those meeting the most difficult health challenges. Wen-Min remembered helping to transport one child in a wheelchair up the stairs to another triplet event. The elevator did not work, so the mother carried the seriously disabled child while Wen-Min carried the wheelchair. "I was in tears; the mom had gone through so much hardship. She must have been burnt out." The child in the wheelchair had cerebral palsy (CP), the most serious mobility disease among newborns.

To my surprise, CP stood out as a key topic at the annual meeting of the Taiwanese Society for Reproductive Medicine (TSRM) in November 2021. "We have probably *created* several hundred CP families," Dr. Kuo-Kuang Lee said in his keynote speech at Taiwan's largest gathering of fertility experts and professionals. Attending TSRM meetings regularly, where participants present and discuss the most advanced research and technical breakthroughs, I seldom heard doctors self-position themselves as being the cause of any inadvertent harm. I could feel the uncomfortable silence of the audience. Dr. Lee asked the TSRM members to imagine the miserable life of a family caring for a child with serious CP for forty years. He stressed that it is the procedure of multiple embryo transfer during IVF, widely practiced in Taiwan to increase the success rate of pregnancy, that increases the prevalence of multiple pregnancy.

And when the number of fetuses doubles or triples, so do the risks to maternal and fetal health. Babies being born too early is the leading complication of multiple pregnancy. Some premature babies may die, some survive well, and some survive but with CP. The CP rate for singletons is roughly 0.2 percent, which rises to 1–2 percent for twins and 4–5 percent for triplets.[2] Based on the incidence rate, Dr. Lee estimated the extent to which Taiwan's IVF cycles have created CP kids. He warned that "there is no reason to increase the chances of CP for the sake of doing infertility treatment." With worrisome data and gloomy scenes of families coping with CP, Dr. Lee asked fertility experts to make a change.

The solution is single embryo transfer (SET). After presenting the international guidelines of countries such as Japan and the US, which recommend SET, Dr. Lee shared his own practice of SET and its clinical outcomes to reassure his listeners that SET can both maintain Taiwan's current pregnancy success rate and prevent the incidence of multiple pregnancy. The skills needed lie in both patient/client selection and embryo selection. Dr. Lee, a former TSRM president, empathized with how doctors may initially feel intimidated about practicing SET rather than MET, so, in order to encourage his fellow members, he revealed his own trajectory from doubting SET to routinely practicing it. His last slide was an image of the phrase "Just Do It," the famous motto of the Nike sports brand. I was laughing with all the others at this funny ending, even though deciding the number of embryos to transfer is certainly not a laughing matter. Does "Just Do It" effectively invite individual doctors to follow in Dr. Lee's footsteps? If not, is the TSRM going to issue a new guideline of SET for its members?

For both Wen-Min and Dr. Lee, making multiple babies is a journey of expecting new life and struggling with life-threatening danger. Having twins or triplets exemplifies the best reward for some and the worst nightmare for others. Assisted reproductive technologies (ARTs) bring hope for those who desire to become parents, yet it is exactly the use of medical intervention to maximize success that magnifies the risk of serious illness and even death. How have people handled the tension between the two? Through what mechanisms do they achieve the best possible future, and whose future is it? In this book I analyze the debates, struggles, and governance over the emergence since the 1980s of increasing numbers of multiple pregnancies/births created through ARTs, both in Taiwan and globally. For several decades this dilemma has haunted parents like Wen-Min, doctors like Dr. Lee, and scientists, activists, and policymakers around the world. It remains an urgent issue because making multiple babies has never been so prevalent in human history as it is today.

The World's Highest Twin Rate

Human beings are producing more twins, triplets, and quadruplets than ever before. Since the 1980s, the global twinning rate has increased by one-third (Monden, Pison, and Smits 2021). Triplets occur in natural conception around once in every ten thousand deliveries, yet by the late 1990s, due to ARTs, this rate had grown fourfold in countries such as England, Australia, and Singapore (Macfarlane and Blondel 2005; Umstad and Lancaster 2005; Imaizumi 2005). Such unprecedented growth in carrying and giving birth to more than one baby at one time is the result of the expansion of medically assisted conception. Some spectacular higher-order multiple births, defined as bearing three or more babies at once, remind us of the extremes that ARTs can create. The best-known case in recent years may be that of the so-called octomom Nadya Suleman of California, who gave birth to octuplets (eight children) conceived by implanting twelve embryos by IVF. Such unusual cases in the history of human reproduction have gradually become a staple on our living-room TV screens. *OutDaughtered*, the reality series on the TLC channel featuring an American family with quintuplet girls conceived due to the use of egg stimulation drugs as an infertility treatment, debuted in 2016. In 2021 I watched its new episode on a "Quints in Quarantine" broadcast in Taiwan. While it was quite amusing to see how the parents managed to homeschool the five sisters during the pandemic, I wondered whether making multiple babies has become normalized and even entertaining. Hopefully not.

Unlike the octuplets and quintuplets who are often reported as a special or even sensational occurrence, twins are common and have become the important target of monitoring. The International Committee for Monitoring Assisted Reproductive Technologies (ICMART)—the leading organization to collect and report worldwide ART data since the late 1990s to better understand the safety of ARTs—regarded the twin rate as one of the key indicators. Multiple pregnancy, including twin pregnancy, has been repeatedly presented as the leading complication of ARTs in medical literature. This may not be evident when we hear that the California octuplets happily celebrated their tenth birthday, or see the quintuplet girls complaining on TV about the boys in their kindergarten class. However, as I have just shown, parents and health professionals who have witnessed the care burden of CP kids may feel alert to the health statistics, which are very telling. It has long been recorded that multiple pregnancy brings serious high risk to both mothers and babies. Women face various complications in carrying multiples, and maternal mortality is higher for them than for expectant mothers who carry a singleton. Babies from multiple pregnancy tend to suffer from premature birth and low birthweight. The chances of having a serious disability such as CP, and of neonatal death, are almost ten times higher than for singletons.

The prevalence of ART-made twins and triplets is uneven around the world. According to the 2011 international data collected by the ICMART, "the highest twin rate from fresh nondonor IVF and ICSI [intracytoplasmic sperm injection] with at least 100 embryo transfers (in a country) was Taiwan at 35.4 percent and the lowest was Japan at 4.2 percent" (Adamson and Norman 2020: 681). In other words, more than one-third of women who became pregnant with "test-tube babies" with their own fresh eggs were bearing twins in Taiwan. If we count by number of babies rather than by number of mothers' deliveries, then twins make up more than half of the tens of thousands of test-tube babies born in Taiwan each year. Out of the sixty-five countries the ICMART surveyed, I selected twenty to demonstrate the variation (see graph 0.1). I present both the twin and the triplet rate per one hundred deliveries (as mothers' statistics), and the multiples rate per one hundred newborns (as babies' statistics). Taiwan stands at the top and Japan at the bottom. Why is the multiple birth rate more than 35 percent in Taiwan and near 30 percent in the US, but less than 5 percent in Japan and Sweden? How do we explain the differences? What has been the trajectory of confronting multiple birth in the world of assisted reproductive medicine?

ARTs such as IVF are not only the way to deal with infertility but also the main mechanism that creates twins, triplets, and those even greater multiple gestations that human beings would never experience without medical intervention. Since the birth of the first test-tube baby, Louise Brown, in 1978, an estimated eight million babies have been born through IVF to date (De Geyter 2018). At least two to three million of that global total are twins, and in some countries, like Taiwan, more than half are twins. This estimate does not include the results of the older ARTs, such as taking egg stimulation drugs with or without intrauterine insemination (IUI), which

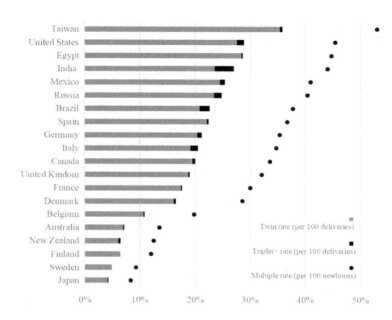

GRAPH 0.1. Twin Rate, Triplet + Rate, and Multiple Rate of Fresh
Nondonor IVF and ICSI Transferred Cycles in 2011, in Selected Countries.
Source: Adamson et al. 2018. © Chia-Ling Wu

Wen-Min went through. Because most of the national data reporting systems focus only on IVF, the multiple birth rate for other ARTs
is less often recorded (e.g., Bardis, Maruthini, and Balen 2005). Still,
whether old or new, ARTs are now almost the primary channel for
making twins.

Viewing multiple pregnancy and birth as the leading complication of ARTs, the international medical world has heatedly
debated this issue. Since the 1980s, leading medical journals on
ARTs, such as *Human Reproduction* and *Fertility and Sterility*, have
published numerous forums and research papers addressing this
leading complication. National and international organizations of
reproductive medicine have formed think tanks, offered advice, and
built guidelines to deal with this compelling issue. The most salient
effort to reduce the incidence of multiple pregnancy is to impose
regulations on the number of embryos transferred (NET). In 1990,
the UK and Germany passed laws to limit NET during IVF. In 1996,
Japan became the first country in East Asia to issue a guideline on
NET, through its medical society. In 2003, Belgium implemented a

subsidy program requiring single embryo transfer (SET) for those wished to receive financial support for infertility treatment from the state. In 2004, Italy attempted to limit the number of embryos by referendum. Still, some efforts work, and others prove to be in vain. When the president of the ICMART, David Adamson, gave an online talk to the TSRM members in 2021, he pointed out this pressing agenda that the world, certainly including Taiwan, needs to take seriously: "Why do higher multiple rates occur with ART? Why is there so much variation globally? What can we do about it?"

Surprisingly, however, compared with the enthusiasm for reducing multiple rates caused by ARTs in the field of reproductive medicine, there are few social studies of ARTs—primarily from the fields of medical sociology/anthropology, gender studies, and science, technology, and society (STS)—and existing studies do not often focus on the health risks of multiple pregnancy and birth. Marcia Inhorn and Daphna Birenbaum-Carmeli (2008) noticed that little research had been done on higher-order ART-assisted pregnancy and proposed it as one of the issues in need of more scrutiny from social studies of ARTs; this book intends to fill the gap. To date, most research has used multiple pregnancy and birth as an example to illustrate the risks that ARTs entail (e.g., Ferber, Marks, and Mackie 2020: 131–34; Franklin 1997: 110; Wu 2012), or as something of less concern than "mundane, day-to-day, adverse reaction" during the treatment of infertile women in Egypt (Inhorn 2003: 190). Risk is crucial, but making multiple babies encompasses more than that. For example, Charis Thompson (2005: 260–62) illustrates how implanting multiple embryos to increase success rates is one of the features of the health economy. Andrea Whittaker (2015: 30–31) shows how multiple birth is viewed positively in Thailand and is associated with how IVF has been viewed as a nationalist pride.

Following Marcia Inhorn's (2020) approach to "think with" the ARTs, I present how making multiple babies provides a powerful lens for examining how a society struggles with unruly technology. These struggles embrace the various domains of social life, including science and innovation, professional work and reflexivity, medical markets and regulation, family making and reproductive labor, and morality and responsibility. I also present in this book how these aspects are gendered. Even though social studies of ARTs to date have seldom engaged with multiple birth as their primary subject, their abundant literature has enriched our understanding of how ARTs and society have shaped each other and has created new theoretical and methodological tools. This has paved the way for this book to examine the clinical procedures of ARTs, the management of increasing multiple births, and women's lived experiences of conceiving and carrying multiples. In doing so, I use "anticipatory regimes" as the overarching framework for analyzing the world of making multiple babies.

Anticipatory Regimes:
Hope Technology or Risky Medicine?

Recent STS literature has been engaged with the conceptualization of anticipatory regimes—the apparatus of power regarding "thinking and living toward the future" (Adams, Murphy, and Clarke 2009: 246)—to capture how we live today. Three major components characterize anticipatory regimes: new knowledge making, being in time, and affective mobilization. The classic example might be climate change. Our increasingly sophisticated modeling foresees the disastrous outcomes, facilitating the urgency of intervention, as a title such as *Fight Global Warming Now* shows (McKibben 2007). Another important area of STS literature researches emerging knowledge-based technology. STS scholars examine how to evaluate and engage with new technoscience, showcasing nanotechnology (see the review of Guston 2014). Research on biomedicalization provides ample insights. Treatment of illness and disease has shifted toward the treatment of risk, being called *Risky Medicine* by Robert Aronowitz (2015). The quest to reduce fear and uncertainty has intensified, due both to our increased capacity to calculate probability and to the impetus of health enterprises to "riskize" the normal so as to create more "patients" (Clarke et al. 2010; Aronowitz 2015; F.-T. Tseng 2017). Anticipatory medicalization burgeons—to "medicalize a condition before a problem or condition has manifested" (Conrad and Waggoner 2017: 95). Even without showing any symptoms, people may feel at risk, gain the identity of being a patient, and begin an invasive treatment, such as the increasing use of mastectomy to reduce the risk of breast cancer (Basu et al. 2021). The sense of urgency to do something for a better future leads to the present action. Due to hope for the desired future or fear of the foreseeable crisis, the affective dimension is mobilized to shape a palpable sense that doing something now for the future is the crucial task.

Making Multiple Babies focuses on "anticipation" as the common thread running through the multifaceted levels of the assisted conception politics and controversy, from clinical innovation and regulation making to the lived experiences of women carrying multiples. Even though the social studies of assisted reproduction seldom adopt "anticipation" as their major concept, much literature has discussed it in different terms. Pioneering scientists *envision* medical break-throughs such as IVF and its ethical concerns (Johnson 2019). The IVF market seizes upon such "promissory capital" to reassure aspiring parents that the new medical intervention will succeed in bringing them new family members (Thompson 2005). Policymakers and activists *estimate* the benefit and cost of ARTs for regulatory reform (Wagner and Stephenson 1993). Infertile couples who regard the latest ARTs as "hope technology"—the answer to their quest to conceive a child—often meet uncertainty and difficulty during the procedure, and many attempts end in failure (Franklin 1997). Social egg freezing as women act upon "anticipating infertility" may best illustrate how their reproductive future is handled in advance (Martin 2010; Brown and Patrick 2018). These important arguments closely link with the literature of anticipation.

I argue that making multiple babies serves as an exemplary site of anticipatory practices. Multiple pregnancy caused by ARTs involves both sides of anticipation—success and failure, hope and risk. Some procedures of ARTs are intended not only to treat the infertility but also to create/increase the success rate. Multiple embryo transfer is the leading example. In the early 1980s, fertility experts found that the more embryos were transferred, the higher the success rate. The result is what Sarah Franklin (1997: 110) calls "too successful," namely, having twins and triplets that these women could not imagine conceiving at the outset. The action to increase the success rate also leads to increasing risk. How to work with this dilemma has been one of the toughest tasks in the world of assisted reproduction. The medical intervention that brings about the most desired outcome may cause the most horrible nightmare, and what do people do with that?

To analyze the anticipatory regimes of assisted reproduction, I highlight two dimensions: "anticipatory governance" and "anticipatory labor."

Anticipatory Governance

I define "anticipatory governance" as the totality of actors, rules, processes, and mechanisms concerned with what to think and how to act now for the future. Diverse stakeholders, evolving technoscience, and enrolling deep emotion are the most salient aspects of anticipatory governance. The conceptualization I build

here was inspired by the literature on technoscientific and reproductive governance from an STS perspective (see the reviews of
Fisher, Mahajan, and Mitcham 2006; Irvin 2008; Jasanoff 2005;
Morgan 2012; and Stilgoe, Owen, and Macnaghten 2013), including
works that directly use the same term "anticipatory governance"
(e.g., Barben et al. 2008; Guston 2014). David H. Guston (2014:
218) defines "anticipatory governance" as "a broad-based capacity
extended through society that can act on a variety of inputs to
manage emerging knowledge-based technologies while such management is still possible." His ideal type is the deliberate democracy
involving public participation in the development of nanotechnology, which has prompted both hope and concerns, much as ARTs
have. Echoing other participatory democracy governance in new
technology development, this approach focuses on the involvement
of the lay public in the stage of innovation. I would like to broaden
the concept to non-emerging technology, since after the "yes or no"
question about investment in promising new technology (to do IVF
or not), the "how" question (such as which embryos and how many
embryos) can still attract contention and engagement from policymakers, scientists and practitioners, and the lay public.[3] Compared
with traditional policy studies, "anticipatory governance" involves
more stakeholders to understand how technoscience is ruled. In
addition to formal policymakers such as the state, congress, experts,
and organized civic groups in the formal policy forum, it investigates
how practitioners, markets, activists, and laypeople shape the moral
landscape involving what to do with technoscience. Therefore, the
governing activities need to incorporate not only formal actions like
congressional debates, public hearings, and administrative negotiations but also informal ethical contentions in clinics and living
rooms. As I show in chapters 1–4, leading scientists, IVF experts,
medical societies, public health officials, pediatricians, feminists,
aspiring parents, civic groups, and media have all become involved
in discussing what to do about the increasing multiples created by
ARTs.

   To capture the contention among stakeholders, "framing"
becomes a useful starting point for examining how different actors
select a particular aspect of anticipation—fulfillment of reproductive
rights or disruption of social order, enhancement of clinical success
or entailment of health risk—to demand certain deeds. Professional
conflicts arise among IVF experts who target the clinical procedures,
pediatricians who handle the dying premature babies resulting from
multiple pregnancy, and public health officials who rely on the

benefit and risk models to evaluate the clinical procedures. Even among IVF experts, there has been much contention; some demand strict regulation by imposing guidelines, whereas others may challenge standardization that harms their professional autonomy. The particular dimension(s) of women, as the essential participants in ARTs, that can be selected for anticipatory attention reveal the spectrum of possible framings. Dimensions selected for highlighting in or erasure from the public forum range from women's strong desire for biological motherhood and the prevalence of complications during twin pregnancy, as well as women's ambivalence about fetal reduction, to the maternal death rate of carrying multiples. The power dynamics among the actors—medical professional dominance, statist intervention, and vibrant activism, including how strongly to put women's welfare in the center, for example—explains why certain framings prevail and others are ignored.

The global diversity of governing multiple pregnancy has been a puzzle, and may push us to generate some explanatory model. While evidence-based medicine and some international organizations such as the ICMART have promoted single embryo transfer (SET) as the most effective method to reduce multiple pregnancy caused by IVF, SET has not been adopted in all countries. The Nordic countries have taken the lead, the US has stayed behind, and Taiwan's law has permitted the transfer of as many as four embryos. This global variation has long been noted in social studies of ARTs. Earlier literature has shown that ART regulations are enormously diverse, comprising a sort of "legal mosaicism" (Pennings 2009), because they are formed in specific cultural, social, and political contexts. For example, scholars have examined how pronatalism in Israel (Kahn 2000; Birenbaum-Carmeli 2004), religion in the Muslim world (Inhorn 2006), political culture in Britain, Germany, and the US (Jasanoff 2005), and stories of ART use told in Demark and Sweden (Adrian 2010) have shaped ART governance. Therefore, both the contextual factors and stakeholder dynamics need to be brought in to explain the global variation.

In addition, I would like to highlight the importance of "national sociotechnical imaginaries," which Jasanoff and Kim (2009: 120) define as "collectively imagined forms of social life and social order reflected in the design and fulfillment of nation-specific scientific and/or technological projects." Counting the world's first and/or a nation's first test-tube baby or other ART-related technical breakthrough has been a trademark way for countries to vie with one another in the arena of global competition (Ferber, Marks, and

Mackie 2020). At the same time, the condemnation of such technologies as causing social chaos never slackens. Therefore, whether IVF is framed as a nationalist glory to achieve a medical breakthrough or as a procedure full of worries for unpredictable outcomes, it turns stakeholders' attention toward looking into the future.

Within the framings that prevail, much anticipatory work evolves. Adele Clarke (2016) convincingly asks us to look into the ample layers of "anticipatory work": hope work, abduction, and simplification. This offers useful guidance for investigating anticipatory governance with the details of the affective dimension (hope work), the back and forth of technoscience making and testing (abduction), and the implementation of effective strategy (simplification). Clarke's anticipatory work echoes the governance approach of regarding technoscience not only as a fixed object that needs to be governed but also as a development that is evolving along with the governance, such as generating new knowledge in order to meet the new requirements of regulation. In the world of assisted reproduction, faced with the increases in multiple pregnancy after IVF, medical societies and the state keep changing NET guidelines along with the innovation of skills, such as growing the embryo to the fifth day in the lab and doing genetic testing for the embryo quality. Fields such as epidemiology and health economics invent new indicators and estimates for the most cost-effective models. International and national professional societies such as the ICMART and the TSRM operate "midstream modulation of technology" to govern from within these professional communities (Fisher, Mahajan, and Mitcham 2006). Engagement of "responsible innovation"—"taking care of the future through collective stewardship of science and innovation in the present" (Stilgoe, Owen, and Macnaghten 2013: 1570)—is salient in the world of reproductive medicine, as seen in the efforts made by Dr. Lee, and also needs critical examination.

Anticipatory governance engages affection. What I would like to adjust in Clarke's hope work here is to incorporate fear work, or the work of revealing the false hope. In literature on new technologies, anticipation is often presented as an either/or situation—namely, either anticipating the good or anticipating the bad. Anticipating the terrible outcomes of climate change, genetic-related cancer, and Covid-19, we act at present to prevent the harmful consequences. Anticipating the good lives promised by vaccines, time machines, and nanotechnology, we invest and we hope, even knowing that counterarguments are certain to arise. Medically assisted reproduction stands out as a case of anticipating both the good and the bad. It is a brave new world in which scientists experiment with human biology, and it is a hopeful technology for people longing to conceive biologically related offspring. At the same time, "[these] treatments for infertility not only have the potential to alleviate infertility but also entail the risk of inducing multiple gestation pregnancies" (Callahan et al. 1994: 244). Expectant parents may regard multiple pregnancy as the best reward—or as shocking news. Practitioners may paper the walls of their offices with all the lovely photos of twins to be proud of, or they may confess—along with Dr. Peter Braude (2006: 3), who led a task force to tackle the problem of multiple birth in the UK—that "it saddens and frustrates me to see [that] so many children born after fertility treatments are denied the best start to life." How such sadness and frustration is an affective force to initiate new action is part of the investigation in researching anticipatory governance. Anticipatory governance is composed of the strong emotions tangled with the data, the formal and informal deliberations of stakeholders, and the devices to make changes for a better future.

Anticipatory Labor

I spotlight women's anticipatory labor as another important dimension of the anticipatory regimes of assisted reproduction. I define "anticipatory labor" in this context as women's thinking and doing, during conception, pregnancy, and childbirth, to achieve the better futures they perceive for their offspring. Again, making multiple babies is an illuminating site of anticipatory labor. First of all, making multiple babies epitomizes the maternal-fetal conflict during decision-making and care management. Achieving pregnancy through ARTs relies on many medical intrusions upon women's bodies. Women must face procedures such as multiple embryo transfer, which may increase the chances of success, but these also raise the question of the extent of health complications of carrying multiples. Some measures to save the mother or the babies from being exposed to risk often entail uneasy anxiety. Fetal reduction may best dramatize this tension. Although doctors advised Wen-Min to reduce one of the three fetuses so that she would carry twins rather than triplets—for better health outcomes for the mother and the remaining fetuses—she worried that the procedure might induce miscarriage, and also felt moral guilt toward the unborn child. Such conflict is best discussed in earlier literature on abortion and fetal surgery (e.g., Casper 1998; Hardacre 1997). I bring in the case of making multiple babies to join the work of these feminist scholars so as to highlight women's struggles between prioritizing their dearly desired children and their own welfare and to problematize how anticipatory regimes put women in such a situation.

Second, making multiple babies reveals the challenging hurdles at every stage of reproduction, from conception and pregnancy to the decision about fetal reduction, the possibility of miscarriage, and (highly likely premature) birth. For each stage, much feminist scholarship has made important arguments. For example, Sarah Franklin (1997) stresses the "reproductive labor" that women go through during the quest for conception to counter the spotlight that IVF experts receive (see also the discussion of embodiment in Inhorn 2003 and of alienation in Thompson 2005). Feminists' studies on pregnancy also emphasize the need to recognize the months of gestation women undergo, involving physical, emotional, and social relationship with the fetus(es) (Rothman 1989; Ivry 2009; Neiterman and Fox 2017; L.-W. Shih 2018). As Rothman (1989: 90) points out, "The pregnancy is thought of as a time of "expecting" for the mother—its future the only thing that counts, its present having meaning only for its future." To underscore the present, Caroline Gatrell (2011, 2013) has coined the term "maternal body work" to highlight the body work that employed pregnant women do in the workplace. I extend this maternal body work from the office to the household and also to medical clinics. As Almeling (2015) argues, the scholarship on reproduction tends to focus on a specific reproductive event (abortion, prenatal testing, or childbirth) rather than exploring reproduction as continuous processes instead (see also Ginsburg and Rapp 1995). Making multiple babies has the great potential to regard all the events involved (the quest for conception, the decision on fetal reduction, the security of a stable pregnancy) as a connected whole. Transferring a high number of embryos at the early stage so as to increase the success rate of clinical pregnancy may lead to hardships to prevent miscarriage at later stages. Making multiple babies thus helps reveal the different and related natures of anticipatory labor during assisted conception, fetal reduction, and pregnancy management.

Anticipatory labor uncovers what the major statistics of making multiple babies fail to present. Biomedical research tends to calculate multiple pregnancy success and risk in terms of live birth rate, or morbidity and mortality; to frame it within a risk/benefit model; and to apply quantitative methods for assessment. By presenting women's anticipatory labor behind and beyond the health statistics, *Making Multiple Babies* shows how laypeople interpret and act in light of success and failure, and therefore participate in the anticipatory regime of ARTs. Women and their families must face a continuum of desired outcomes and uncertain risks: physical, emotional, and social. I locate their navigation and negotiations within their specific sociocultural contexts, including their economic resources, social welfare, religious beliefs, and gender norms. In the context of Taiwan, the lack of public financing for most ARTs, combined with delayed parenthood due to late marriage and the gender division of childcare, may all contribute to women's framing of having multiples. Why Wen-Min decided to stop intrusive procedures at some point, preferred a twin pregnancy, and worried about carrying triplets needs to be considered within the broader social milieu of how reproduction, gender, and care are organized in Taiwan. Anticipatory labor highlights how women, under such constraints and with such opportunities, coordinate heterogeneous technical, legal, financial, emotional, ethical, political, and gender elements around hope and fear, life and death.

Global Comparison and the Case of Taiwan

Making Multiple Babies traces international regulatory debates, explores East Asian ART politics, and uses Taiwan as an extreme case in elaborating anticipatory ART regimes. Although most IVF ethnography and histories are nation based, there have been important efforts to compile global IVF history (e.g., Ferber, Marks, and Mackie 2020) and to advocate for a globally comparative approach (see the review and advocacy of Franklin and Inhorn 2016). With respect to making multiple babies, globally collective efforts to tackle the issue are evident, from the international surveys of IVF practices by the International Federation of Fertility Societies (IFFS) and the global data collection and reporting by the ICMART, already mentioned, to evidence-based medicine to find the causes and solutions to multiple pregnancy caused by IVF. Still, great global variety exists precisely because local complexity exists. Therefore, to fully understand how the world is facing the challenge of making multiple babies, I incorporate different levels of investigation—those of global governance, national comparison, and one exemplary case.

For anticipatory governance, I focus on the characteristic procedure involved: the number of embryos transferred (NET) during IVF. Although the use of fertility drugs also causes multiple pregnancy, the most visible exertion in anticipatory governance is how to handle NET. After the birth of the first test-tube baby in 1978, the world awaited the second, the third, and more, only to discover that it was not that easy. And when efficacy consisted not simply of one successful event but of an acceptable successful rate, IVF experts needed to find a new recipe for success. Multiple embryo transfer became the key to boosting success rates to meet the expectations of aspiring parents and the competitive IVF industry. When increasing multiple pregnancy came up, some tragic events and alarming statistics in Europe, Australia, and the US attracted risk framing from the state, reflexive expertise, international regulatory agency, and feminist activism. Number governance—imposing three, two, or just one embryo to transfer by law or by voluntary guideline—is never an easy battle. Data, new techniques, moral responsibility, money, and the joy and the tears of sorrow of the families involved all became entangled in considering the action of simplification (reducing to one embryo or two, or doing nothing). The global variation, as I discuss in chapters 1–2, including the diverse contrasts among East Asian countries, illustrates how local reproductive politics interact with global evidence-based medicine and policymaking.

Taiwan's rich and specific features contribute to this field both empirically and theoretically. The international statistics on ARTs, which first became available in 1998, reveal that Taiwan has the world's highest number of multiple embryos transferred during IVF, followed by the US and South Korea (IWGRAR 2002). In 2007, Taiwan enacted the Assisted Reproduction Act, limiting the number of embryos transferred to fewer than five—the most lenient globally. As an extreme case, Taiwan thus provides abundant data on the regulatory debates. As a latecomer to number governance, why did Taiwan generate such a permissive regulation, which has inevitably led to the highest multiple birth rate, as shown in graph 0.1? Taiwan's extreme case needs to be understood within the global context. In chapters 3–4, I propose three interrelated aspects that reveal the "global in the local" analytical framework based on the case of Taiwan: (1) the power relationships among stakeholders, (2) the selected global form that involved actors drew upon, and (3) the recontextualized assemblage made of local networks.

To illustrate the anticipatory labor involved, Taiwanese women's experiences provide rich data, somewhat sadly. The first test-tube baby was born in Taiwan in April 1985. IVF was widely welcomed as a medical breakthrough to treat infertility, limited to married couples through various stages of regulation. Before that, women in Taiwan already experienced higher chances of bearing mul-

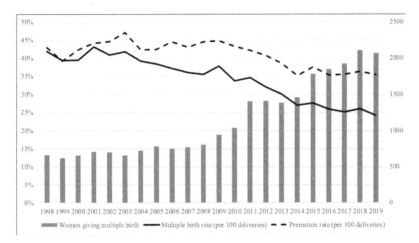

GRAPH 0.2. Number of Women Giving Multiple Birth, the Multiple Birth Rate, and the Premature Birth Rate after IVF in Taiwan. Sources: ROC Ministry of Health and Welfare 2021a, 2021b. © Chia-Ling Wu

tiples due to the use of egg stimulation drugs. After IVF became a medical option for conceiving children, it was largely privatized until very recently, so people needed to pay for IVF out of pocket. Still, the treatment cycles in Taiwan increased from seven thousand cycles in 1998 to forty-four thousand cycles in 2019, largely due to the increasing delayed parenthood (ROC Ministry of Health and Welfare 2021a). Since the 2000s, Taiwan has had one of the lowest fertility rates in the world and one of the highest average maternal age when first giving birth. Late parenthood drastically enhances the use of ARTs. After IVF became an option, the number of women experiencing multiple pregnancy due to IVF increased as well. Graph 0.2 shows that more and more women who used IVF gave birth to twins, triplets, and quadruplets. In 1998, the year that registry data first became available, it reveals that more than 40 percent of such women were pregnant with twins or more. The rate would have been higher if some of them had not used fetal reduction to reduce a higher-order multiple pregnancy. Although the multiple birth rate in Taiwan subsequently declined, the most recent data show that roughly one-fourth of women in Taiwan who undergo IVF still give birth to twins. This is far above some policy goals, such as less than 10 percent in the UK, or the 3 percent that Taiwan's neighbor Japan is proud of. Another warning sign is that around 40 percent of Taiwanese women pregnant through IVF give birth before the thirty-seventh week, most of them because of carrying multiples. Women face challenges hurdle by hurdle, from the great hope promised by ARTs to failure of embryo implantation, possible miscarriage induced by fetal reduction, and preterm birth due to multiple pregnancy. Taiwan has become a fruitful site for probing the strenuous anticipatory labor women must do at different reproductive stages.

Data and Methods

The research design of *Making Multiple Babies* was born of a broad project on IVF. I conducted four waves of research on IVF development in Taiwan and East Asian countries: in 1999–2001, 2006–8, 2010–12, and 2015–21. In 1999–2001 and 2006–8, I investigated the gender politics of ARTs in Taiwan, focusing on how the sociotechnical network of infertility treatment and sperm banking shaped the gender order there. In 2010–12 and 2015–21, I focused on the controversy of making multiple babies through ARTs and compared the governance among East Asian countries. The data I use most in this book come from those collected since 2010. However, the earlier research projects helped me build a long-term understanding of how stakeholders work and transform, as well as how the diverse users of ART include married heterosexual couples, single women, and lesbians and gays.

The data for this book include archival documents, participant observations, in-depth interviews, and registry statistics. Combing both archival data and fieldwork, I pursued a multisited ethnography to trace various stakeholders' governing and laboring activities. Data on the anticipatory governance to standardize and regulate embryo transfer include actors' testimony at public hearings, discussions during regulatory meetings, negotiating processes with other actors, opinions on media stories on the subject, related public education, and proposed solutions. Since regulating activities occur at different sites, I followed these activities through different methods. Archival data used to follow these activities include newsletters and reports of related organizations, conferences, academic research, and governmental documents and newspapers, globally and particularly in East Asian regions. Interviews and fieldwork were conducted in Taiwan, and a few in Japan and South Korea, including more than a hundred interviews with and observations of relevant actors, such as government officials, IVF specialists and technicians, NGO activists, legislators, journalists, and scholars of bioethics, about their practices of multiple embryo transfer and participation in policymaking. I attended the annual meetings and continuing education sessions of several medical societies in Taiwan over the past fifteen years and gave about twenty talks to practitioners in different institutions to exchange ideas. Cross-national comparison helps to identify how anticipatory governance differs. In this book, while the analysis of global governance is mainly based on archival data, I conducted interviews and fieldwork in Japan between 2015 and 2019, which became the second richest data source I have for analyzing anticipatory governance.

The data on anticipatory labor were mainly interviews with more than a hundred Taiwanese women (and a few men) who had experiences of assisted conception, fetal reduction, and/or multiple-fetus pregnancy from 1999 to 2021. I used a snowballing technique to find interviewees, and some came from support groups for parents of twins and triplets, or for lesbians, gays, and single women who often need to go abroad to use ARTs. I had two overlapping groups of interviewees. The first sample consists of women (and their families) using ARTs to achieve pregnancy, ranging from women such as Wen-Min, who turned out to have triplets through IUI, to others who withdrew after several attempts. This group's reproductive trajectories reveal their diverse anticipation trajectories toward becoming parents. I analyzed how the social, cultural, financial, and legal situations in Taiwan shaped their framing of ARTs and of making multiple babies. The second sample includes women carrying multiples, whether spontaneously or through ARTs. No matter whether women conceive multiple fetuses "naturally" or by IUI and IVF, they are categorized as a high-risk group, in contrast to those pregnant with a singleton. These women faced the decision of whether or not to undergo fetal reduction during their second or third month of pregnancy, and often made efforts to prevent premature birth in the second and third trimesters. Combining experiences from the two samples shows the different layers of anticipatory labor women undertake, from before conception through to the end of their nine-month pregnancy (or less, in many preterm cases).

Overview of the Book

The first part of *Making Multiple Babies* traces the global anticipatory governance of ARTs. Chapter 1 delineates the anticipatory practices of IVF since the 1970s, centering on the clinical procedure of multiple embryo transfer. I examine historically how different framing actors selected specific dimensions of anticipation and developed their anticipatory tools. In the early years of IVF development, a singular successful event—such as the birth of Louise Brown in the UK, or the birth any other nation's first test-tube baby—could meet the expectations of a medical breakthrough. A pioneering British team used women's "natural cycle" to take one egg during the menstrual cycle, develop one embryo in the lab, and achieve a successful pregnancy. Soon after such widely publicized events, leading IVF teams faced the new anticipation that they would be able create acceptable success rates for IVF clients, which led to multiple embryo transfer (MET) standing out as the solution. This solution led to a sharply increasing incidence of multiple pregnancies, bringing new health risks to both mothers and infants, criticized by feminists, public health experts, pediatricians, and some reflexive IVF doctors. Since the late 1980s, fetal reduction has been a new solution to manage the crisis, even though it has generated new physical, psychological, and moral troubles. The global IVF community therefore began to impose new guidelines to limit the number of embryos transferred, but there was no standardization: in 1998, for example, while the UK recommended that only two embryos be transferred, the US allowed as many as five.

Number governance arrived at the proposal of elective single-embryo transfer (eSET). Chapter 2 describes the anticipatory practices of eSET, proposed by some as the only effective solution to dealing with the skyrocketing incidence of multiple births after IVF. Some reflexive medical communities identified the misleadingly high clinical success rate of MET as creating "false hope," asserting instead that the "real hope" that expectant parents needed and deserved lay in the "take a healthy baby home" rate. I compare and contrast the ways Belgium and Japan have successfully built an eSET network by integrating the resources from the state, the medical societies, the international community, and civil society. The global anticipatory governance of IVF involves both international collective efforts and highly diverse national practices.

Chapter 3 discusses the anticipatory governance in Taiwan. Taiwan's first birth of a test-tube baby was widely perceived as a nationalist glory and hence restrained the state from rigorously supervising the medical community. I illustrate how the contrasting national sociotechnical imaginaries of emerging IVF between Taiwan (glory) and Japan (controversy) influenced the dominant dimension of anticipation in each of the two countries—namely, achieving success in Taiwan and preventing risk in Japan. In

Taiwan, it has been the protests from NGOs concerning the increasing numbers of premature babies caused by ARTs and the feminist health movement concerning maternal health that have framed multiple pregnancy as a public problem. Still, these critical framings of health risks have not led to an effective solution.

Chapter 4 analyzes the making of the world's most lenient guideline on number of embryos transferred (NET): Taiwan's "fewer than five" was stipulated in its Assisted Reproduction Act in 2007. Although some reflexive medical doctors, engaged governmental officials, and concerned activists have endeavored to restrict the clinical procedure of IVF in order to handle the health problems caused by making multiple babies, the disconnected patchwork of these efforts has led to an ineffective legal restriction to prevent the health risk that had been well discussed in the international community of reproductive medicine by the year 2000. This chapter shows that Taiwan, as a latecomer in regulating IVF, selected a certain global form to meet the local anticipation. Although some actors may select the governing practices in the UK, Japan, and the Nordic countries to model, it is the US that has become the crucial reference point for local Taiwanese medical societies to follow.

Making Multiple Babies then turns to exploring Taiwanese women's anticipatory labor—their various making and doing during conception and pregnancy to achieve their reproductive goals. I focus on how women pregnant with twins, triplets, or quadruplets calculate, act, and "live in preparation" (Clarke 2016: 90). Chapter 5 presents women's (and a few men's) optimization of ARTs for their reproductive ideals. Advanced medically assisted conception serves as the tool to reach one's best possible future, but people anticipate their futures differently. I sketch four trajectories of anticipation to demonstrate why people may perceive reaching multiple pregnancy as "winning the lottery," as efficient family building, as a worrisome outcome, or as fulfilling reproductive justice. The sociodemographic trend of late marriage, the gender order, and the social organization of reproductive care in Taiwan are the major contextual dimensions for understanding women's optimization within their disrupted reproduction.

Fetal reduction in the first trimester and bed rest after the second trimester are the two most challenging tasks when women carry multiples. Based on women's experiences in deciding to undergo fetal reduction and on pregnancy management to prevent premature birth, chapters 6 and 7 present women's anticipatory labor during pregnancy: navigating information, maternal body work, and negotiation between production and reproduction. Comparing different tasks and hurdles women meet at different reproductive stages, I elaborate upon how the responsibility to reach their reproductive goals gradually narrows down to women alone.

Making multiple babies is a crucial arena in which IVF experts, policymakers, activists, and aspiring parents advocate for their ideal futures and battle for various intervention options. In the conclusion, I return to the theoretical themes of anticipatory regimes and argue for the importance of thinking with anticipation. Based on the research findings, I offer some policy recommendations, especially for Taiwan, the country with the world's highest twin rate caused by ARTs.

Notes

1. All names are pseudonyms except those of public persons.
2. The prevalence of CP that Dr. Lee used was not based on the data in Taiwan but on textbook data based on studies in the UK and Australia in the 1980s and 1990s (see Pharoah 2005).
3. For example, the UK built one of the most complete regulations on IVF, viewing itself as the creator of the world's first test-tube baby (Jasanoff 2005). But the governance continues. To handle the high multiple birth rate after IVF treatment, an expert group composed of scientists, practitioners, and lay civic groups produced a report titled *One Child at a Time* (Braude 2006). The new guideline to promote elective single-embryo transfer (eSET) has become the important anticipatory governance since then.

Chapter 1

MULTIPLE EMBRYO TRANSFER
ANTICIPATING SUCCESS AND RISK

A t the news conference right after the birth of Louise Brown in 1978, Patrick Steptoe, the British gynecologist who played the key role in making the world's first test-tube baby, said that he believed that "several thousand women a year could *soon* be benefiting from it" (Beresford 1978, emphasis added). However, women did not benefit from IVF so quickly. The second live birth of IVF by the British team came a half year later. Robert Edwards, the IVF pioneer of the same team, knew well that the scientists' anticipation of success differed from that of patients:

> I think, frankly, that we have brought hope to thousands of couples and interest to millions of others watching from the sidelines. The new advances we have made in the treatment of infertility are perhaps *sufficient in themselves, sufficient reward for all our efforts.* We must *improve our success rate* though, make our work more realistic for the hundreds of patients on our waiting lists. (Edwards and Steptoe 1980: 185, emphasis added)

For scientists, the success of Louise Brown said it all, proving the efficacy of the invention and new theory, and confirming their scientific efforts. For such innovation, the single event of IVF pregnancy was worth reporting in the earliest breakthrough. However, what aspiring parents looked forward to was an acceptable success rate, so they could utilize the medical breakthrough to achieve their reproductive desire. What did these leading scientists and doctors do to meet the new expectation? One of the answers is multiple embryo transfer, the spotlight of this chapter.

This chapter delineates the trajectory of anticipatory practices in IVF since the late 1960s. Multiple embryo transfer emerged to meet the change of the expectations, but new risk—the increasing multiple pregnancy—came along with it. The foreknowledge of possible danger entailed a new dimension of anticipation to work with. Facing a combination of hope, success, and risk, more stakeholders joined the medical community to participate in framing certain aspects of anticipation (success, risk, and/or their balance) and come up with new conceptualizations, clinical practices, and regulations.

Scientists of ARTs are often key actors in providing "vanguard visions" (Hilgartner 2015). The following analysis begins by tracing the leading IVF experts' anticipatory practices—namely, their words, images, and graphs presented in science journals, science meetings, public hearings, and media communications—as well as how they designed their clinical practices, organized their medical societies, and announced their achievements. Other actors quickly enrolled to echo, challenge, confront, or transform the anticipation that swirled around IVF. Public health experts, feminists concerned about women's health, doctors who treated infertility with other methods, pediatricians who cared for the premature babies born through IVF, and governments concerned with the controversies all reframed and reconfigured the anticipation of IVF. It was not long before people realized that transforming this anticipation would require a wide-scale re-coordination of the IVF network.

Anticipating the World's First Success

Success in the Lab but Failure in Pregnancy

Hope was a prime ingredient from the very beginning. The pioneering British IVF team led by Robert Edwards had made various scientific breakthroughs since the late 1960s. Their success in the maturing of human oocytes in vitro was reported in the leading science journal *Nature* (Edwards, Bavister, and Steptoe 1969). At the press conference for this scientific breakthrough, Robert Edwards and Patrick Steptoe pointed out that the possible benefit was to help women with some type of infertility. This became headline news in major newspapers, and the keyword was "hope": "Test-Tube Fertility Hope for Women" (*The Times* 15 February 1969: 1), and "New Hope for Childless" (*The Guardian* 14 February 1969: 1).

Hope sprang, and concern rose. "The first successful fertilization of a human egg in a test tube" (*The Times* 15 February 1969: 8) triggered anxiety about the next step. One concern was the slow application of IVF to making babies. The media expected steady progress on the new ladder of success—from fertilization in the test tube to test-tube babies—but the gap seemed large. A *Guardian* article titled "Limitations on Test Tube Babies" (Ezard 1969) emphasized that, according to scientists, the breakthroughs to "allow childless women to have babies were 'a long long time ahead.'" The concern was about scientists' manipulation of life. The editorial comment "What Comes after Fertilization?" published in the same issue of *Nature*, was fully aware of the different public responses:

> These are not perverted men in white coats doing nasty experiments on human beings, but reasonable scientists carrying out perfectly justifiable research. One of the possible benefits of this research could be the treatment of some forms of infertility. ... There is, for work like this, a real need to explain that the purposes of scientists are very different from those of Big Brother in George Orwell's *1984*. Unless this is done, *there is a danger that the public may come to lose faith in science.* (Anonymous 1969: 613, emphasis added)

The "danger" of this work lay in scientists' new ways of controlling life, which had been heatedly debated in the early days of reproduction research in the UK as well as other parts of the world (Clarke 1988; Mulkay 1997).

With more scientific breakthroughs, expectations remained high. New findings continued to appear in *Nature*: fertilization of eggs with sperm, and cleavage in vitro (Edwards, Steptoe, and Purdy 1970); use of a laparoscope to retrieve preovulatory human oocytes (Steptoe and Edwards 1970); and embryos reaching the stage of blastocysts in culture in the lab (Steptoe, Edwards, and Purdy 1971). Scientists expressed their excitement about "magic culture fluid" and "beautiful blastocysts," as documented in Robert Edwards's memoirs (Edwards and Steptoe 1980). Hope mobilized the essential resources: more and more women volunteered to participate in this experiment. Frustration occurred when experiments failed. Joy abounded when the pioneering scientists saw the vibrant growth of embryos in the lab. By the mid-1970s, human embryos had been made in the lab for more than five years, but no woman had successfully become pregnant with an IVF baby. This became a continuous worry because the anticipation of success had long shifted focus from creating an embryo *outside* a woman's body (i.e., IVF) to implanting embryos *inside* the womb, leading to pregnancy and birth (i.e., a test-tube baby). The team repeatedly inserted one or more cleaving embryos into a woman's womb, but the in vitro fertilized embryos kept failing to implant in the uterine wall.[1] No "womb pregnancy" occurred; frustration lingered.

The team eventually figured out that the use of hormone drugs to stimulate egg production might be preventing successful implantation of the embryos. These IVF pioneers routinely used the egg stimulation drugs because they needed more eggs with which to create embryos in the lab for the goal of in vitro fertilization. Egg stimulation was also often used for the earlier infertility treatment method—artificial insemination—for women having problems producing an egg. In addition, with the use of hormone drugs, scientists could control the timing of ovulation, and hence fertility practitioners could manage the working time for the oocyte pickup procedure to fit in with the working time in the clinic, for "the use of fertility drugs also makes organization of the procedure considerably easier" (Wood and Westmore 1984: 60). Nevertheless, the use of hormone drugs such as human menopausal gonadotrophin (hMG) and human chorionic gonadotrophin (hCG) seemed to "*upset* the normal rhythm of the ovary and the uterus" (Edwards, Steptoe, and Purdy 1980: 743, emphasis added). To resume the rhythm, the team decided to try a new route: "back to nature" (Edwards and Steptoe 1980: 134–40).

Following the Natural Cycle

The new attempt in IVF was to follow a woman's natural menstrual cycle. This meant not using any egg stimulation drug, and hence being able to retrieve only the one egg that is naturally produced in each cycle. Scientists had not needed to consider the natural cycle when the anticipation was located in making embryos rather than in making babies. Now, with the anticipation changed to pregnancy, making the optimal womb environment was essential, and hence the idea of "back to nature" emerged. Still, retrieving the egg needed to be done. The new task was, then, to figure out when the ovulation happened, i.e., to observe the luteinizing hormone (LH) surge and retrieve the single egg at the right time. A Japanese product called Hi-Gonavis worked well to determine the timing by testing the urine. Dr. Steptoe, famous for his laparoscopy to retrieve eggs, had gained skill and confidence in retrieving them successfully, even when only one was available for fertilization.

Leslie Brown was their second patient to follow the natural cycle. During the retrieval procedure, her single egg was described as "beautiful" and "excellent" by the technicians (Edwards and Steptoe 1980: 148). According to Steptoe, when Leslie Brown awoke from the anesthetic, they had the following exchange (ibid.: 149):

> "Did you get an egg?" she asked me softly.
> "Yes, a very nice egg. You can go back to sleep."

The conversation focused on "an egg." It was a natural cycle, so only a single egg was retrieved. The single egg was inseminated by Mr. Brown's sperm in the lab for fertilization, bypassing Mrs. Brown's blocked fallopian tubes and making conception outside the body possible. When the embryo reached the eight-cell stage, Steptoe described it as "beautiful: eight rounded, perfect cells" (ibid.: 150). The single embryo was transferred to Leslie Brown's womb—the step of embryo transfer (ET). When the urine and blood samples showed the pregnancy hormones, Edwards later wrote: "My blood started racing" (ibid.: 154). Leslie Brown was pregnant. Unlike the pregnancies of the other three out of seventy-nine women who had volunteered for IVF, which had failed (Edwards, Steptoe, and Purdy 1980), Leslie was doing well.[2] The media eventually heard the news and started following the Browns as well as Oldham General Hospital.

Louise Joy Brown was born on July 25, 1978, receiving international attention. To reach this stage, scientists had to overcome many technical obstacles, including the capacity to retrieve an egg through laparoscopy, fertilize it in the lab, and implant the cleaving embryo into a woman's womb. The scientists themselves were well aware that what they had built was a sociotechnical network—the financial support for doing the research, the sources of experimental materials, the labor they had to devote, the participation of women, the ethical concerns, and the moral debates. No wonder Edwards referred to "the bumpy road" to IVF in the title of an autobiographical article (Edwards 2001) when he received the Laster Clinical Research Award in 2001; he later won the Nobel Prize in 2010.

The British success with the natural cycle inspired the Australian team, and Australia became globally recognized as the second country to succeed at an IVF birth.[3] The IVF team from Monash University in Melbourne "took up the bait and began routine natural cycles in most cases" (Leeton 2004: 496). Ian Johnston honestly stated that, "from a logistics point of view," using the induction drug had made it easier to "manipulate the actual time a woman is going to ovulate, to fit in with the normal pattern of a hospital," but that "we could never get a pregnancy going that way" (*The Canberra Times* 1980).

Therefore, they opted for the natural cycle. In Australia's earliest clinical report, its natural cycles led to two pregnancies as a result of fourteen embryo implantations (Lopata et al. 1980). Australia's first IVF birth in June 1980 was also a singleton. Linda Reed was called a "miracle mum," and Dr. Johnston, who delivered the baby, Candice Elizabeth Reed, told the media that "it's just miraculous!" (*The Australian Women's Weekly* 1980: 2).

Compared with other procedures, the "natural cycle" has seldom garnered media attention, even though it clearly played a crucial role in making the earliest IVF pregnancies possible.[4] As Steptoe noted: "It was a wonderful feeling to be so confident about our new approach (i.e., natural cycle). Despite the extra work, the inconvenience, I wished we had dispensed with the fertility drugs earlier" (Edwards and Steptoe 1980: 163). However, the "extra work," "inconvenience," and new anticipation of IVF soon made the natural cycle method outdated. Fertility drugs again dominated the procedure, mainly due to the new anticipation of a higher success rate.

Calculating the Success Rate

As these successful events attracted couples who suffered from infertility, the anticipation moved from proving the theory right to realizing a successful birth for the zealous scientists, and then to being able to "take baby home" for patients suffering infertility. In contrast to the miracle discourse on IVF in the media, the majority of cases failed. Infertile couples now faced the discrepancy between the hope springing from the scientific breakthrough and the reality that most of them could not yet take a baby home from the clinics. Sarah Franklin, based on her fieldwork in the late 1980s and early 1990s, characterized the gap "between the representation of IVF as a series of progressive stages and the experiences of the procedure (for the majority of couples) as a serial failure to progress" (1997: 10). The gap was even wider in the early 1980s.

After the 1980s, calculating the "success rate" became a new task for the leading IVF teams, starting with the pregnancy rate. IVF was organized within the medical team, so that the data showing performance were first presented by the clinics or hospitals. What the early scientists presented was the success of the procedures, such as the "rate of aspiration" and "rate of embryo transfer." These "success rates" were important for scientists in terms of measuring the perfection of their procedures, but they were not the most relevant measures "for the hundreds of patients on our waiting lists" whom Edwards kept in mind (Edwards and Steptoe 1980: 185). The "pregnancy rate" was therefore a new start in view of patients' anticipation.

Calculating the "pregnancy rate" itself was a luxury. It could be done only when the IVF team had more than one case for reaching pregnancy. In the earliest stage, the single event of pregnancy was worth reporting. For "pregnancy rate," the nominator was pregnancy, so it did not make sense to present it when it was only one. For the British team, the second successful test-tube baby was born in 1979, in another hospital. In the earliest report on the IVF "success rate" by the British team, only four pregnancies were achieved among seventy-nine women (Edwards, Steptoe and Purdy 1980); no percentage is presented, probably because it was far too low. The world-famous team recognized that "this method becomes a realistic approach to the alleviation of human infertility.... . The success rate of the method clearly needs to be improved" (ibid.: 751–52). And when the Australian team presented their first few successful cases, they were listed one by one, without being presented in the statistical form of a "rate" (see Lopata et al. 1980; Wood et al. 1985). Therefore, when Ian Johnston told the media in 1980 that "the success rate now was about 1 percent" (*The Canberra Times* 1980: 8), this was more a symbolic way of saying that the rate was very low than a statistic based on clinical data. As Australia's leading IVF expert, Johnston promised that, with more research, the success rate could reach 10–15 percent in the next two or three years.

The British team first presented a pregnancy rate as a percentage in *The Lancet* in 1983, five years after the birth of Louise Brown (Edwards and Steptoe 1983). More than twelve hundred women had been implanted with embryos over those five years, and the report showed that the "clinical pregnancy rate" had risen from 16.5 percent in the early period to 30 percent in 1983.[5] Although 30 percent sounds promising for this new technology, the method used to calculate the success rate requires some scrutiny. The denominator was embryo replacement, so only embryos that reached the stage of embryo transfer were counted. If the team had chosen "treatment cycle," defined as the start of egg stimulation, the rate would have been much lower. Those who began egg stimulation might not obtain any usable eggs. And those who did retrieve eggs might meet obstacles in making embryos in the lab. Therefore, those who had

embryos to transfer became the "survival group" who had passed
the hurdles in the previous stages. In addition, the nominator was
"clinical pregnancy," not "live birth." Since miscarriage happened
quite often after showing the sign of early pregnancy, many clinical
pregnancies might not reach the outcome of live birth that women
really anticipated. Public health experts challenged the usual way of
presenting success in the IVF community:

> Doctors have defined success as pregnancy. The infertile woman's
> goal is a healthy baby, and for her, a successful outcome is a live birth
> or preferably a "take-home" baby. Because of the high incidence of
> pregnancy loss after IVF, however, these two success rates are quite
> different. (Wagner and Stephenson 1993: 8)

The live birth rate per treatment cycle was what women needed
to know for their decision-making. Of all the combinations of nominators and denominators, the live birth rate per treatment cycle
would be the lowest, while the pioneering UK team's clinical pregnancy per embryo transfer would be the highest.

Some early survey data did show the live birth rate per treatment cycle as the different success rates and found that it was most
often under 10 percent. For example, a large survey conducted
in 1987, covering more than fifty thousand cycles from eighty-six
IVF centers in several countries, reported that the pregnancy rate
per treatment cycle was 11.6 percent and the live birth rate was
7.5 percent (Schenker 1993: 28). The gap between the pregnancy
rate and the live birth rate in the survey shows that the miscarriage
rate was high. The UK reported similar outcomes. The Voluntary
Licensing Authority showed that in 1986 the live birth rate per
treatment was 8.5 percent. Two doctors challenged this low rate as
"the most disappointing and expensive of all treatments" (Winston
and Margara 1987: 608). Recalculating published US data shows the
live birth rate per treatment cycle as 6.6 percent in 1985 and 7.8
percent in 1986.[6]

Whether 7.5 percent in the global survey, 7.8 percent in the US
data, or 8.5 percent in the UK, these success rates were perceived as
too low by the medical community. Finding a formula to increase
these rates was an urgent agenda item for the community of reproductive medicine because the new technology was leading to wide
expectation. The leading teams began to figure out the main factors.
And "multiple embryo transfer" quickly emerged as an essential
way to increase success.

Finding a Successful Formula:
Multiple Embryo Transfer

In the earliest days of IVF, only one embryo was available. The model of the "natural cycle" retrieved only one oocyte. In addition, the poor results of egg stimulation, fertilization, and embryo cleavage thus often led to only a single embryo being available for the treatment cycle. However, as various techniques improved, the embryo availability increased. IVF experts started to abandon natural cycle and test multiple embryo transfer. One reason was that following women's natural cycle was difficult under hospital management. For example, the Australian team stated that because different women ovulate at different times in their cycles, to follow every individual woman meant "literally working seven days a week, 24 hours a day" (*The Canberra Times* 8 December 1980: 8). Perhaps more importantly, most teams failed to achieve success with natural cycles and thus needed to try other methods (Seppala 1985).[7] More teams started to report successful cases by using egg stimulation drugs to obtain and transfer one or more embryos. For example, unlike in the UK and Australia, in the US the first test-tube baby was born with the use of a stimulation drug for retrieving more eggs.[8] Dr. Howard Jones told the media that "I think this day is a day of hope" (Cohn 1981). The team emphasized that with the egg stimulation procedure, it was easier for the medical staff to estimate the best time for implantation and be ready for the procedure (Sullivan 1981).

The leading British team and Australian team did not stick to the natural cycle either. When Robert Edwards and Patrick Steptoe reported their 833 cases between October 1980 and December 1982, following the "natural cycle" only accounted for 30 percent (Edwards and Steptoe 1983); the other practices used the egg stimulation drug clomiphene and human chorionic gonadotropin (hCG). With the increased possibility of retrieving eggs, leading to an increasing availability of fertilized embryos, doctors implanted two, three, or even four embryos into a woman's womb. Improvements followed in terms of drugs used, culture media, aspiration needles, catheters, ultrasound monitoring, and lab staff management. Multiple embryo transfer quickly became the common practice.

Doctors promptly found the pattern: the more embryos transferred during IVF, the greater the likelihood of pregnancy. The British team found: "Pregnancy was more likely ... when two embryos were replaced in the uterus, and even more so when three embryos, rather than one, were replaced after clomiphene/LH" (Edwards and Steptoe 1983: 1266). The success rate for single embryo transfer (SET) by natural cycle was 15 percent, but for some egg stimulation drugs with two or three embryos, the rates were over 30 percent. Around the same time, the American leaders also found a clear pattern that "the best chance to improve results for IVF lies in the ability to recruit more fertilizable eggs and to transfer more concepti per cycle" (Jones et al. 1983: 732). The Australian team documented 1,530 treatments from 1979 to 1983 and found that "the chance of pregnancy *increased dramatically* with the number of embryos transferred, ranging from 7.4 percent with one embryo to 28 percent with three" (Wood et al. 1984: 978-979, emphasis added). The Melbourne team did find many factors that might influence the results, including women's age, but concluded that "the most important factors *determining* pregnant rates were the number of oocytes collected and the number of embryos transferred" (Wood et al. 1985: 245, emphasis added). All the forerunners found that multiple embryo transfer was the magic factor to increase success. Some global surveys of IVF clinics (e.g., Henahan 1984; Seppala 1985) and national reporting data (e.g., Stanley and Webb 1993) all showed that the more embryos transferred, the higher the pregnancy rate.

The practice of transferring more embryos to increase the success rate became prevalent. For example, the US registry data show that in 1987 the most common number of embryos to transfer was four and that there were cases of implanting seven, eight, or nine embryos (Medical Research International and the Society of Assisted Reproductive Technology of the American Fertility Society 1989). The registry data from Australia and New Zealand also showed that 68 percent of the IVF pregnancies in 1985 resulted from implanting at least three embryos (Stanley and Webb 1993: 66). By 1985, single embryo transfer was even questioned by the Australian team, because its low success rate might cause risk and harm to patients: "Are the costs and risks to the patient of laparoscopy, general anesthesia, and hospital care justified if only one embryo is transferred, the success rate being only one third of that when two or more embryos are transferred?" (Wood et al. 1985: 250). Success rates needed to be high to compensate for all the costs and health risks borne by the aspiring parents. Multiple embryo transfer became the solution, with the interests of women in mind. However, it soon became apparent that what the success formula brought was not simply pregnancy but multiple pregnancy.

The World's First Test-Tube Twins, Triplets, Quadruplets, and Quintuplets

"Test-Tube Twin Has Heart Surgery" was the headline on the front page of *The Canberra Times* on 7 June 1981. The baby, named Stephen, was one of the world's first IVF twins, born in Melbourne's Queen Victoria Hospital, Australia. Stephen and his twin sister Amanda were the world's seventh and eighth test-tube babies. At the press conference, doctors emphasized that they were not identical twins because two separate embryos had been transferred to their mother's womb. The twins had been born three to four weeks prematurely, the common situations for twins. Amanda, weighing just over five pounds, was categorized as low birthweight but reported to be very healthy. Stephen was "born blue" and sent to the incubation ward for his "serious conditions." He had heart surgery later on the day of his birth, and gradually improved. With all the joy of a miracle by IVF, the Australian IVF twins' "serious condition" nevertheless marked the beginning of a new challenge that IVF had to confront: multiple pregnancy and multiple birth.

This was not new for an infertility treatment. Since the late 1950s, the increasing use of egg stimulation drugs, particularly for women having problems with ovulation, had led to more frequent multiple pregnancy and multiple birth. In a detailed review, it was found that the incidence of multiple pregnancy caused by different types of ovulation-inducing drugs ranged from 2 percent to 54 percent in more than twenty-five medical reports between 1958 and 1980 (Schenker, Rarkoni, and Granat 1981). The review article listed eighteen case reports of "high plural births," from quadruplets, quintuplets, and sextuplets to septuplets, octuplets, and nonuplets, mostly with the use of hMG and hCG. These statistics reports and cases came from the UK, the US, Australia, New Zealand, Germany, Israel, and so on. Some cases were heartbreaking, such as that of septuplets in the US who all died within twelve hours of being born. Some cases were called a "success," such as the "successful quintuplet pregnancy" described in a *Lancet* article presenting the care of a woman pregnant with five fetuses in New Zealand (Liggins and Ibbertson 1966). Before the use of IVF, the medical community had already faced these adverse outcomes of infertility treatment.

The "high plural births" caused by these ovary-stimulating drugs created a media spectacle. Doctors from the University College Hospital in London gave a detailed report in the *British Medical*

Journal on a sextuplet (six fetuses) pregnancy and birth in 1969; in addition to the treatment, pregnancy, and delivery, the report recorded medical practitioners' efforts to "maintain the secrecy necessary to protect the patient from publicity and harassment" (Lachelin et al. 1972: 789). The strategy was to tell other patients and most of the staff that triplets were expected. At the end of the report, the doctors claim to have been "successful in avoiding publicity before delivery," though they nevertheless faced several hundred journalists afterward and had to handle forced entry into the obstetric hospital by some reporters (ibid.: 790). The reports published in the leading English medical journals seldom included cases from East Asia, which had some sensational stories of multiple births as well. For example, in 1976, the birth of quintuplets in Kagoshima was widely reported throughout Japan (*Yomiuri Shimbun* 2 February 1976: 19). The mother had been given an ovary-stimulating drug, which led to the births of two boys and three girls. Although there were some concerns about the side effects of the new infertility treatment at the time, most media reports followed the story with curiosity and joy.

The multiples created by multiple embryo transfer prompted a new wave of attention to IVF. More and more cases of the world's or a given country's first IVF twins, triplets, quadruplets, and quintuplets started to emerge. The world's first IVF triplets were born in Australia in June 1983. The family named one of the babies "Chenara," after their physician Dr. Chen, to show their appreciation. The media portrayed a happy story:

> Mrs. Guare named first-born Chenara Jade Elizabeth after Dr. Chen. "I felt nothing but joy, I saw them all born," she said, beaming at her triplets.[9]

The world's first IVF quadruplets were also born in Australia, in January 1984. The medical team had implanted four embryos into the mother's womb. All four newborns weighed less than five pounds each, but were reported to be healthy and needed no intensive care. The world's first IVF quintuplets were born in London in March 1986. Every "successful case" of first IVF multiples made headlines. In addition to world records, national records were highlighted and reported by the media. For example, the UK's first quadruplets were born in May 1984, due to retrieval of four eggs, leading to four embryos, resulting in four babies. By 1985, when South Korea announced its first successful IVF case, it was twins.

The team from Seoul National University had adopted the American model of using egg stimulation drugs and implanting more than one embryo when available. The twins, a baby boy and a baby girl, each weighed more than twenty-five hundred grams (five pounds and eight ounces), the cutoff for low birthweight. The doctor announced to the media that they were very healthy (*Chosun Ilbo* 13 October 1985: 1). Indeed, quite a few healthy IVF twins came to the world, bringing joy to their parents and other family members.

As Robert Edwards reported, dealing with multiple pregnancy was "a routine aspect of our work" (quoted in Price 1988: 161). The first effort to collect global data in 1984 already noted that "an impression was that, in the hands of experienced teams, replacement of multiple embryos increased the number of multiple pregnancy" (Seppala 1985: 562). This "impression" turned into statistics as more data were collected. One global data collection done in 1985 showed that of 1,195 IVF births, 19.3 percent were multiple births (Cohen, Mayaux, and Guihard-Moscato 1988). The national data from Australia in 1986 showed that 25 percent of IVF pregnancies were multiple pregnancies, and that among them, 15 percent were triplets or quadruplets (Bartels 1993: 79). In 1988, out of all the IVF cycles, Australia, France, and the UK had around 20 percent that resulted in twin pregnancies and 3–5 percent that led to triplet or higher-order births (Cohen 1991). One decade after the birth of the first test-tube baby, about one in five women who became pregnant through IVF procedures bore two or more babies. Multiple pregnancy has long been viewed as high risk for mothers and babies. Solving the problems of infertility involved facing the new worry of conceiving too many babies.

Confronting Hazard

The consequences of multiple pregnancy and birth were worrisome. Early global data on IVF outcomes showed the high miscarriage rate, premature delivery, and low birthweight (i.e., less than twenty-five hundred grams), mostly resulting from multiple pregnancy (Cohen, Mayaux, and Guihard-Moscato 1988). National registry data documented that prematurity, low birth rates, and neonatal and perinatal mortality for twins, triplets, and higher-order births were much higher than in the general population. For example, data from Australia, France, and the UK showed that 55–60 percent of twins and 95 percent of triplets (and higher-order multiples) weighed less than twenty-five hundred grams (Cohen 1991: Table VII). Some IVF twins were born healthy and full term, but some needed to be sent directly to incubators for intensive care.

The adverse outcomes of IVF had already begun to gain attention when IVF procedures became prevalent, and among them the health risks of multiple pregnancy and birth were not a new issue for the medical community.[10] Previous research, both of natural and assisted multiple pregnancy/birth, had revealed its health consequences. Multiple embryo transfer was added to the list of fertility treatments that had dramatically increased the incidence of multiple births since the 1980s (Botting, Macfarlane, and Price 1990). Women pregnant with multiples have increased incidence of toxemia, bleeding, hypertension, diabetes, obstetric hemorrhage, and maternal mortality (Wennerholm 2009). Psychological effects became another dimension for infertility treatment in general, and for multiple pregnancy in particular. Early research systematically showed that the contrast between the high expectation of medical breakthrough and the low success rate led to mental suffering for many women and their families (Johnston, Shaw, and Bird 1987; Koch 1993). The media seldom presented cases of failure, and women and their families who underwent the treatments felt strong distress about the uncertainty of every procedure (Johnston, Shaw, and Bird 1987). IVF twins and triplets had a higher than usual probability of needing to be admitted to a neonatal intensive care unit (NICU) and often required extra care after being discharged from the hospital. The worry and burden of care often created distress for the babies' mothers, in contrast to the "miracle" image presented in the mainstream media.

Newborn multiples suffered various adverse health outcomes and began to gain much visibility. Photos of tiny babies struggling in incubators created a strong impression of facing death and saving life. All the textbooks agreed that "multiple birth babies have much higher rates of perinatal mortality, neonatal morbidity and long-term neurological impairment than singletons" (Wennerholm 2009: 13). Being "very low birthweight," under fifteen hundred grams, was a particularly serious warning sign. The early data in Australia showed that 11.6 percent of IVF babies were very low birthweight, compared to 1 percent of all babies (Bartels 1993).

Medical practitioners who worked in NICUs were sensitive to the increasing number of IVF babies in their care. Neonatologists in a Paris hospital found that the numbers of IVF babies admitted to their NICU increased from 7 percent in 1987 to 17 percent in 1989, therefore demanding more labor and resources for neonatal care (Relier, Couchard, and Huon 1993). Some multiple births, such as that of the Halton septuplets born in the UK in 1987, none of whom survived their first month after birth ("Seventh Septuplet Dies" 1987), raised awareness of the suffering of their families as well as of the burden of neonatal care. Professional conflicts between neonatologists and IVF experts often intensified the controversy: IVF specialists had made such pregnancies possible, yet it was the staff of NICUs who cared for the tiny infants. In the UK, it was complaints from neonatologists about IVF creating more very high-risk babies that helped speed up the regulation of ART practices (Price 1990).

It was not only the burden of care (for mothers, family members, and health practitioners) but also the cost of that care that alarmed many policymakers. Women with multiple pregnancy were identified to be at high risk, so antenatal visits, laboratory tests, ultrasounds, medical drugs, and care from medical staff all increased greatly. The twins and triplets often need intensive neonatal care, which is costly. A study in the UK in the mid-1980s showed that the average National Health Services (NHS) cost for the pregnancy/birth/neonatal care of twins was five thousand pounds, and for triplets it was twelve thousand pounds—60 percent of which was, in both cases, for neonatal care (Mugford 1990).[11] At the beginning of the IVF era, patients paid the costs out of their own pockets. Part of the reason the medical community wanted to increase the success rate by using multiple embryo transfer was to reduce out-of-pocket expenses for infertile couples who longed to become parents. However, multiple embryo transfer led to the even higher costs of caring for multiple babies. In some countries, such as the UK, the cost was often absorbed by public medical resources, but in other countries it became a crushing financial burden for individual families.

Morbidity, mortality, burden of care, and financial cost were the main concerns for the increasing numbers of multiples. Some doctors downplayed the financial cost and emphasized the risks of health problems and even death:

> The practice of reproductive treatment is associated with a wide range of *complications* that may *endanger* the patient.... . Many of us consider cost as an important factor of assisted reproduction practices. We believe that the main problem is not cost but the complications of this mode of treatment, which may result in *permanent damage* or *even death* to patients who otherwise are healthy. (Schenker and Ezra 1994: 418, emphasis added)

The anticipation of IVF thus gradually shifted from an expectation of success and a "miracle" to an awareness of hazard and risk. For those who focused on anticipating adverse outcomes, one radical new proposal included abandoning the technology.

Eliminating the Hazard:
Anticipatory De-medicalization

In addition to some doctors who reflected on the risk of ARTs, public health experts and feminists addressed these adverse outcomes and offered some new solutions. Some renowned public health experts—such as the World Health Organization (WHO) representative in the Regional Office for Europe, Marsden G. Wagner, and his co-researchers—asked to "shift from the individual focus of the clinical model to the group approach of the public health model" (Wagner and Stephenson 1993: 10; see also Wagner and St. Clair 1989). Feminists were another group to fundamentally challenge the use of ARTs in general, and IVF in particular, if it created unnecessary danger for women and their babies. In what follows, I highlight the feminists' criticism to present the anticipatory practices of the whole spectrum.

Since the 1970s, the feminist movement had been cautious about the medicalization of reproduction, including pregnancy and childbirth. The "medicalization of infertility" became an important touchstone for feminists offering critical perspectives and action in the face of admiration of the scientific breakthrough as the solution to women's childlessness. The Feminist International Network for Resistance to Reproductive and Genetic Engineering (FINRRAGE), established in 1984 by activists from Australia, the UK, and the US, voiced its concerns loudly and widely (for the history of FINRRAGE and its feminist standpoints, see Mottier 2013). For example, Janice G. Raymond contended that "much of technological reproduction is brutality with a therapeutic face" (Raymond 1993: xix). Her long list of "medical violence against women" includes ovarian hyperstimulation syndrome (OHSS), fetal reduction, maternal death, multiple pregnancy, and much more. Raymond used the birth of the Frustaci septuplets (seven babies), born in Los Angeles in 1985, as a textbook case of how the dangerous fertility drug could go wrong. Four of the infants died within months of their birth, and three survived with serious disabilities. The family sued the fertility center for malpractice and settled for six million dollars.

In addition to the health risks, both public health and feminist perspectives tried to highlight the following factors: (1) the efficacy of the treatments, and (2) the social causes of infertility. First of all, efficacy was the key measure for public health officials and feminists who were assessing ARTs. Feminist journalists Gena Corea and Susan Ince reported in 1985 that IVF clinics and hospitals in the US manipulated the reporting of success rates (Corea 1988). Half of the fifty-four IVF clinics they surveyed had not yet had a single live birth, despite claiming that they were providing IVF services. Others had produced only a few babies, and these often used implantation rate or chemical pregnancy rate, not live birth rate, as their measure of success to boost the accomplishment of ARTs. Scholars also criticized the calculation of success rates, pointing out that when a clinical pregnancy was defined as a success, possible later spontaneous abortion, stillbirth, or preterm birth could all be counted as success (Stanley and Webb 1993). Many raised the fact that IVF had not gone through randomized clinical trials (RCT) like other medical procedures before being put into wide use, so that its efficacy and safety were in question (Price 1990). Efficacy was also related to another competing "treatment": after surgery to make their fallopian tubes work again, women could regain the reproductive capacity to become pregnant. Early IVF experts may have presented cases of women who had lost their fallopian tubes completely, such as Leslie Brown, to justify the need to practice IVF to produce babies. However, as the indications to use IVF widened, debate arose as to whether those who underwent IVF would or could have become pregnant through this other long-available technology. In other words, other medical options, such as tubal surgery, could reinstate some couples' capacity to achieve conception.

The practice of multiple embryo transfer during IVF highlighted the intersection of efficacy and safety. Increasing the number of embryos meant increasing the success rate. However, the very procedure used to boost efficacy raised the new problem of safety. For the feminists, all the adverse outcomes were not necessarily evil but did constitute an iatrogenic burden for women. "Multiple pregnancy" was one of the conditions that demonstrated the suffering that women had to go through, and the concept of "iatrogenic multiple pregnancy"—i.e., physician-made complications—questioned the use of the MET procedure to increase success rates at the expense of women and children's safety.

Second, feminists highlighted the social causes of women's troubles to argue that their exposure to these hazards was not necessary. It is the social norm of ideal motherhood within heterosexual marriage that may pressure women to seek infertility treatment. Alternative situations such as adoption or voluntary childlessness were underrepresented both in the media and in self-help books (Franklin 1990; Laborie 1993). Some public health experts offered similar viewpoints. With the low success rate and high adverse health outcomes of multiple embryo transfer, Wagner and Stephenson offered social options such as adoption, foster care, and childlessness as measures to deal with infertility (Stephenson and Wagner 1993: 12). Furthermore, the top priorities should be preventing the causes of infertility—including sexually transmitted diseases (STDs), which often led to infertility for both men and women—and also enhancing general reproductive healthcare.

Therefore, the risk to women's lives, low success rates, and indignity for women undergoing such an invasive infertility treatment led feminists and women's health activists to view ARTs as "violence against women" (Raymond 1993: xix). Given the strong criticism of the potential harm that IVF brought, one proposal was to abolish the new reproductive technology:

> I contend that the best legal approach to reproductive technologies and contracts that violate women's bodily integrity—such as IVF and its offshoots, egg donation, sex predetermination, fetal reduction …— is *abolition*, not regulation. The starting point for the protection of women's bodily integrity is the abolition of technological reproduction by penalizing its vendors and purveyors and by *preventing women from being technologically ravaged*. (Raymond 1993: 208, emphasis added)

I call this proposal of "abolition" a matter of "anticipatory de-medicalization." Peter Conrad and Miranda Waggoner see "anticipatory medicalization" as "defining and/or treating a putative potential problem with medical intervention because it may pose a risk in the future" (Conrad and Waggoner 2017: 98). The exemplar case is preconception care to "reduce the (future) risk of adverse pregnancy and birth outcomes, such as preterm birth, low birth weight, and infant mortality" (ibid.: 99; see also Waggoner 2017). For exactly the same goal, other measures, such as "abolition" of ART itself, were proposed by some radical feminists such as Janice G. Raymond. Such advocacy can be called "anticipatory de-medicalization," namely, defining the problem as nonmedical or even as being caused by medicine itself, and treating this problem with elimination of the medical intervention because it may pose a risk in the future.

Balancing Benefit and Risk

The abolition proposal was not adopted in reality; rather, it was the risk management model that commanded the world of reproductive medicine. Raymond insisted on the abolition model and remained cautious about the risk management model on the grounds that it is "the kind of regulatory legislation [that] intends only to *manage the risks* to women, *not to eliminate those risks*" (Raymond 1993: 208, emphasis added). In a broader context, the discourse and model of "risk" management and assessment had emerged to evaluate hazard, danger, and threat since 1970 in environmental and technological controversies (Winner 1986; Lupton 1999). Critics argued that three types of transformation occur when a discourse and related action move from hazard to risk (Winner 1986; Lupton 1999). First, the "cause and effect" moves from being a clear source to being a possibility. Instead of identifying the source of the threat, research is needed to calculate the chances of creating adverse outcomes, and this brings in the idea of uncertainty. Second, the assessment is linked to "gain and benefit." Instead of emphasizing the action's adverse outcomes, assessment needs to weigh and balance the good and the bad. Third, for action, the hazard model means removing the danger, while the risk model yields calculations and leaves space for individual choice. The new risk model, rather than the hazard model, dominated the discussion about the increasing numbers of multiple pregnancies and births caused by ARTs.

The early assessment of multiple embryo transfer fit into this new risk model. Looking at the first few scientific articles by IVF pioneers shows that a "benefits and risks" model had been offered since the 1980s by the leading IVF practitioners to analyze the issue of multiple pregnancy. Benefits were put before risks. Assessing "benefits and risks of multiple embryo transfer"—as demonstrated in the title of a paper published in *Fertility and Sterility*— highlighted these concerns (Speirs et al. 1983): the benefits were higher pregnancy rates, and the risks were multiple births. Probably due to the birth of the world's first IVF twins, the Melbourne team also released the first few series of health risk assessments for multiple embryo transfer. For example, the IVF team from Queen Victoria Medical Center of Monash University, where the world's first IVF twins had been born, singled out the number of embryos transferred as the key factor to boost the success rate. The data show that in 1983, the pregnancy rate for single embryo transfer was 7.4 percent—much

lower than the 21.1 percent for two embryos transferred—and that
the rate was 28.1 percent for three embryos. The team thus concluded that "the much lower pregnancy rate after the transfer of one
embryo [rather] than two embryos (7 percent v 21 percent) may *be
sufficient reason to accept the risk of twins* (about 2 percent)" (ibid.: 797,
emphasis added).

"Acceptable risk" became a new way of understanding. With
more data, the Australian IVF community concluded that the risk of
twins "was far outweighed by the relative poor result after transferring a single embryo" (Wood et al. 1984: 978). The term "acceptable
risk" came from the couples surveyed in this clinical report. The IVF
team represented the patients' voices as follows: "*Our couples more
readily accepted the risk of twins* because of the limited chance of conceiving repeatedly by in vitro fertilisation and embryo transfer and
a reduced span of reproductive opportunity by virtue of increased
age" (ibid.: 979, emphasis added). What was selected to balance out
the increased risk posed by multiple birth was, in a word, failure—
repeated failure of IVF, and the possible loss of best timing.

Twins may sound all right to many prospective parents, but what
about triplets? In addition to the thirteen sets of twins, the 1984
Wood et al. report showed that four sets of triplets had been born
in 1983. The Melbourne team recognized that because of "the risks
of multiple pregnancy, including the psychological and physical
complications in the mother and child, *couples are now advised* to
restrict the number of embryos transferred to two or three" (ibid.,
emphasis added). Again, it implied that couples had a great deal of
say in deciding the number of embryos transferred, and that it was
not unusual for them to prefer more embryos than was appropriate.

While the benefit and risk model for IVF focused on the number
of embryos transferred, for the egg stimulation drugs—the older
method used to cause multiple pregnancy—the medical community
had no clear solution to achieve success and prevent risk. Dr. Joseph
G. Schenker and his team in Israel evaluated the consequences of
egg stimulation drugs in the early 1980s and concluded that "there
is no absolute means for preventing multiple pregnancy while still
achieving a reasonable pregnancy rate" (Schenker, Yarkoni, and
Granat 1981: 118). The complications were obviously serious, but
the prevention measures, such as reducing the dose of the drugs,
all proved ineffective, especially when the goal was to achieve
pregnancy. Schenker's review lists only some methods, such as
monitoring the estrogen level of the patient, to judge whether it is
appropriate to use egg stimulation drugs.

IVF was a different story. The number of embryos needed seemed to be clear-cut: if only one embryo was implanted, it was almost impossible to have twins. Therefore, limiting the number of embryos stood out as an easy and feasible strategy. Again, for IVF experts, the goal was not simply to reduce the risk of multiple pregnancy; the primary reason to start the IVF cycle was to achieve pregnancy. As mentioned earlier, to increase the possibility of success, the usual "natural cycle," which only produces one egg and one embryo, quickly gave way to multiple embryo transfer. The natural cycle was mentioned again as "an attractive alternative, since it poses fewer risks to the woman and her children" (Schenker 1993: 27; see also Wagner and Stephenson 1993: 8). However, in the early days of struggle with the low success rate, the natural cycle was rarely in practice. What other efforts were made to mitigate the reproductive risk?

The Emergence of Fetal Reduction

"Fetal reduction" has emerged since the mid-1980s as a new intervention measure to deal with the risk of multiple pregnancy. This clinical procedure reduces the number of fetuses *during* a woman's pregnancy. Fetal reduction did *not* begin for the multiple pregnancy caused by ART, but after prenatal genetic testing of twins.[12] It was first developed for termination of the genetically abnormal fetus in a pair of twins in order to help the healthy one survive after the co-twin received a prenatal diagnosis of a serious genetic disease such as Hurler disease in Lund, Sweden (Aberg et al. 1978), Down syndrome in New York (Kerenyi and Chitkara 1981), and Tay Sachs disease in Virginia (Redwine and Petres 1984). Reports often showed that it was the pregnant mother's strong request to keep the healthy twin that led to the experimental procedure.[13] To deal with the "twin discordancy," these pioneering doctors developed different procedures of "selective termination of an abnormal twin" instead of aborting both fetuses, as would previously have been done.[14]

In the mid-1980s, the procedure began to be applied to the situation of "grand multiple gestation" (Evans et al. 1988: 289); in practice, "grand" meant triplets to octuplets. Several methods were developed to conduct the fetal reduction, which could be roughly categorized as three types: transcervical suction aspiration, transabdominal reduction, and transvaginal reduction (see the review of Berkowitz et al. 1996). Each method had an affinity with a related medical practice, i.e., suction abortion, amniocentesis, and egg retrieval, respectively. Diverse specialists such as ultrasound technicians and amniocentesis experts joined infertility treatment practitioners to deal with the serious problems of higher-order multiple pregnancy.

One of the earliest papers on fetal reduction for multiple pregnancy described the practice of "transcervical aspiration," which was similar to the procedure of suction abortion, or vacuum aspiration. A French team first reported fifteen cases of three to six fetuses in a woman's womb, caused by ovarian hyperstimulation (Dumez and Oury 1986). With the assistance of ultrasound, the fetuses that were closest to the cervix were aspirated through suction.[15] The practice was soon followed by a US team, but was abandoned after the third case due to an incident of serious complications (Berkowitz et al. 1988).[16] What was not discussed in the English medical literature was that in 1986, Dr. Yahiro Netsu, an obstetrician and gynecologist in Japan, performed fetal reduction to reduce four fetuses to two, leading to the birth of healthy twins (Netsu 1998).[17]

Some other teams started to report another procedure: the abdominal approach, which was similar to amniocentesis. A Dutch team first published a case of selective termination in quintuplets in *The Lancet* (Kanhai et al. 1986). A team from Israel reported a case of reducing quintuplets to triplets, caused by implanting six embryos due both to a lack of embryo cryopreservation and a prohibition on destroying unused embryos due to ethical and religious concerns (Brandes et al. 1987). Similar to the earlier cases of terminating fetuses with severe genetic diseases, doctors inserted the needle transabdominally into each fetus and terminated it by different methods, including injection of potassium chloride (KCl) (Evans et al. 1988; Berkowitz et al. 1988). Dr. Netsu from Japan claimed that after learning the transabdominal method from Mark I. Evans's team by reading papers published in medical journals, he switched from transcervical aspiration to the transabdominal approach in 1988 (Netsu 2015).

Some other teams practiced the transvaginal procedure with the assistance of the advancement of transvaginal ultrasonography (e.g., Itskovitz et al. 1989; Shalev et al. 1989). These teams claimed that the advantages of the so-called transvaginal approach, compared to the transabdominal approach, included the better imaging of the vaginal probe, the shorter route to inserting a needle into the fetus, and the earlier time period in which to do fetal reduction (Timor-Tritsch et al. 1993). For IVF practitioners who practiced egg retrieval through the vagina, transvaginal fetal reduction shared some similar procedures (Shalev et al. 1989: 419; Berkowitz et al. 1996: 1267). However, several studies that collected data from the US and some European countries found that practitioners' preferences and experiences tended to determine which method they used, and that fewer and fewer practitioners were using the transvaginal approach (Evans et al. 1994, 1996). Later studies showed that the transvaginal approach had a higher pregnancy loss rate, so some suggested that it should be saved for women who could not undergo the transabdominal approach due to obesity or abdominal scars (Timor-Tritsch et al. 2004). Overall, the preferred method gradually converged on transabdominal reduction, which came to be called "fetal reduction" or "multifetal pregnancy reduction" (MFPR) (Malik and Sherwal 2012).

These pioneering doctors recognized that this was a "third option" (Berkowitz et al. 1988: 1045; Evans et al. 1988: 292). Like the dilemma that women faced with one healthy twin and one abnormal one after genetic testing, women who found they were pregnant with triplets, quadruplets, quintuplets, sextuplets, septuplets, and even octuplets faced the "either/or" trouble: either keep them all or abort them all. To keep the higher-order pregnancy meant an "extremely poor prognosis" (Evans et al. 1988: 291). However, to abort all the fetuses and try for another pregnancy was, for these infertile women, "a particularly difficult and tragic choice" (Berkowitz et al. 1988: 1405). In addition, doctors mentioned that these women who had undergone infertility treatment for years were typically older, and thus they may well have doubted whether they could become pregnant again after aborting all the fetuses.

"Last Resort" or "Safety Net"?

The medical community again adopted the benefit and risk model to evaluate fetal reduction. The whole reason for employing the clinical practice was to "enhance the probability that a healthy infant (or infants) will be born" (Wapner et al. 1990: 90), especially by preventing premature delivery due to multiple pregnancy. However, this entailed several levels of risk. The one most evaluated by the medical community was pregnancy loss, miscarriage, or what was called "complete abortion." Mark I. Evans, a leading American doctor in the field, collaborated with other centers to document the outcomes of fetal reduction, and the main concerns were pregnancy loss (Evans et al. 1994; Evans et al. 1996). Data from thousands of cases showed that miscarriage rates before twenty-four weeks of gestation improved from 16.4 percent in the late 1980s to 11.7 percent in the early 1990s. In the 2000s, although the risk of miscarriage still existed, Dr. Evans and his team were confident that the pregnancy loss rate might be under 10 percent after years of technical improvement and experience (Evans, Ciorica, and Britt 2004).

In addition, fetal reduction entailed moral risk. Research shows that some women faced emotional disturbance when making the decision (Collopy 2002, 2004). Some regretted having their doctors implant too many embryos and thus causing multiple pregnancy, even though sometimes this had been a last-ditch effort after several failures. They did not experience the joy of pregnancy but immediately faced the dilemma of whether or not to assent to fetal reduction. For those who believed that life begins at conception, the decision was even more difficult to make (Britt and Evans 2007a). Furthermore, the moral risk increased when fetal reduction was viewed as abortion and became entangled with the legal controversies over abortion rights. The media reported the ethical dilemma widely. The issue of fetal reduction appeared in the *New York Times* as early as 1988, under the headline "Multiple Fetuses Raise New Issues Tied to Abortion" (Kolata 1988). Right after the publication of twelve fetal reduction cases in the *New England Journal of Medicine* (Berkowitz et al. 1988), antiabortion activists asserted that "fetal reduction is the thinly veiled killing of unwanted babies," as reported in *Time* magazine (Grady 1988). There was public debate as to whether or not this new practice was legal according to abortion laws (Brahams 1987). Even though, at least in the UK and the US, it was justified as acting in the best interests of the women, the controversy lingered (Pinchuk 2000).

Fetal reduction gradually became "an integral part of infertility therapy" (Evans et al. 2004: 609). Evans's collaborative team of eleven centers reported more than three thousand cases between 1988 and 1998, revealing how commonly fetal reduction was practiced. To monitor the practice, some countries' registries began to report the prevalence of fetal reduction. For example, the first annual report of the European Society of Human Reproduction and Embryology (ESHRE) recognized the importance of recording fetal reduction as part of the complications of ARTs, but it wasn't until four years later that data became available. In the report for 2000, fetal reduction joined OHSS, complications of oocyte retrieval, bleeding, infection, and maternal death in the published table. Among 21 European countries, 8 reported 256 cases of fetal reduction in total,

4 did not have the data available, and the remaining 9 countries claimed zero (Nyboe Andersen et al. 2004). The practice of fetal reduction continued. The registry for European countries shows that at least hundreds of fetal reductions have been done each year since 2000. The latest data show that 35 countries together perform a total of more than 500 fetal reductions annually for prevention of multiple births, and the European IVF-Monitoring (EIM) Consortium is aware that the numbers are underreported (Wyns et al. 2020).

The availability of fetal reduction has *not* dramatically reduced ART-related multiple pregnancy. Considering the complex risks of fetal reduction discussed above, it is not surprising that not all women with multifetal pregnancy use this "last resort." The American Society for Reproductive Medicine (ASRM) has recognized the limitations of fetal reduction and lists three reasons why fetal reduction "does *not completely eliminate the risks* associated with multiple pregnancy" (Practice Committee of SART and Practice Committee of ASRM 2004, emphasis added): (1) fetal reduction may result in losing all the fetuses; (2) it causes a psychological burden; and (3) many women do not perceive it as an option. Fetal reduction was not an ideal solution; the IVF multiple pregnancy continued to prevail.

Instead of viewing fetal reduction as the last resort, some critics argued that it became doctors' "escape route" and "safety net" (Murdoch 1998). Some doctors tended to achieve pregnancy first, by transferring multiple embryos, and then reduce multiple pregnancy later, by employing fetal reduction. And it is not a reliable "safety net." Fetal reduction was invented to handle the risk of multiple pregnancy, but it entails many other risks. By comparison, preventive strategies were proposed. Debating the number of embryos to transfer became the regulatory battlefield.

Number Governance

Limiting the number of embryos transferred (NET) *before* implantation stood out as the most important measure to deal with "the tension between maximizing pregnancy rates and increasing the risk of multiple birth" (Katz, Nachtigall, and Showstack 2002: S31). Risk had been highlighted, yet success could not be compromised. Medical teams, medical societies, and governments started to work on arriving at the "primary number" for the local centers' principles, national guidelines, and even global recommendation. The clinical question—how many embryos put into a woman's body—thereby became a collective decision rather than an individual judgment.

Number governance began with the number three. At the early stage, some teams established their own individual principle. For example, the UK's Bourne Hall group shared with international colleagues that they limited the number of embryos to "no more than three embryos per cycle except in very special circumstances" (Henahan 1984: 878; see also Edwards and Steptoe 1983). In addition, some medical societies started to issue recommendations, often based on registry data. For example, as early as May 1987, the Voluntary Licensing Authority (VLA) in the UK announced that for IVF, no more than three embryos should be transferred, and for gamete intrafallopian transfer (GIFT), no more than three eggs. If there were some exceptional clinical reasons, up to four were allowed.

Several formal regulations, including laws on ART, began regulating NET, again centering on the number three. Germany stipulated as early as 1990 that the number of embryos transferred should be fewer than three (Federal Law Gazette 1990). In the UK, the first edition of the Code of Practice "rule book" of the 1990 Human Fertilisation and Embryology Act (HFE Act) limited the number of embryos transferred to three or fewer. The Japan Society of Obstetrics and Gynecology (JSOG) announced its code of ethics for multiple pregnancy in 1996, instructing careful use of ovary-stimulating drugs and limiting the number of embryos transferred to three or fewer—the first such restriction in East Asia. This was due in part to a controversial local case of fetal reduction (Yanaihara 1998), as well as to a keen desire to follow the international trend. By 1998, according to a survey done by the International Federation of Fertility Societies (IFFS), at least nine countries had legislated limitations on the number of embryos transferred (Jones and Cohen 1999).

Age-specific guidelines quickly emerged. Further data have shown that the IVF success rate is sensitive to a woman's biological age: the older she is, the less the chance of success. Therefore, to maintain the success rate, only those who had a higher success rate, such as younger women, had to limit the number of embryos to two. In 1990, based on national registry data, France proposed transferring *two* embryos to women under thirty-five years old and *four* embryos to women over thirty-nine years old. The data seemed to indicate that with this guideline it would be possible "to obtain the same eventual pregnancy rate without the risk of triple pregnancies and the risk of twin pregnancies is reduced by 50 percent" (Cohen 1991: 617). The success rate could not be compromised even though "multiple pregnancies must be avoided" (ibid.).

Deciding on the number of embryos to transfer is what Timmermans and Berg (2003: 5) categorize as "procedural standards." When a medical society or the state started to build this standard, scientific evidence was provided, including some evidence-based medicine datasets, such as the Cochrane Library (Pandian et al. 2005). Indeed, the Cochrane review did not publish any discussion until 2004, when it compared the effects of two-embryo transfer and single-embryo transfer. Thus, even though the medical community may share published scientific findings, there is no global standardization.

Maximum Two (UK) versus Up to Five (US)

To illustrate how scientific evidence is mobilized to build the guideline, I compare the guidelines from the medical societies in the UK and US. In 1998, the British Fertility Society (BFS) issued a "recommendation for good practice" for embryo transfer, which stated that "it should be the usual practice to transfer *a maximum of two embryos* in each treatment cycle" (emphasis added). The British researchers utilized the national registry data collected by the Human Fertilisation and Embryology Authority (HFEA) and found that transferring just two embryos would not decrease the live birth rate for women who have more than two embryos ready to transfer, thus indicating that the selection of good embryos was feasible (Templeton and Morris 1998). This important research provided strong evidence for practicing *elective* double-embryo transfer (eDET). Once again, the success rate could not be and was not compromised: "Transfer of only two embryos will not diminish the woman's chance of becoming pregnant" (Templeton and Morris 1998: 577). The key is found in the lowercase "e" in eDET: namely, electively choosing the embryos of high quality, not the "leftovers." The British researchers stressed that implanting three embryos did not increase the success rate but did increase the rate of multiple pregnancy. Thus, they offered clear suggestions for clinical practices: when more than four embryos were available, implanting two would not only result in a success rate similar to implanting three or four but would also reduce the risk of multiple birth—a win-win situation.

In contrast, the medical societies in the US published their first embryo transfer guideline in 1998, allowing implantation of up to five embryos. Instead of a single number, such as two or three, the US advises an age-specific and prognosis-centered recommendation. The 1998 guideline recommends that the maximum number of cleavage-stage embryos to transfer be three (for women younger than thirty-five years old), four (thirty-five to forty years old), and five (more than forty years old) for "patients with above average prognosis." Although the three-four-five guideline, regardless of any age group, is already higher than the "two" in the British guideline, it is specifically for women who have an "above average prognosis." In the revised 2004 US guideline, this term is changed to those with "the most favorable prognosis"—i.e., women who are undergoing their first IVF or have already been successful with IVF, and who have good-quality embryos or an excess of good-quality embryos.[18] The 1998 US guideline was very much aware of how it differed from those in other countries:

> Strict limitations, such as a maximum number of three embryos replaced by law in the UK, do not allow individual variation according to each couple's circumstances. These guidelines may be varied according to individual clinical conditions, such as patient age, embryo quality, and cryopreservation opportunities. (ASRM 1998)

These "strict limitations" meant two things: that the guideline was legally binding, as in the mandatory NET limits set in the UK, and that it specified an exact number, such as three. By comparison, the SART-ASRM guideline was voluntary, and the recommended number could be as high as five as long as the woman had a good prognosis. The three-four-five US guideline was undoubtedly the most lenient one in the world at the time.

The rationale behind the lenience was to "allow individual variation." This individualization included two parts: one concerning the individual characteristics of patients, and the other concerning the data from individual programs. The ASRM guidelines in 1998, 1999, and 2004 all state that "individual programs are encouraged to generate and use their own data regarding patient characteristics and the number of embryos to transfer." The US has collected national data since 1992. The national data in the US have consistently shown that multiple pregnancy has led to increased risk for mother and fetuses. Still, individual clinics' situations were greatly respected. In an evaluation of the effects of the voluntary 1998 guideline, the percentage of clinics that most frequently provided multiple embryo transfer to women younger than thirty-five years of age decreased from over 50 percent in 1996 to under 20 percent in 1999 (Stern et al. 2007). Despite the fact that the impacts of the guideline were evident, the researchers recognized that "even the latest guideline (published in 2006) will not eliminate the multiple births and allow us to reach our goal of the delivery of a single healthy child for all patients" (ibid.: 208). The 2006 ASRM guideline further distinguishes cleavage embryos from blastocysts for recommendation, in addition to a woman's age and prognosis. Still, for women over forty years old, the medical society maintained five embryos as the upper limit. This was soon found to be problematic because "almost all multiple birth (93.4 percent) ... resulted from ETs [embryo transfers] that were performed in accordance with ASRM/SART guidelines: 94.1 percent of twin births and 72.1 percent of triplet and higher order births" (Kissin et al. 2015). Lenient guidelines like those issued by the ASRM do not significantly reduce the problems they would like to solve.

This "legal mosaicism" (Pennings 2009)—that is, enormous diversity in the regulation of ART—echoes Jasanoff's (2015) argument that within seemingly shared scientific findings, specific regulation regimes shape different scientific governance. As the social studies of standardization have shown, standardization is a complicated social act (Clarke and Fujimura 1992; Timmermans and Berg 2003; Timmermans and Epstein 2010). Deciding the NET is more than the claim of evidence-based medicine (EBM): "the conscientious, explicit, and judicious use of current best evidence in making decisions about the care of individual patients" (Sackett et al. 1996: 71).

The fertility experts offer similar explanations. After comparing the 1998 UK and US guidelines, one such expert argued that "the differences ... do not appear to be based on scientific fact but probably reflect the different cultural and political environments in each country" (Murdoch 1998: 2669). Another US team also pointed out that the problem of multiple birth "will require that we also address the socioeconomic issues that pressure patients and physicians to transfer more embryos" (Stern et al. 2007: 282). The medical community knows well that social, cultural, and political factors reign. In chapter 2, I discuss the factors that lead to different trajectories in making guidelines. After all, the debate did not stop at the magic number two. The medical community moved to single embryo transfer (SET).

Conclusion:
Anticipating Risk without Compromising Success

This chapter has highlighted "multiple embryo transfer" in the history of IVF anticipation. In the early IVF development, the singular successful event of the birth of a test-tube baby fulfilled people's anticipation of a scientific breakthrough. The repeated failure to achieve pregnancy was overcome by the method of following the woman's "natural cycle," which meant single embryo transfer. After zealous reporting in the media, IVF anticipation shifted from scientific circles to the general public. IVF was viewed as an infertility treatment rather than just an eye-opening scientific finding. Achieving a high success rate became the new expectation. IVF experts quickly found that multiple embryo transfer was the key to increasing the success rate. However, the practice immediately led to a higher incidence of multiple pregnancies and births. This brought rising health risks to both mothers and infants, and some cases were catastrophic. Fetal reduction was one newly invented clinical intervention to manage the crisis, but it entailed additional risks—physical, psychological, and moral. Facing much criticism from the public, both medical societies and governments began to work toward a new expected goal: reducing the risk of multiple pregnancy without compromising the IVF success rates. Limiting the number of embryos transferred became the salient effort for anticipatory governance. Table 1.1 shows the changing anticipatory framing of IVF, along with corresponding tools to meet the selected dimension of anticipation.

When anticipation involves both sides—success and failure, hope and risk—it provides a powerful lens with which to examine how actors frame that anticipation and why certain anticipatory tools are mobilized. Table 1.1 shows that different main actors tend to emphasize different specific aspects of IVF anticipation. The feminist health movement tends to underline women's health risk, whereas competitive IVF clinicians prefer to publicize IVF's high live birth rate. Medical societies may either take the responsibility of stipulating NET limits for their members, so as to reduce risk, or adopt a laissez-faire stance toward risk that puts success rates first and foremost. By the same token, a government can take part in framing anticipation and subsequently decide either to get involved in legislating guidelines or to do nothing. Therefore, tracing the trajectory of anticipation helps reveal the contours of a given society. For instance, while the American Society for Reproductive Medicine

TABLE 1.1. Framing In Vitro Fertilization (IVF) Anticipation. © Chia-Ling Wu

Dimension of anticipation	Main framing actors	Exemplar tools to meet the selected anticipation
Successful birth	Vanguard scientists; media	Women's natural cycle
Success rate	IVF clinics; infertile couples	Multiple embryo transfer (MET)
Risk of multiple pregnancy	Public health experts; feminists; neonatologists	Fetal reduction; reducing number of embryos transferred (NET)
Reducing risk without compromising success rates	Reflexive medical society; government	NET guideline

allows five embryos for women over forty years old in its 2004 guideline (Practice Committee of SART and Practice Committee of ASRM 2004), the Nordic countries have moved toward elective single-embryo transfer (eSET) since the early 2000s.

In the next chapter, I explain the emergence of and resistance to eSET in the IVF world. The standard two-embryo transfer in several European countries has proven to reduce the number of triplet pregnancies but not the number of twin pregnancies. This has prompted main actors to advocate eSET as a way to effectively remove the risk of multiple pregnancy. But what about the success rates of eSET? Are there new tools to invent with which to face this new anticipation?

Notes

1. One pregnancy happened in 1976, but it was a "tubal pregnancy," a type of pregnancy that can sometimes be fatal to the pregnant woman (Steptoe et al. 1976).
2. Reading the early reports on IVF (in vitro fertilization) as an infertility treatment, "failure" rather than "success" is the keyword. Among the seventy-nine women admitted to the Oldham General Hospital between

1977 and 1980, for example, there were eleven "patients sent home without laparoscopy," twenty-three who had "failure to collect preovulatory egg," ten with "failed fertilization," three with "failure of cleavage," twenty-eight with "failure of embryos to implant," and only four who reached the stage of "pregnancies" (Edwards, Steptoe, and Purdy 1980: table IX). This failure to establish full-term human pregnancies stood in stark contrast to the scientific progress in IVF in the lab that had prompted a "miracle" discourse in the media since the 1960s.

3. A few months after the birth of Louise Brown, Dr. Subhas Mukerji in Calcutta, India, announced that the world's second test-tube baby had been born. This became controversial partly because of a lack of scientific reports in accredited circles. For the detailed discussion, see Bärnreuther (2016) and Bharadwaj (2016).

4. For example, the "natural cycle" method was not mentioned in the special exhibition of the fortieth anniversary of IVF in the Science and Industry Museum in the UK. See https://blog.scienceandindustrymuseum.org.uk/baby-launched-test-tube-revolution/ (retrieved 4 December 2020).

5. For the so-called clinical pregnancy rate in Edwards and Steptoe's 1983 paper, the nominator was clinical pregnancy, defined as "those with endocrinological and clinical evidence of pregnancy" (ibid.: 8362), which differed from "biochemical pregnancy," referring to a two- or three-day delay in menstruation and rise in some hormone indication, or simply to a positive pregnancy test. Or, in another definition, clinical pregnancy meant "positive fetal heart documented by ultrasound" (Medical Research International and the American Fertility Social Interest Group 1988: 213).

6. Of all the combinations of nominators and denominators, the live birth rate per treatment cycle was probably least preferred by some IVF clinics and medical societies. As a result, it was sometimes *not* selected for presentation to the public. For example, the medical society in the US started to collect data on IVF outcomes in 1985. Although they collected the numbers about treatment cycles and live births, these data were *not* used for the calculation of success rates. Like Edwards and Steptoe, what the medical society presented was the clinical pregnancy rate per embryo transfer cycle, which was 14.1 percent in 1985 and 16.9 percent in 1986 (Medical Research International and the American Fertility Social Interest Group 1988). Based on the published data, I calculate the live birth rate per treatment cycle as 6.6 percent in 1985 and 7.8 percent in 1986. Clearly, the success rate that best showed the efficacy of the technology and interests of its users was *not* selected for presentation to the public.

7. A report collected in 1984 found that, out of sixty-five teams, seven had tried the natural cycle. Of these seven, only the Bourne Hall team reported successful cases, whereas the other six had zero success (Seppala 1985).

8. Drs. Howard and Georgeanna Jones and their team had originally followed the UK's natural cycle approach but failed forty-one times in 1980 (Garcia et al. 1983). Natural cycles did not work for the US pioneers. They then followed the new experiences from Australia and moved to experimenting with the egg stimulation drugs in 1981, which led to the first successful pregnancy cases in the US.

9. "The Doctor Who Delivered the World's First Test-Tube Triplets ...," UPI Archives, 9 June 1983, retrieved 10 January 2021 from https://www.upi.com/Archives/1983/06/09/The-doctor-who-delivered-the-worlds-first-test-tube-triplets/3659423979200/

10. Fertility drugs have been well researched as the major factor causing multiple pregnancy. Public health expert Patricia Stephenson reviewed nearly two hundred scientific papers and systematically presented the risk of ovulation induction. Different from the major clinical research, which often separates the use of egg stimulation drugs, artificial insemination, and IVF, Stephenson's work put them under the bigger umbrella of "fertility drugs" (Stephenson 1993). Indeed, egg stimulation drugs such as clomiphene citrate and hMG can be used either for the medical treatment of infertility (e.g., for women with ovulation problems) or for the preparation procedures of artificial insemination (e.g., for infertile men with few sperm) and IVF (e.g., for women with obstructed fallopian tubes). The "known adverse effects"—with strong evidence from diverse data reports—include multiple pregnancy, pregnancy waste (perinatal mortality), and ovarian hyperstimulation syndrome (OHSS). France's first report on IVF complications showed that 23.4 percent of all IVF cycles had OHSS (Cohen 1991: 617–18). In other studies, OHSS was estimated to have 3–4 percent incidence, including 0.1–0.2 percent incidence of severe cases that can lead to the death of the pregnant woman. There was also some worry about cancer from use of the drug. Moreover, the procedures of IVF involved various complications from the injuries and injections caused by the egg retrieval procedure. The risks related to pregnancy include increased rate of spontaneous abortion, ectopic pregnancy, and multiple pregnancy.

11. Another study, based on the billing done by a hospital in Boston, revealed that the charges for the healthcare for twins were more than $30,000, and for triplets, more than $100,000 (Callahan et al. 1994).

12. For example, amniocentesis and chorionic villus sampling have moved from experiments to routine procedures since the late 1970s in some European and American countries (Cowan 1993).

13. The first published report came from the hospital in Lund, Sweden, in *The Lancet* (Aberg et al. 1978). A woman went through genetic testing during prenatal care because of her previous child having Hurler disease. She was pregnant with twins. The amniocentesis found that one twin showed abnormal signs and the other was in the normal range. According to the doctors' report, it was at the woman's request

that the doctors invented the procedure to "avoid abortion of unaffected co-twin" (ibid.: 990). As the title of the report shows, doctors
used "cardiac puncture" to stop the heart of the twin diagnosed with
serious genetic disease during the twenty-fourth week of pregnancy.
The mother had labor contractions in the thirty-third week. The dead
fetus was delivered vaginally, and the healthy twin was born by cesarean section due to the transverse position. The report ends by noting
that "mother and child are in perfect health." Similar procedures were
performed in Denmark and the US (Kerenyi and Chitkara 1981). The
case in Sweden seems to have inspired a mother in New York who
had a history of infertility after one of her twin fetuses was diagnosed
with Down syndrome and the other was healthy. Again, the mother
requested "selective termination of an abnormal twin" instead of aborting both fetuses (Kerenyi and Chitkara 1981). This was presented as
a new option for parents, who until this time could only abort all the
fetuses or continue the pregnancy for them all.

14. The naming of the procedure varied from "selective abortion," "selective termination," or "selective feticide" to "selective survival" and
"selective birth."

15. The procedure was similar to suction abortion, so the French team
called it "selective abortion" in the paper title (Dumez and Oury 1987).

16. This US team, based in New York, reported fifteen cases from 1986,
calling the procedure "selective reduction" (Berkowitz et al. 1988). The
team followed the French team in using transcervical aspiration for
the first three cases, and one woman had excessive bleeding and had
to terminate the entire pregnancy. As a result, doctors changed to the
method of transabdominal injection, using a needle to inject potassium
chloride, a poison, into the fetal heart. Most cases reduced the fetuses
to two, and around half of the women successfully gave birth to twins
after the reduction.

17. The method Netsu used was also transcervical abortion, which caused
heated debates, and I discuss it in chapter 2.

18. For the 2004 US guideline, patients are divided into four age groups,
each with a different recommended number range based on prognosis:
women younger than thirty-five (one to two embryos transferred),
thirty-five to thirty-seven (two to three transferred), thirty-eight to
forty (three to four), and more than forty years old (no more than five).

Chapter 2

ESET

ANTICIPATING NEW SUCCESS AND RE-NETWORKING IVF

"Who's afraid of single embryo transfer?" In 1998, two Belgian doctors posted this question on the debate forum of *Human Reproduction*, the official journal of the European Society of Human Reproduction and Embryology (ESHRE) (Coetsier and Dhont 1998). Single embryo transfer (SET) sounds straightforward: transferring only one embryo can only result in a singleton birth, thus reducing if not eliminating multiple pregnancy created by IVF. Chapter 1 has explained the "number policy" that started in the late 1980s with "three"—transferring no more than three embryos—and then moved to "two," the so-called double embryo transfer (DET), to reduce the chances of triplet or quadruplet pregnancy. Starting in the late 1990s, however, some policymakers and members of the medical community noticed that DET was inadequate. The triplet rate declined with DET, but the percentage of twins remained high or even higher. The laboratory and clinic practices continued to improve, so as the pregnancy rate increased, so did the twin rate. For example, the European data in 1998 show that, among more than thirty thousand deliveries after IVF and ICSI (intracytoplasmic sperm injection), the multiple birth rate was 26.3 percent, including 23.9 percent twin deliveries, 2.3 percent triplets, and 0.1 percent quadruplets (Nygren, Nyboe Andersen, and EIM 2001). If counting number of babies rather than number of deliveries, some global data show that almost 50 percent of IVF kids are born from multiple birth (ESHRE Task Force on Ethics and Law 2003). Test-tube babies used to betoken miracles; now they foretell multiples.

Single embryo transfer was proposed to handle the overwhelmingly high percentages of multiple pregnancy and birth. SET has different faces. The "natural cycle" used in the case of the first "test-tube baby," Louise Brown (see chapter 1), entailed single embryo transfer. Without egg stimulation drugs, women usually produce one egg per month for retrieval and therefore have at most one embryo in the lab for transfer. Even when an egg stimulation drug is used, it is likely that only one embryo will be available for transfer. This is called "compulsory SET," or cSET (Gerris et al. 2009: 56–57). cSET often means a poor result from egg stimulation, retrieval, or fertilization, which leads to the making of only one embryo in the lab—an unwelcome result for both practitioners and patients. Since the late 1990s, what IVF experts have promoted as the best risk-prevention policy is neither the natural cycle nor cSET but "elective single-embryo transfer" (eSET). The US Society for Assisted Reproductive Technology (SART) defines eSET as "an embryo transfer in which more than one high-quality embryo exists but it was decided to transfer only one embryo" (Practice Committee of ASRM and the Practice Committee of SART 2012). It refers to the practice of choosing a single embryo for transfer—hopefully the best one—among several available candidates.

Who is afraid of eSET? The provocative question asked in 1998 indicates the fear about what could happen if single embryo transfer became real:

> We ... need to consider an individualized embryo transfer policy: *elective transfer of a single embryo* in patients at risk for multiple gestation and a more liberal attitude for those with a less good prognosis. Would this *reduce significantly the number of multiple pregnancies without dramatic fall in overall success rates*? Can we in fact *anticipate the effect* of such a strategy on our IVF results, in terms of the overall pregnancy rate and multiple pregnancy rate? (Coetsier and Dhont 1998: 2663, emphasis added)

A new anticipation arose. The desired future was not only to achieve pregnancy and live birth but also to avoid the risk of multiple pregnancy. It is clear that the promotion of eSET was meant to further reduce the risk of multiple pregnancy, yet the leading concern was a decline in the "success rate." The balance between risk and success, as shown in chapter 1, continued. Implanting just one embryo even though several were available was indeed a "never-before zone" in the world of IVF. In 1998, only around 10 percent of IVF cycles in Europe were SET (Nygren, Nyboe Andersen, and EIM 2001), and most of these were probably cSET, not the ideal eSET.

In this chapter, I present the anticipatory practices of eSET. What has been done to make eSET work? How can eSET become a new routine of IVF? Who are the leaders to make eSET possible? I start with the useful framework of "anticipatory work" articulated by Adele Clarke (2016): hope work, abduction, and simplification (see the introduction to this book). I illustrate what kind of anticipatory work is needed for implementing eSET. I argue that practicing eSET entails re-networking IVF, both globally and locally. While the international IVF epistemic community does build an important foundation for eSET, national contexts matter. The state, medical societies, and civic groups intertwine in different ways to shift eSET from an experimental to a routine practice.

New Hope Work: Redefining Success

IVF has been promoted as a hope technology (Inhorn 2020). The hope is to enable infertile couples, and sometimes single women and same-sex couples, to have genetically related children. The chance of fulfilling that hope is often measured by the "success rate." Multiple embryo transfer (MET) was part of hope work by IVF experts to increase the success rate. The multiple births resulting from MET are sometimes celebrated as an unexpected blessing. However, if the mother and babies suffer complications and even death, the miracle can become a nightmare. If the babies are in critical condition, this can hardly be regarded as hope being fulfilled.

In light of the risk associated with IVF, various stakeholders started to develop a new hope work focused on redefining success. The ideal goal is not to become pregnant or "take a baby home" but to "take a *healthy* baby home." To reach this best possible future that IVF can bring, it was necessary to clarify what the future should be and how to reach that ideal. This new hope work is therefore composed of two aspects: identifying false hope and advocating a new ideal future. I will show how IVF scientists, medical societies, and policymakers have been working to articulate the new hope of IVF and justify the need for eSET.

Identifying False Hope

Challenging the mainstream definition of "success" was the first step in identifying false hope. As chapter 1 shows, "success rate" is the primary criterion for evaluating the effectiveness of IVF. In the early period of IVF, success was defined as chemical pregnancy and the clinical pregnancy rate. This meant that a positive pregnancy test or an ultrasound showing a fetus counted as success, regardless of whether miscarriage or stillbirth occurred later. Pennings (2000: 2466) has paraphrased the old saying about surgical operations ("The operation was a success. Regrettably, the patient died") to point out the irony of "success" in multiple pregnancy by IVF: "The establishment of the pregnancy was successful. Regrettably, the children are handicapped and the mother suffers from depression." Clearly, success needed to be redefined.

Thus we can see that, even though clinicians and medical societies may prefer to reveal the pregnancy rate from IVF because it is higher than the live birth rate, this creates false hope. Leaders of the International Committee for Monitoring Assisted Reproductive Technologies (ICMART) observed that in the early period "both national and international reports have focused on *markers of efficacy*, while issues of access to treatment and *safety* have not been addressed" (Adamson et al. 2001a: 1284, emphasis added). What to report reflects the central value of the monitoring system—namely, what we should care about: success (markers of efficacy) or risk (safety). The typical way to identify "false hope" was to present the adverse outcomes along with "success" rates.

The independent regulatory body in the UK, the Human Fertilisation and Embryology Authority (HFEA), does this in its annual reports, which began in 1991. The very first table in each report shows the live birth and multiple birth rates for IVF, ICSI, and donor insemination. For example, the table published in 1998 presents the multiple birth rates (around 27 percent) right next to the live birth rates (around 15 percent). This indicates the shadow (multiple birth) that casts a pall over the goal (live birth). In addition, the number of embryos is cross-tabulated with live birth rates, multiple birth rates, and stillbirth and neonatal birth rates. Although live birth rates increased with number of embryos transferred (NET), adverse outcomes also did so. The juxtaposition of the success of live births with the tragedy of deaths and complications yielded an important warning. The HFEA's data reporting illustrates what the research has shown: "Success, however, has come *at the expense* of an increased incidence of multiple gestations, along with their inherent maternal, neonatal, and pediatric complications" (Stern et al. 2007: 275, emphasis added).

International medical organizations often include safety as an important part of hope. They present multiple birth rates across countries to compare the degree of false hope. In 1997, the ESHRE began to present the data reported by European countries, with multiple births being presented after the pregnancy/delivery rates (Nygren and Nyboe Andersen 2001). This revealed that the overall multiple birth rate of 29.6 percent in Europe was lower than the 37 percent in the US and Canada. Moreover, it highlighted that Sweden and Denmark had reduced their triplet rate to 0.4 percent, whereas the UK still had 3.3 percent and Spain 11.9 percent. Similarly, the ICMART yields data on safety and presents the global trend. The International Working Group for Registers on Assisted Reproduction (IWGRAR, later transformed into the ICMART) showed in its first world report that Taiwan had the highest number of embryos transferred during IVF, followed by the US and South Korea (Adamson et al. 2001b). In presenting the data collected in 2000, the ICMART quickly realized the serious consequences of multiple birth in the US, Middle East, and Latin America. Singleton babies became minorities: the figures show that "in Latin America, only 48.7 percent, and in the Middle East, only 44.1 percent, of the newborns [from IVF] were singleton babies" (Adamson et al. 2006: 1606). Some regions still transferred four or more embryos. The ICMART's annual reports have shown that Taiwan and South Korea *continue* to have some of the highest NET, leading to the highest multiple birth rates, while Japan has the lowest rates in East Asia (Dyer et al. 2016).

Reporting the neonatal outcomes of IVF works directly to highlight the false hope it can offer. The ESHRE has listed stillbirths and miscarriages from the beginning but has not included detailed data on birth rates and prematurity. Such follow-up data require a stronger monitoring system. Taiwan is one of the few countries that has reported low birthweights from the very beginning of the ART registry in 1998 (Wu, Ha, and Tsuge 2020). The earliest report, based on the state-run registry, showed a high prevalence of premature babies among those of low birthweight, with triplets suffering the most. The warning sign of low birthweight is also included in the annual report, but the official report failed to point out that this is a serious health problem and thus did not link it to a call for action. I discuss below how to translate data related to the new hope work, so as to prompt changes in IVF practices.

Representing the Real Hope: "Taking a Healthy Baby Home"

In addition to revealing the false hope for a healthy baby that could result from IVF, the medical community struggled to present the real hope. In 2001, the ESHRE convened a special task force to address the complications of IVF and listed ten points to explain why the problem of multiple pregnancy in IVF had not yet been solved (ESHRE Campus Course Report 2001). Two of the ten points are about the definition and presentation of "success":

- The success of IVF is too often expressed in terms of pregnancies instead of healthy newborn children per cycle.
- There is a lack of enforcement by journal editors to express results in terms of singleton pregnancies and healthy children. (ibid.: 791)

Both these points challenge the traditional calculation of success rates, which did not accurately represent the real hope: taking a healthy baby home. And both points propose a new way to measure success: counting the healthy singletons. Johannes L. H. Evers (2002: 158), the chair of the ESHRE, reviewed the benefit and risk of IVF and declared in *The Lancet*, "The most appropriate outcome variable of all assisted reproduction procedures ... is not pregnancy rate, but singleton livebirth rate per cycle started." The leading journals on assisted conception also agreed to require standardized terminology in reporting success in clinical studies (Barlow 2004).

Some doctors and scholars have similarly called for new indicators to peg the quality of ART. To reach the standard of "taking a healthy baby home," some propose that efficacy should focus on "singleton delivery" (Adamson et al. 2001a) or "delivery rate of singleton, normal weight and live birth" (Min et al. 2004) as the success rate. Such data are not easy to collect. A division of labor exists: IVF experts aim to make women pregnant, obstetricians are in charge of maternal care, and pediatricians care for the test-tube babies. As a result, IVF experts may not see the full outcomes of birth. Women may not give birth in the IVF clinics, so tracing IVF outcomes requires additional efforts. What is more, the ESHRE Campus Course report (2001) points out that IVF experts tend to pursue the pregnancy rate without viewing the adverse outcomes that multiple embryo transfer brings, and thus they fail to feel responsible. Therefore, counting the live birth rate itself involves strongly mandating the reporting system. When a national registry system is built, "live birth rate" and "singleton birth rate" must become the routine calculation of success rates.

The most challenging new hope work is to prioritize the outcome of "taking a healthy baby home." This outcome takes into account not only a successful live birth but also the health condition of the newborn baby. Some innovative terms were therefore created. The IVF center at Monash University in Melbourne proposed the measure of "the singleton, term gestation, live birth rate per cycle initiated," dubbing it BESST (Birth Emphasizing a Successful Singleton at Term) statistics (Min et al. 2004). Not only does the numerator in this measure reflect the value of taking a healthy baby home but the denominator counts the start of treatment, rather than the date of embryo transfer, to recognize the length of the process that aspiring parents may undergo. Jason Min and colleagues presented their clinical outcomes with the BESST calculation. This report is believed to be the first to valorize the new hope of "taking a healthy baby home." The success rates decreased progressively from preclinical pregnancies (24.8 percent) to viable pregnancies (19.6 percent) to live deliveries (17.0 percent) to live singleton deliveries (12.4 percent) to term gestation (11.1 percent). This meant that at the Monash IVF center, the aspiring parents' "prospect of a singleton, term gestation, live birth of a baby per cycle begun was 11.1 percent" (Min et al. 2004: 7). Even though 11.1 percent is much lower than the conventional success rates, the team claimed that "this is precisely what a subfertile couple wishes to know" (ibid.: 6).

The US is probably the only country that stipulated a law specifically on success rates. The Fertility Clinic Success Rate and Certification Act was enacted in 1992. Since then, the Centers for Disease Control (CDC) and the SART have required each ART clinic to report its performance data and have published those data annually by clinic. In 2013, a new success rate came forth: the "term, normal weight & singleton live births" rate. This new item highlights the births of singletons born no sooner than thirty-seven full weeks and weighing at least twenty-five hundred grams (five pounds eight ounces). This "term, normal weight & singleton live births" rate is calculated per transfer cycle rather than per treatment cycle as advocated by the Monash IVF team. Still, this rate is lower than the "singleton live birth" rate, "live birth rate," and "pregnancy rate." For example, in the 2013 report (CDC, ASRM, & SART 2015), for women who were between thirty-five and thirty-seven years old with fresh embryos from nondonor eggs, the rate of taking a healthy singleton baby home was 19.6 percent—much lower than the live birth rate (31.6 percent) and almost half of the pregnancy rate (38 percent). This low rate may not be what clinicians would like to present, but the state mandates that the data be presented on what the couple is hoping for.

Incorporating adverse health outcomes and innovative indicators in national registries is not an easy task. Different stakeholders (physicians, counselors, policymakers, and patients) may place emphasis on different indicators (Dancet et al. 2013; Thompson 2016). Establishing better indicators also requires that demanding infrastructure changes be made. Tracking health outcomes of babies is challenging work because women may go to different clinics for ART and for childbirth. To account for whether single embryo transfer leads to better health outcomes, cycle-based data for individual patients are needed rather than clinic-based data, which are aggregates. A shift to care-centered data reporting requires information technology reform, new regulatory requirements, and sometimes consensus mobilization (Wu, Ha, and Tsuge 2020). IVF clinic websites also became a new challenge for presenting success. Some countries like Australia and the UK started offering guidelines on how to present success rates on clinics' websites and social media.[1]

Abduction: Testing eSET

How do we achieve the new hope—namely, "take a healthy baby home"? The answer involves abduction work. Adele Clarke (2016: 90–91) defines abduction as "tacking back and forth multiple times between the empirical information collected … and new theorizings about that data to generate new conceptualization—and adding a future-orientedness to its utility." In the late 1990s, several new trials began to test ways to fulfill the new hope of healthy singleton babies. A prestigious evidence-based Cochrane review provided the answer in 2005.

The Cochrane review produced a recommendation on number of embryos transferred after IVF and ICSI. The principle was to find the balance: "While the most effective way to minimize multiple pregnancy is to limit the number of embryos transferred, such a policy has to be balanced against the risk of reducing the overall pregnancy rates in IVF" (Pandian et al. 2005). We have seen this pattern repeatedly: success rates cannot be compromised. eSET was assessed as to whether or not it was meeting this principle. The authors of this Cochrane review combined four studies, from Belgium, Finland, the Netherlands, and Sweden, to compare the results of single and double embryo transfer. They were all randomized controlled trials, viewed as the highest standard of evidence. The review concludes that "a single embryo transfer policy involving a fresh followed by a frozen embryo transfer *reduces the risk of multiples while achieving a live birth rate* comparable with that achieved by transforming two fresh embryos" (Pandian et al. 2005: 2682, emphasis added). The evaluation equally weights both the success (live birth rate) and the risk (multiple pregnancy rate). Evidence-based medicine recommends that implanting one embryo each time for two times could reach the same live birth rate as implanting two embryos at one time, while significantly reducing the multiple pregnancy rate. One plus one equals two, and the risk would be reduced too.

The Cochrane review pointed to a new course of action for IVF clinicians. The data collected for testing eSET yields "probabilistic anticipations of the future that in turn demand action in the present" (Adams, Murphy, and Clarke 2009: 255). One Cochrane review did not change the whole IVF world. Its authors suggested that to make the policy work, it must identify women who have higher chances of twin pregnancy, such as those who are younger than thirty-five and have some good embryos for future use. The authors also admit that this is only clinically effective, and also needs to consider cost-effectiveness and acceptability (Pandian et al. 2005: 2686). Even the clinical effectiveness needs a lot of new refinement, particularly about how to select the embryos.

Abduction continues on how to make eSET feasible. One new invention is the "cumulative success rate." Like what the Cochrane review shows, the success rates of two "eSET" equal those of one "DET." This requires a new conceptualization of calculating success. The traditional method of calculating success rate "per cycle" would *not* reflect the efficacy of eSET. "Cumulative live birth rate" takes two or more transfer cycles to present the outcomes. The Cochrane review counts one fresh eSET and one frozen eSET embryo as the denominator. This usually leads to an equal or even better live birth rate than that rate produced by one DET. Due to the maturity of cryopreservation, clinicians tend to choose the best embryos in early cycles and then freeze surplus embryos (and sometimes eggs) for future use. This also reduces the need to do additional intrusive egg-retrieval procedures, thus lowering women's health risk. Therefore, the egg retrieval cycle can count as one cycle for the new success rate.[2]

eSET starts with selecting the "best" embryo, but what is the best? The question of how to select the best embryo has opened up a new wave of research. The "how" question therefore moves from balancing success and risk to pursuing best quality. Abduction expands. The IVF community has often reflected on its inadequacy in judging embryo quality. The ESHRE team on reducing multiple birth of IVF (ESHRE Campus Course Report 2001: 790–91) listed the three major technical limitations:

- Lack of efficiency of IVF, necessitating the transfer of more than one embryo.
- Poor predictability of embryo survival and implantation potential.
- Overall poor results of cryopreservation programmes.

The IVF medical community is aware that to make eSET feasible, it needs to develop various techniques. For instance, it needs to know how to select a good prognosis group for practicing eSET; it needs to improve the lab technique to decide whether to implant day three embryos or those that will develop to the blastocyst stage (day five or six); and it needs to stabilize cryopreservation so that frozen embryos can be safely used in later transfer cycles (also see Gerris et al. 2009).[3]

New techniques continue to evolve and be subject to deliberate debate. Time-lapse imaging has been used to record the development of embryos within the embryo incubator, seeking to provide better visual information to embryologists when selecting and deselecting candidates for embryo transfer (Herrero and Mesequer 2013). Embryologists' observation has been shown to vary greatly, so artificial intelligence (AI) is now used to increase the accuracy of embryo assessment (e.g., Bormann et al. 2020). Preimplantation genetic testing (PGT), used for monogenic diseases, began to be applied to embryo selection in the mid-2000s. Aneuploidy, the most common type of chromosome abnormality, has been regarded as the leading cause of implantation failure and miscarriage for IVF. Therefore, PGT for aneuploidies (PGT-A) is used to select embryos based on their genetic composition, hoping to improve implantation and reduce miscarriage, and thus enhance eSET (Lee et al. 2015). However, opponents remain. Since the error rate of PGT-A is not zero, PGT-A can risk wasting a good embryo. If counting by the cumulative success rate, "survival of the fittest" may achieve good outcomes as well as "no embryo left behind" (Munne et al. 2016). According to the latest survey by the International Federation of Fertility Societies (IFFS), more and more countries regard PGT-A as an established medical practice, but some, including Japan, still list it as experimental (IFFS 2019). IFFS and ASRM statements all ask for more research to test its efficacy (IFFS 2019; Practice Committee of ASRM and Practice Committee of SART 2018; for the difficulty of building evidence-based medicine for these "add-ons" to IVF, see Perrotta and Geampana 2021). Abduction continues.

Simplification: SET Guidelines

Setting a guideline for eSET is the simplification work needed to anticipate "taking a healthy baby home." As Clarke (2016: 96) argues, "Simplification is necessary because of TMI (too much infor-mation)—the increasingly common situation in which there is too much information, too much data to manage—or too much affect." Embryo selection and patient selection both involve complicated conditions. To effectively implement policy to reduce the risk of multiple births, some medical societies and national/regional regu-latory agencies have offered either voluntary or legally mandatory guidelines on the number of embryos transferred for IVF practices. Although the content of these guidelines varies, simply transferring *one* embryo is usually the major statement.

The first guideline mandating single embryo transfer came from Sweden. The complete registry data in Sweden made the agenda evident. Sweden started its registry in 1982, the year the country's first IVF baby was born. A group of scholars revealed the striking increases in multiple births, congenital malformations, and low-birthweight/high-risk babies that IVF created and published these findings in *The Lancet* (Bergh et al. 1999). The Swedish doctors recog-nized that eSET was the major strategy to reduce the risk (Hazekamp et al. 2000). To prevent adverse outcomes, double embryo transfer (DET) has been promoted in Sweden since the 1990s. In 2001, 81.6 percent of cycles were DET, the highest in Europe (Nyboe Andersen et al. 2005). However, twin pregnancy remains high—23.3 percent in 2001, for example. In 2002, the South Swedish Health Care Region required that all IVF cycles offered in public hospitals must adopt SET, except under circumstances that justified the use of DET (Saldeen and Sundstrom 2005). IVF is included in the public healthcare in Sweden, and risk prevention and cost management are important parts of this agenda. The regulatory agency in Sweden is regional, so the reform started in local districts. The local policy soon led to the national mandate requirement. In 2003, the Swedish

National Board of Health and Welfare issued a new guideline stating that, except when the risk of twinning is low, all public-health-supported IVF treatments must be SET.

Sweden's innovative policy is straightforward. The major rationale is to reduce health risks and lower the costs of neonatal care (Bhalotra et al. 2019). The confidence to issue the guideline came from research findings confirming that the cumulative success rates of SET do not differ from those of DET. Data from several pioneering research studies in other Nordic countries also confirmed the feasibility of practicing SET. The abduction work continued. The mandatory SET policy in Sweden was evaluated, showing promising outcomes: the SET rate increased from 25 percent one year before to 73 percent one year after; the multiple pregnancy rate decreased from 23 percent to 6 percent; and the clinical pregnancy rate remained unchanged (Saldeen and Sundstrom 2005). Risk decreased and success remained. The Swedish team announced that the SET policy is "the most reasonable way to solve the problem of the high incidence of multiples after IVF" (ibid.: 7).

Although the Swedish policy reform has been well reported in the global IVF community, it has not traveled easily to other countries. By 2007, the IFFS reported the "resistance to eSET" (Jones et al. 2007: S19). Among the twenty-six countries that have some legal regulation or guideline on number of embryos transferred (NET), most still had three embryos as the maximum, and a few had two as the rule. The magic number of only one embryo transferred became part of law only in Sweden and Belgium. Finland claimed that SET was the norm in practice without any law or guideline. Some countries, such as Australia and the US, included "one" in their guideline only for specific conditions, such as young maternal age and high embryo quality. Howard Jones and Jean Cohen claim that for the 2007 IFFS report, "the most striking finding is the great diversity in these laws and guidelines" (ibid.: S5). This certainly is true of the regulation of NET.

The anticipatory work shown so far—new hope work to redefine success, and abduction work to test various clinical skills—is often shared globally, through journal publications, international medical societies' recommendations, and evidence-based medicine. However, the practice of simplification—issuing a guideline to implant only one embryo in most circumstances—varies greatly among nations. To fully grasp the implementation of SET requires that we turn our attention to the national contexts. Which contexts?

Promissory Capital and Redistributing Cost

Why do some countries demand eSET while others ignore it? The IVF community is keenly aware that many factors are involved (Jones et al. 2007: S19–S22; Adamson 2009; Maheshwari, Griffiths, and Bhattacharya 2011; Ezugwu and Van der Burg 2015; Adamson and Norman 2020). They argue that the capacity for embryo selection and cryopreservation varies among labs, and that having the expertise to reach a certain pregnancy rate is the precondition for trying eSET, especially when the competition among clinics is aggressive. Some also argue that patients may prefer twins, or even triplets, because they are more efficient, so that they hesitate to accept eSET. Among the different explanations for resistance to eSET, however, the financial factor is the usually the crucial one.

The way IVF is financially organized shapes the dimensions of anticipation. In chapter 1, I presented the multiple dimensions of anticipation that are framed by specific stakeholders: for example, feminist groups highlight the risks of IVF, whereas pioneering scientists focus on the opportunities for successful birth. The never-before-clinical practice of eSET intended to reduce risk without compromising success rate. The public health sector has the strongest sense of the need to act on the foreseeable risk, precisely because the health of mothers and infants is endangered by multiple birth and the cost of care is increasing. Thus, when IVF is incorporated as part of public healthcare, the high multiple birth rate tends to ring a warning bell and solicit action to change more urgently in the public health sector than in other sectors.

Some note that the early pattern shows that an eSET policy is only feasible in Europe, where a few countries offer a subsidy program for IVF (Pandian et al. 2005). For example, the UK's National Health Services (NHS) fund some IVF cycles, and most neonatal care services receive public financing. The increasing multiple births from IVF have therefore increased the burden on NHS resources for neonatal care. The HFEA, the monitoring agency for IVF in the UK, started the eSET policy in 2007 with the slogan "One at a Time." In 2009, the guideline became of part of the licensing requirement, but this was later removed due to a legal challenge arguing that eSET reduced success rates and increased patients' emotional burdens.[4] Still, due to the continuous efforts from the medical societies of embryologists and IVF doctors, eSET has been encouraged. The rate of multiple birth in the UK decreased from 26.6 percent in 2009 to

16.3 percent in 2013, but remained far from the goal of lower than 10 percent. Both the HFEA and the medical societies continued to promote "One at a Time" clinical practices and provide the best possible clinical evidence for embryo selection, patient selection, data reporting, and public communication to achieve eSET (Harbottle et al. 2015). The 10 percent multiple birth target for all age groups was first reached in 2018 (HFEA 2020).

For most other countries, where IVF is highly privatized and *not* integrated into the public healthcare system or covered by national health insurance, eSET needs subsidy programs if it is to be implemented. As mentioned earlier, aspiring parents pursue quick success to save money, so clinicians pursue high success rates, often with the tacit promise of multiple embryo transfer to attract clients. The competitive environment of the IVF business, combined with the emotional and financial burdens that IVF users face, therefore make transferring more embryos for a higher success rate sound rational.

This IVF market follows the "logics of capital" in anticipation (Adams, Murphy, and Clarke 2009: 260). IVF promises a new family with kid(s), as long as you invest money to start the treatment. What Charis Thompson (2005: 258) calls "promissory capital" in the IVF enterprise is raised with the expectation of "something that unfolds over time in the future." Presenting a high success rate is a major predictive guarantee that renders the investment less speculative. eSET threatens the promise if it decreases the success rate or requires more cycles to reach the same cumulative success rate as that of multiple embryo transfer (MET). It is worth noting that the expectation in IVF differs from other expectations in the promissory bioeconomy. For example, commercial umbilical cord blood banks also operate within the promissory economy, encouraging parents to store their newborns' cord blood for its stem cells, thus securing a "what if" in the future (Martin et al. 2008). Even if the investment is never put into use for regenerative therapy, parents may still feel thankful because this means their child is healthy. IVF is different. Not reaching the goal of having a baby means loss of expectation. Even if the failure could be attributed to the patients themselves being too old, too fragile, or coming to the clinics too late, never seeing a positive sign on the pregnancy test is still viewed as a bad investment.

To implement eSET, the new agenda is to provide public financing for privately paid IVF—in other words, to redistribute the cost, and hopefully reassemble IVF. In most countries IVF is paid for out of pocket, whether fully or partially. Whether IVF should receive

TABLE 2.1. Guidelines on Number of Embryos Transferred (NET) for Countries with and without Public Financing for In Vitro Fertilization (IVF). Sources: Keane et al. 2017; IFFS 2019. © Chia-Ling Wu

Countries		NET		Total	Guideline for Women < 35 Years Old				
		Yes	No		One embryo	Two embryos	Three embryos	Four embryos	Average (N)
Public Financing for IVF	Yes	27 (84%)	5 (16%)	32 (100%)	7	10	10	0	2.11 (27)
	No	16 (53%)	14 (47%)	30 (100%)	1	7	6	2	2.56 (16)
Total		43	19	62	8	17	16	2	43

public funds involves complicated debates, with the rationales ranging from equal access and reduction of health risk to pronatalism (Neumann 1997; Mladovsky and Sorenson 2010; Keane et al. 2017; Wu et al. 2020). Not all countries with public financing bind subsidies to SET, but almost all that do practice SET do so with public financial support. Table 2.1 shows that, among those countries with public financing, 84 percent have required limiting the number of embryos. And among them, seven countries ask for SET for women under thirty-five years old. In contrast, for those who do not provide any public financing for IVF, only one country— Colombia—requires SET for young women.

In the US, even when scientists proposed eSET to lower the risk of multiple pregnancy, "improved insurance coverage" was often mentioned as the broader context to support the clinical procedure (Davis 2004: 2442). But little has been done.[5] For example, in the ASRM guideline recommended in 2004, only women under thirty-five years old with embryos of cleavage stage were recommended for NET of one to two embryos. Studies show that such a guideline was far from an ideal eSET policy and that it did not reduce multiple birth (Stern et al. 2007).

Next, I present two cases to illustrate how redistributing the cost of IVF can work for practicing eSET: the well-known Belgian Project, and the less known JSOG Project. The two cases shed light on how anticipatory work needs to reassemble the money, but in diverse ways. Most studies of promissory capital or bioeconomy focus on how the market is built (e.g., Waldby and Mitchell 2006;

Petersen and Krisjansen 2015; Krolokke 2018). Here I present ways the twenty-year-old IVF market may be able to change.

The Belgian Project:
Anticipating with Cost-Effective Rationing

On 1 July 2003, Belgium started to finance IVF with a strict limit on the number of embryos transferred (NET) during IVF. As table 2.2 shows, Belgium reimburses up to six IVF cycles in exchange for restriction of NET. For younger women to receive the reimbursement, the guideline requires that the first cycle be SET and the second be eSET. Bundling SET with financial support became a model solution for reducing multiple pregnancy. Willem Ombelet, the president of the Flemish Society of Obstetrics and Gynecology (VVOG) from 2001 until 2004, proudly called this "The Belgian Project." How did it start?

The reshaping of the financial allocation began in 2001. The Belgian government wanted to change the reimbursement of IVF and asked for the policy design. IVF in Belgium had been regulated by the state, first with a data-reporting system in 1993 and then with standard requirements and quality control of IVF hospitals and clinics. The state also appointed members of the College of Physicians in Reproductive Medicine to monitor ART. The state has been involved in all aspects of IVF regulation. Its reform to reduce multiple birth was carried out by the country's two major medical societies: the government-appointed Belgian College of Physicians in Reproductive Medicine and the Belgian Society for Reproductive Medicine.

The path toward "doing something" was also paved by academic research. To begin with, Belgian IVF specialists had actively experimented with eSET since the late 1990s (Coetsier and Dhont 1998; Gerris et al. 1999). Research teams from Ghent and Antwerp reported a series of studies showing that eSET could reach the same success rate as DET for young women. "It took a lot of clinical courage to launch the study altogether," the Antwerp team claimed, because it involved extending the use of eSET to women up to thirty-seven years old (ESHRE Campus Course Report 2001: 797). The Belgian doctors attempted to prove that as long as there were embryos of good quality to transfer, eSET could result in the same, or even better, pregnancy rate and live birth rate as DET. The myth that two embryos are a better guarantee than one was dismissed by these pioneers. These doctors also worked actively to transform their

TABLE 2.2. The Belgian Regulation on Number of Embryos Transferred (NET) in In Vitro Fertilization (IVF) in 2003. © Chia-Ling Wu

Age	Number of Embryos Transferred (NET)		
	Cycle 1	Cycle 2	Cycles 3–6
<36	1	1 or 2*	Maximum 2
36–39	Maximum 2	Maximum 2	Maximum 3
40–42	No restriction.		

*Two embryos are allowed if embryo quality is not sufficient.

scientific findings into clinical practices, asking colleagues to take eSET as "the ideal to which we should strive, taking into account the many objectives and subjective variables that give our work its human depth" (ESHRE Campus Course Report 2001: 799).

The anticipated outcomes included money saving. By the time the financial reform started, the Belgian National Health Care system already covered 50–70 percent of medication, clinic visits, and treatment monitoring. What was not covered included laboratory costs, for which couples needed to pay 1,000–1,250 euros. The proposal to the government bundled clinical practices with money: namely, reimbursement for up to six cycles of IVF and ICSI in exchange for a strict guideline on NET, with the goal of reducing twin pregnancies by 50 percent. The reimbursement did not cover women over forty-three years old, showing that the agenda was focused more on cost-effectiveness than on fairness.

The medical societies presented a simple "before and after" graph, highlighting the gain through the cost reduction (Ombelet et al. 2005: 10). The evidence-based policymaking mobilized both the experiment data (to show the efficacy of eSET) and the registry data (to calculate health outcomes and cost). The calculation was based on Belgium's registry of IVF since 1991 and the perinatal data on all births in Flanders since 1988. In terms of "short-term benefit," it shows that in 1997, with 28 percent of IVF births as twins and 5 percent as triplets, the care cost of the neonatal ICU was 11.875 million euros. With implementation of the new reimbursement and new guideline, it was estimated that by 2003 twin deliveries would decrease by half (to 14 percent) and triplets would be only 0.5 percent, so that the money needed for healthcare of premature

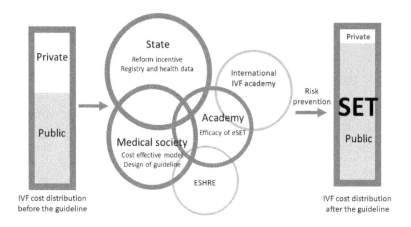

FIGURE 2.1. Anticipatory Governance of In Vitro Fertilization (IVF): The Belgian Project (SET = single embryo transfer; eSET = elective single-embryo transfer). © Chia-Ling Wu

babies would be 7.25 million euros—close to the amount needed to reimburse the cost of seven thousand IVF cycles. The public money spent on IVF would therefore be the same, but the need for neonatal care would be reduced significantly.

In terms of "long-term benefit," the money saved on the lifetime costs of caring for severely handicapped children due to multiple birth could be as much as 52.5–70 million Euros. Never before had the financial cost of the creation of lives (IVF) and the care of lives (neonatal care) been so simply and clearly presented. Taking reproduction as a continuous process (e.g., Almeling 2015), the redistribution of cost can lead to a win-win-win situation: the state budget might be decreased, the financial burden on the family could be relieved, and the health of mothers and babies would improve. To carry out the anticipatory work of implementing eSET, Belgium therefore employed an integrated triple helix of the state, the academy, and the medical society. The promissory capital was transferred into public funding, with scientific calculation to optimize the outcomes in terms of healthcare cost. Figure 2.1 shows my conceptualization of the Belgian model.

The effect of the new regulation was immediate and obvious—namely, a "sharp decrease in multiple pregnancy rate" (Van Landuyt et al. 2006). In just fifteen months, the multiple pregnancy rate for women less than thirty-six years old decreased from 28.9 percent to

6.2 percent. And for all the patients, the rate decreased from 29.1 percent to 9.5 percent. The practices of SET became the model practices, from around 15 percent in early 2000 to around 50 percent since 2004 (De Neubourg et al. 2013). All the research shows that the overall pregnancy rate did not change much (Gordts et al. 2005; Van Landuyt et al. 2006; De Neubourg et al. 2013). For the cost, a study analyzing hospital bills showed that after three years of the SET guideline, the multiple birth rate had decreased by half and the health cost was reduced by 13 percent (Peeraer et al. 2017).

This model is a distinguished way to reduce the health risk of multiple birth by reallocating public money. In retrospect, the Belgian leader of IVF gave the credit to the reimbursement program:

> Although Belgian infertility specialists were aware of the twin epidemic and knew about the possible advantages of single embryo transfer (SET) many years before the reimbursement policy was launched in 2003, a significant drop of twins could only be observed from 2004 on, which means that *only a financial incentive made the difference.* (Ombelet 2016: 190, emphasis added)

While noting the importance of financial support as the crucial aspect, the Belgian expert singled out Japan as an exception:

> One of the exceptions is Japan. In this country ART practices seem to be regulated by *the rules and moral policy* of a society without any stringent regulation. It is surprising that Japan obtained 86 percent of SET in 2012, compared with 59.6 percent in Belgium. (Ibid., emphasis added)

What rules? What moral policy? Compared with the "Belgian Project," the "Japanese Project" is seldom presented in the English literature. Since the primary agent to promote SET in Japan is the Japan Society of Obstetrics and Gynecology (JSOG), I will call it the JSOG Project here. The JSOG Project utilizes a different re-networking model, in which the three elements of registry-finance-guideline were reorganized to pave the road to SET in Japan.

The JSOG Project:
Anticipating with Avoidance of Controversy

Japan announced its SET guideline in April 2008, the strictest in East Asia. Unlike Sweden and Belgium, where the local and national governments issued the regulation, it was the medical society, the

JSOG, that recommended the new practice. The JSOG's guideline states that single embryo transfer (SET) is the primary principle. Double embryo transfer (DET) can be considered only for women thirty-five years or older for whom the first two SET cycles fail (table 2.3). The voluntary guideline in Japan is stricter than the legal regulation in Belgium, where there is no limitation on NET for older women. As shown below, with its guideline Japan has one of the highest SET rates and one of the lowest multiple birth rates for its IVF practices.

The case of Japan illustrates another social context of the anticipatory work to implement eSET. In what follows, I argue that the SET guideline is shaped by each country's sociopolitical context and by the national "sociotechnical imaginary," which Jasanoff and Kim (2009: 120) define as "collectively imagined forms of social life and social order reflected in the design and fulfillment of nation-specific scientific and/or technological projects." In other words, the eSET network building in Japan (aka the JSOG Project) needs to be understood through two waves of controversy: the social concerns over IVF in Japan in the early years, and the interprofessional conflict between Japanese IVF doctors and neonatologists.

Social Concerns over IVF

Beginning in the late 1970s, worries about IVF triggered the Japanese medical community to actively govern the newly developed technology (Wu, Ha, and Tsuge, 2020). During the early period, several surveys of patients seeking fertility treatment showed that fear of having a child with a malformation was one of the common reasons for refusing to undergo IVF (Iwaki et al. 1979; Iwaki, Tachibana, and Ogura 1983; Suzuki 1983). Some Japanese ob-gyns expressed feeling in the early years that IVF "is not natural" (Tsuge 1999). Some leading doctors and governmental officials voiced strong anxiety about the possibility of producing a "deformed child" (*kikei-ji*) through IVF, or about the high level of compensation that could be involved if this occurred, while noting medical professionals' responsibility for the health of babies (Yamaguchi et al. 2005; Mori 2010). Although similar worries surfaced elsewhere, in Japan they remained loud and strong. The discourse of doubt around Japan's IVF development was related to other highly publicized controversies on topics of technology and health, such as Minamata disease (linked to environmental pollution) and Wada heart transplants (leading to debates on brain death). The technological optimism that had accompanied Japan's economic miracle faced new challenges

TABLE 2.3. The JSOG Opinion on Number of Embryos Transferred (NET) in In Vitro Fertilization (IVF) in 2008. © Chia-Ling Wu

Age	Number of Embryos Transferred (NET)		
	Cycle 1	Cycle 2	Cycles 3–
<35	1 as the principle		
≥35	1	1	Maximum 2

in dealing with these widely reported controversies, lawsuits, and requests for high-fee compensation.

To reduce the worries about the new technology, not only from the public but also from their medical colleagues, three university-based IVF teams adopted the strategy of self-regulation along with their experimental practice (Suzuki 2014; Tanaka 2015; Yui 2016). This included establishing a new nationwide medical society on ART and setting up ethics committees at the university level to codify ethical guidelines. These decentralized ethical institutions helped individual medical teams demonstrate their capacity for self-regulation in order to gain social trust.

Moving from self-monitoring of individual medical teams to national health surveillance, the various ethical measures were eventually combined at the old JSOG, which had existed since 1949. In the early 1980s, with leaders from the three major universities holding important positions in the society, the JSOG announced its guidelines on IVF, started the clinic registration system, and initiated Japan's voluntary registry. The JSOG has maintained its autonomy of ART governance ever since, with only some governmental interference through ART subsidy programs after the mid-2000s (Tsuge 2016). Without a national law to regulate ART in Japan, the governance of IVF largely remains under the JSOG's jurisdiction.

Risk prevention to avoid controversy has been a major agenda item. For example, in the early reports of registry data, "risk" was the main theme. The reports emphasized the high miscarriage rate, high multiple pregnancy rate, and the possibilities of abnormalities in the newborns, and presented these as important factors in the evaluation of ART. The reports also made comparisons with "normal reproduction," where the miscarriage rate and multiple pregnancy rate are much lower. Although not using the exact term "taking a healthy baby home," the very first report strongly emphasized the same goal and tied it to the very action of collecting data:

> The higher incidence of miscarriage and *multiple pregnancy* for ART than for natural conception means there is risk for both mothers and babies. We need to deal with the problems of the high-risk pregnancy ..., the abnormal newborns, and the follow-up of children's health. The main goal of this technology is not pregnancy only, but the birth of a healthy baby. For this purpose, we need to collect better and richer data in the future. (JSOG Science Committee 1990: 397; emphasis added)

"Better and richer data" meant following up on the health of infants. The abnormal cases soon became a routine list in the annual report. The JSOG advocated improving data quality so as to better evaluate the prevalence and causes of risks and thereby ensure the care quality of IVF.

The controversy over fetal reduction strengthened the concerns about ART. Fetal reduction was first practiced in Japan in 1986 to deal with the problem of a quadruplet pregnancy caused by ovary-stimulating drugs. Dr. Yahiro Netsu performed the fetal reduction to reduce the four fetuses to two, leading to the birth of healthy twins (Netsu 1998). The experiment came from a painful lesson he had learned. In 1982, a woman pregnant with quadruplets due to the egg stimulation drug came to him for advice. Multiple pregnancy due to the infertility treatment had increased in Japan since the 1970s, and the media often reported on it with curiosity and joy. At that time, people had no choice but to abort all the fetuses if they wanted to avoid multiple pregnancy. The woman decided not to do this, and started a tough journey. With intensive prenatal care, she gave birth to three healthy babies and a fourth baby with cerebral palsy (CP). When Dr. Netsu later encountered a similar case, he decided to experiment with fetal reduction surgery, which resulted in a successful story.

However, the event led to a series of attacks from the Japan Association of Obstetrics and Gynecology for Maternal Protection (JAOGMP), which was in charge of abortion practices among doctors. Abortion had been legalized in 1948, but fetal reduction raised questions about what does and does not constitute "ethical boundary-work" (Wainwright et al. 2006). The JAOGMP and other opponents mobilized some contents of the law to claim that Dr. Netsu might have violated the abortion regulation. Although the case was eventually settled, media zeal made it a public issue or, as it was often phrased, "a scandal."

The JSOG started conducting a series of surveys to better understand the practices of fetal reduction. The earliest survey was done by Dr. Takumi Yanaihara (1998), who worked for the ethics committee of the JSOG and criticized Dr. Netsu's practice seriously. The survey found that, of the 197 institutions for infertility treatment, 15 practiced fetal reduction, which had resulted in 87 cases in 1996. For cases of women pregnant with three or more fetuses, 30.3 percent adopted fetal reduction to reduce the fetuses to two or one. Among the 69.5 percent who continued the multiple pregnancy, 10.9 percent had health problems. The need to prevent the incidence of multiple pregnancy became more urgent.

In 1996, the JSOG announced the first code of ethics to prevent multiple pregnancy. It instructed its members in the careful use of ovary-stimulating drugs and limited the number of embryos transferred to three or fewer—the first such restriction in East Asia. The 1996 guideline reduced the incidence of quadruplets and triplets, but the registry data show that the prevalence of twins remained high. The registry data helped identify ovary-stimulating drugs as the cause of half of the higher-order pregnancies, followed by multiple embryo transfer (MET) (Irahara 2002). In addition, JSOG leaders surveyed international trends and recognized that limiting MET further would be the more effective measure to reduce multiple pregnancy (Irahara and Kuwahara 2003).

It is worth noting that Japan's feminists became an important pressure group to monitor IVF. The Japanese branch of the international feminist organization FINRRAGE was established in Tokyo in 1991. It started from a small reading group of feminist literature on ARTs, and expanded to thousands of members in its heyday in the late 1990s. This became an important source of critical voices representing women's experiences. In 2000, the group published *New Report on Infertility: The Survey of Real Experiences of Infertility Treatment and Reproductive Technologies* to voice the women's worries about the health risk, safety, and financial burden of seeking ARTs (FINRRAGE no kai 2000). In addition, feminist scholars such as Azumi Tsuge (1999) have published research to challenge the medical model of treating infertility since the 1990s. The JSOG and related medical societies sometimes invited FINRRAGE leaders and feminist scholars to their forums to incorporate diverse voices when discussing ethical issues, enhancing their capacity to be engaged with public debates.

However, the direct impetus to make the JSOG take further action came from other medical professionals.

Interprofessional Conflict

Almost all the Japanese doctors I interviewed agreed that it was pressure from pediatricians/neonatologists that made ob-gyns change their ART practices. One of the JSOG leaders vividly described how neonatologists urged the organization to take action:

> [Around 2002 to 2004] we met very strong criticisms from the neonatologists, many times and at many conferences, because at that time Japan's health care system did not have enough personnel in the neonatal intensive care to handle the situation. ... They asked us to make a big change to reduce the pre-term labor and low birthweight, or they could not continue the neonatal intensive care unit. ... As representatives of JSOG, we were invited to attend the symposium held by the society of prenatal care. They always accused us. *But it was not my fault. We were just collecting data. That is the direct reason we established the cycle-based data of the registry.* Because we did not know enough about the reasons causing the high rate of multiple pregnancy. (Dr. J-K interview, Taipei, April 2018, emphasis added)

The JSOG's registry data, which did not include information such as the percentage of low-birthweight IVF babies, were not adequate to reveal these problems. The government did not associate the data on neonatal outcomes with the development of IVF. Therefore, the neonatologists' face-to-face pressure and strong emotion were required to convince JSOG leaders to take further measures to reduce the health risks to newborns.

The interprofessional conflict between those who transfer embryos to make women pregnant and those who care for fragile premature babies is not about the jurisdiction of medical expertise or professional autonomy (Abbott 1988) but about the unacceptable burden created by the division of labor. The 2001 ESHRE report points out why multiple pregnancy was less recognized by IVF experts: "Infertility specialists are frequently not involved in obstetric care and hence have no direct feedback from the obstetric outcome of their treatment successes" (ESHRE Campus Course Report 2001: 791). When neonatal care units face personnel shortages, such as occurred in Japan, confrontation may arise.

These JSOG leaders worked on both the registry and the ethics committees, which helped them translate the neonatologists' anger into new codes of practice. The first step was to change the registry system from site-based to cycle-based in order to provide evidence with which to evaluate IVF practices.[6] The second step was to build a new guideline. In 2008, after discussion and evaluation, the JSOG announced its recommendation of single embryo transfer (SET) for women under thirty-five years old to solve the problem of multiple pregnancy. By that time, Sweden and Belgium had built the SET guideline, and Japan became the first in Asia to follow. The acceptance of the SET guideline in Japan involved many factors, including improvements in the technical process of embryo selection, the refinement of data reporting for policy evaluation, and the partial subsidy program initiated in Japan in 2004 to boost the low fertility rate.

Unlike Sweden, Japan did not make IVF part of the public healthcare system. When the first test-tube baby was born in 1982 in Japan, comprehensive health insurance had already been established, but the Japanese government did not include IVF due to its low success rate (Semba 2005). Unlike Belgium, Japan did not initiate a subsidy program aiming to reduce health risk. The financial subsidy of IVF was initiated by the Japanese government as a pronatalist policy. In 2002, when the total fertility rate reached the record low of 1.3, some local governments began to offer a subsidy program to promote a higher birth rate. The national policy started in 2004 for couples under a certain economic threshold, and only 15 percent of IVF cycles received a subsidy. The subsidy was later extended, partially due to strong lobbying from the Fertility Information Network (FINE), an NGO aiming to relieve the financial burden for infertile couples to receive medical treatment.[7] By 2016, a new age limit—up to forty-three years old—was established, and resources were increased to cover 32 percent of cycles for about 39 percent of the cost (Maeda 2019).

Thus it was the JSOG, not the government, that set up the SET guideline. In doing so, JSOG leaders utilized the opportunity created by the government subsidy program to increase the birth rate in ways that support SET. With strong agreement among JSOG members, the SET guideline has reached almost full compliance. Data show that the use of SET increased rapidly after the JSOG's 2008 guideline, from 46.5 percent in 2007 to 82.2 percent in 2018—close to the rates in Sweden, Australia, and New Zealand, and much higher than those in Belgium and the UK, not to mention in those countries without a strict SET policy, such as Taiwan (graph 2.1). And in Japan, all the perinatal health risks, such as stillbirth, cesarean section, preterm birth, and low birthweight, decreased significantly (Takeshima et

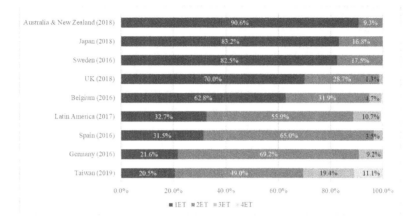

GRAPH 2.1. Number of Embryos Transferred (NET) by Selected Countries. (1ET = one embryo transferred; 2ET = two embryos transferred; etc.) Sources: HFEA 2019; JSOG Science Committee 2020; Newman, Paul, and Chambers 2020; ROC Ministry of Health and Welfare 2020; Wyns et al. 2020; and Zegers-Hochschild et al. 2020. © Chia-Ling Wu and Wei-Hong Chen

al. 2016). Osamu Ishihara—the key person who promoted upgrading the registry in the JSOG and a devoted representative in the International Committee for Monitoring ART (ICMART)—has successfully used Japan's high-quality data to present Japan's approach in international comparative studies (e.g., Chambers et al. 2014). Japan has been singled out in ICMART reports as a successful case of practicing SET (e.g., Adamson et al. 2018).

Unlike the integrated triple helix of the state, academy, and medical society in Belgium, the JSOG was the reform engine that did the main anticipatory work to implement eSET in Japan. Although the Japanese government's subsidy program was intended to boost the birth rate, the JSOG recognized it as a timely tool for reducing the financial burden of practicing SET for practitioners and patients alike. The JSOG allied with the international IVF academy to provide research findings on eSET, and with international IVF societies such as the ICMART for guidance on reducing risk through data reporting. The JSOG Project also shows that redistributing cost was only part of the momentum driving SET as a routine practice (figure 2.2). I argue that it was the waves of controversy—from (a) the early social concerns about IVF to (b) the intraprofessional disputes among IVF pioneers about fetal reduction to (c) the interprofessional conflict between IVF doctors and neonatologists about neonatal care—that

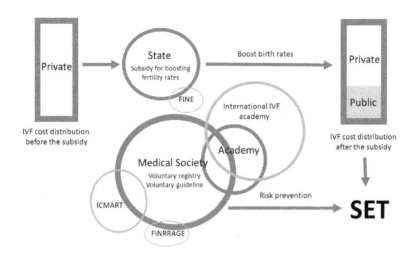

FIGURE 2.2. The Japanese Society of Obstetrics and Gynecology (JSOG) Project. (FINE = Fertility Information Network; FINRRAGE = Feminist International Network for Resistance to Reproductive and Genetic Engineering; ICMART = International Committee for Monitoring Assisted Reproductive Technologies; IVF = in vitro fertilization; SET = single embryo transfer.) © Chia-Ling Wu

step-by-step intensified the ethical responsibility of JSOG leaders and members to act on preventing the risk posed by multiple birth.

Conclusion: Building an eSET Network

This chapter has analyzed the intensive anticipatory work required for the routine practice of eSET to reduce multiple pregnancy/birth in IVF. The "hope work" involved centers on redefining success. The international IVF community has promoted the use of the live birth rate, and the singleton full-term live birth rate, to present the value of "taking a healthy baby home." The abduction needed to test the efficacy of eSET involves much biomedical innovation, from calculating cumulative success rates to improving embryo selection accuracy, thus building the foundation for eSET practice. SET has started to work as a simple and straightforward guideline in some countries. Hope work, abduction, and simplification altogether make eSET desirable and feasible.

Anticipatory work enacts eSET only in some countries. Graph 2.2 shows that Sweden, Belgium, and Japan all had a sharp rise

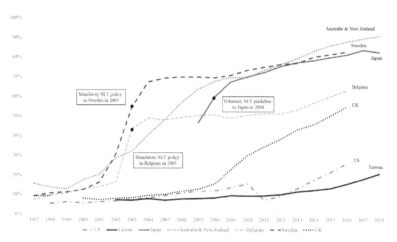

GRAPH 2.2. Percentage of Single Embryo Transfer (SET) in All In Vitro Fertilization (IVF) Cycles for Selected Countries. Sources: *Australia and New Zealand*: Lancaster et al. 1995, 1997; Hurst et al. 1997, 1999, 2001a, 2001b; Dean and Sullivan 2003; Bryant, Sullivan, and Dean 2004; Waters, Dean, and Sullivan 2006; Wang et al. 2006, 2007, 2008, 2009, 2010, 2011; Macaldowie et al. 2012, 2013, 2014, 2015; Harris et al. 2016; Fitzgerald et al. 2017, 2018; Newman et al. 2019, 2020; *Belgium, Sweden, and UK*: Nygren, Nyboe Andersen, and EIM 2001, 2002; Nyboe Andersen et al. 2004, 2005, 2006, 2007, 2008, 2009; Mouzon et al. 2010, 2012; Ferraretti et al. 2012, 2013; Kupka et al. 2014; EIM for ESHRE et al. 2016a, 2016b, 2017, 2018, 2020a, 2020b; *Japan*: Saito et al. 2017; Ishihara et al. 2018, 2019, 2021; *US*: CDC, ASRM, SART, and RESOLVE 2000–2002; CDC, ASRM, and SART 2003–18; and *Taiwan*: ROC Ministry of Health and Welfare 2021a. © Chia-Ling Wu and Wei-Hong Chen

in practicing SET in the years they issued their SET guidelines. The contrast is seen in the low percentages of SET practiced in the US and Taiwan, where there is no strong recommendation on, or regulation of, SET. SET policies work in different ways. Most countries that establish a SET guideline combine the guideline with public financing, as in the Belgian Project. The international IVF community has repeatedly contended that reorganizing promissory capital is essential for the routine use of SET (Pandian et al. 2005; Davis 2004). However, Japan stands out as a different case, in which sociotechnical imaginaries of IVF have been infused with concerns and conflicts. This shaped the framing of anticipatory work in Japan primarily in terms of risk prevention. The result is that, with reflexive leaders of Japan's medical society to articulate the diverse anticipatory work needed, SET has become routine in Japan even without much public financing from the government.

Comparative analysis of the Belgian Project and the JSOG Project demonstrates the different national formations of eSET. The new invention of calculating success, the evidence shown in Cochrane reviews (Pandian et al. 2005; Glujovsky et al. 2016), and the recommendations by the ICMART and the IFFS are important resources and are shared globally. Yet, locally, it is the state (Sweden), dual cooperation of the state and medical societies (Belgium), or the medical society (Japan), depending on the IVF governance, that designs the different programs for implementing eSET. The anticipated crisis of IVF—the increasing adverse outcomes due to multiple pregnancy/birth—has prompted a variety of responses. I have shown, via the actions of the JSOG Project, that the sociotechnical imaginaries of IVF guide the direction of anticipation. In the case of Japan, avoidance of controversy led to adoption of eSET. In chapter 3, I present the different sociotechnical imaginaries of IVF in Taiwan, which direct an anticipatory regime that still welcomes multiples today.

Notes

1. The Reproductive Technology Accreditation Committee of Australia published a guideline in 2017, titled "Public Information, Communication and Advertising: Australian Clinics," on how to present success rates on websites and social media. Even though the guideline recommends that clinics report "per cycle started" as the denominator of success rates, none of the thirty surveyed clinics did so (Goodman et al. 2020).

2. For example, ten eggs may be retrieved from a single procedure, resulting in eight embryos for future use. The doctor would choose a "best" fresh embryo to transfer. If it does not lead to pregnancy, then the available frozen embryo is used for the next transfer. As long as the woman reaches pregnancy and live birth with one of these first two transfers, or within transfers of her eight other embryos, the process counts as a success. In other words, if the woman becomes pregnant from the third attempt at implantation, this counts as success (1/1), whereas in the old calculation, the first two cycles would be counted as failures (1/3). In addition, for those clinics promoting natural-cycle IVF, cumulative success rates are preferred in presenting the results. For example, the famous Kato clinic in Japan shows that the cumulative live birth rate for women thirty-five to thirty-seven years old is 51 percent by the completion of four cycles, compared to 17 percent after the first cycle (Bodri et al. 2014).

3. Take the assessment of embryos as an example. The so-called grading system of embryos has transformed greatly but does not always reach consensus. Much research explores how to grade and score embryos (see the review of Van Blerkom 2009; Harbottle et al. 2015). Traditional scoring relies on morphological assessment, including the development and appearance of embryos. However, there have been no national or international efforts to reach a consensus, so "numerous grading schemes evolved which varied in both complexity and efficacy" (Bolton et al. 2015: 157). The blastocyst stage of embryo development, five or six days after the insemination of sperm into eggs in the lab, once met the standard for high-quality embryos in the guideline of the ASRM (Practice Committee of ASRM and Practice Committee of SART 2013) but also raised new concerns because couples could lose all the embryos for use (Harbottle et al. 2015). A Cochrane review of twenty-eight randomized control trials showed no difference in cumulative pregnancy rates between blastocyst transfer groups and cleavage-stage (days 2–3) transfer groups (Glujovsky et al. 2016).

4. For the UK debates on implementing eSET, see "The UK Human Fertilisation and Embryology Authority's 'One at a Time' Campaign," Centre for Public Impact, 7 January 2019, retrieved 17 February 2021 from https://www.centreforpublicimpact.org/case-study/uk-human-fertilisation-embryology-authoritys-one-time-campaign.

5. Historically, IVF has not been on the healthcare priority list in the US. For example, in the famous 1991 Oregon priority-setting list, IVF was listed as number 701 out of 714 conditions (Dixon and Welch 1991). Low birthweight (defined as 750–999 grams in this program) was ranked 123 out of 714, in the top 20 percent, whereas extremely low birthweight (< 500 grams) was ranked 713, the lowest in the priority ranking. This implies that the general public is willing to spend public resources on neonatal care, but not on improving IVF so that it no longer increases the need for neonatal care. When the Clinton administration in the US proposed the Health Security Act in 1993, IVF was among the medical packages that were explicitly excluded from the standard coverage list (Neumann 1997). Groups of infertile couples were the major force lobbying for coverage of infertility treatment in the US, but reducing health risk was not the major concern (King and Meyer 1997).

6. The early data came from the clinics' report of their annual aggregate data: the total number of cycles; distribution of NET; total cases of miscarriage, live birth, and stillbirth; and so on. This type of data cannot reveal how NET is associated with twin and triplet births. The cycle-based reporting system, in contrast, requires that clinics report every single case to a new online reporting system. This yields data for evaluation of clinical practices. In addition, the new registry data add the new items: the neonatal health outcomes. Every cycle needs to

report the newborn's sex, length of term, birthweight, and abnormal outcomes, and it must also follow the situation to twenty-eight days after the birth. Some IVF clinics told us that the new registry system requires one or several full-time staff to make the records and do the follow-up work.

7. The feminist group FINRRAGE in Japan collected infertile women's opinions and found that financial burden was the major obstacle infertile couples faced during treatment. However, the major action of FINRRAGE in Japan was to challenge unnecessary treatment rather than ask for a public financing program.

Chapter 3

WHEN IVF BECAME
A NATIONALIST GLORY

In April 1985, the first test-tube baby in Taiwan, "Baby Boy Chang," was born in the Taipei Veterans General Hospital. Mr. and Mrs. Chang, a lieutenant colonel and an accountant, had been married for six years and suffered from infertility. Mrs. Chang sought treatment and was recruited into the IVF experiments, starting in April 1984. Dr. Sheng-Ping Chang, who happened to share the same last name as the family and who was later crowned the "father of the test-tube baby," recalled that when the IVF team decided to move from the lab to the clinic, they expected "repeated experiment, failure, frustration, and disappointment" (S.-P. Chang 1985). By August 1984, when Mrs. Chang became the first volunteer whose hormone test showed early signs of pregnancy, thirty-nine women had undergone the new IVF attempts at Taipei Veterans General Hospital. The IVF team announced the news of her pregnancy in late 1984, so the media followed Mrs. Chang's due date closely.

The first successful IVF birth was a highly anticipated event. The newborn Baby Boy Chang and the making of a test-tube baby in Taiwan were in the headlines in all the newspapers, and follow-up stories appeared for an entire week. The event was widely celebrated under headlines such as "Made in Taiwan Champion" (*China Times* 11 April 1985: 3) and "Turn a New Page in Medical History" (*Central Daily* 17 April 1985: 1). IVF was applauded as a nationalist glory. One doctor I interviewed vividly described the pride of learning how to perform IVF at that time: "It was heatedly discussed. Achieving an 'Asia's First' was really an honor. Doing ART became a hot preference among us medical students" (Dr. F, 2010 interview). Baby Boy Chang was *not* in fact Asia's first test-tube baby, but Dr. F rightly recalled the zeal of competition at the time. As described further below, gaining international visibility through medical achievement has gradually come to constitute one of Taiwan's national sociotechnical imaginaries.

This chapter examines how IVF was perceived as a nationalist glory in its early development in Taiwan and how this also shaped the trajectories of framing IVF anticipation. Which dimension of anticipation stood out—success or failure, hope or risk, or some type of hybrid? Which actors gained the most credibility for directing the anticipation? Facing the major complication of IVF—multiple pregnancy—what governing strategies were at work, and what were their consequences?

"Achieving First"

Two layers of "achieving first" discourses stimulated the IVF experiments in Taiwan. One is "first in Asia." Many countries referred to the success of a first test-tube baby as achieving a nation's "position in the technology-driven modern world" (Ferber, Marks, and Mackie 2020: 91). For example, when Israel presented its first successful IVF birth in 1982, only weeks after the US, the media portrayed the medical progress as "lagging only slightly behind powerful countries like the USA" (Birenbaum-Carmeli 1997: 526). In the case of Taiwan, newspaper editorials advocated developing ART to "elevate Taiwan's status in the world" (S.-C. Li 1982a) and warned against Taiwan being seen to "lag behind" (S.-C. Li 1982b). After the first IVF baby was born in Singapore in 1983, an editorial in Taiwan's *Min-Sheng Daily* claimed that "we once thought that our technical competence was second only to Japan, so it was a surprise to learn that Singapore is ahead of us" (S.-C. Li 1982a).[1]

Taiwan's zeal to become technologically competitive emerged in part from efforts to overcome international political isolation. Taiwan had suffered several major diplomatic setbacks since the 1970s. It had withdrawn from the United Nations in 1971 and faced a diplomatic break with the US in 1979. Achieving a "first in Asia" became a way to present Taiwan's national power, whether through competing with other Asian countries in terms of economic growth rate, winning gold medals in sports, or making a medical breakthrough. Achieving medical miracles gained new energy when

National Taiwan University (NTU) Hospital surgically separated con-
joined twins in 1979, a twelve-hour procedure that was broadcast
live on TV in Taiwan (D.-J. Tsai 2002: 247–55). Doctors checked
the international medical records to confirm that this was a "first in
Asia" and the second successful case globally. Chang-Gung Hospital
performed a liver transplant in 1984, highlighting it as the first in
Asia (*United Daily News* 4 April 1984: 3). These events helped Taiwan
regain confidence and shed its "Orphan of Asia" identity. IVF joined
the wish list of ways to demonstrate national power by achieving a
medical miracle. After successful cases in Singapore and Japan, the
timetable for Taiwan to achieve ART became more and more urgent.

Several hospitals in Taiwan made IVF a goal, and doctors began
learning and training internationally. Ferber, Marks, and Mackie
(2020: 84–85) found that Bourne Hall in the UK and Monash
University in Australia became a "little scientific 'empire,'" but for
Taiwan the center of acquiring skill in IVF was the US. Ethnic ties
with Taiwan-educated Taiwanese American scientists established
an important learning route. Both the US policy since 1965, which
attracted highly skilled immigrants, and the tendency of elite
students in Taiwan to study in the US—to obtain a better graduate education and career and to escape political instability (from
Communist China and also the local authoritarian Nationalist government)—facilitated the so-called brain drain in engineering and
science (S. L. Chang 1992; Ng 1998; J.-Y. Hsu and Saxenian 2000).[2]
The brain drain nevertheless became an important ethnic network
that enabled the newly established IVF centers in Taiwan to acquire
cutting-edge knowledge and skills. Taiwanese Americans (and a few
Taiwanese Canadians) either offered direct assistance on the latest
expertise or built bridges between leading pioneer IVF experts in
the US and medical centers in Taiwan. One distinguished example is
Helen Hung Ching Liu, who received her undergraduate degree in
chemistry in Taiwan, her PhD in biochemistry in the US, and then
worked with Howard and Georgeanna Jones in Norfolk, Virginia,
in the early 1980s (e.g., Rosenwaks et al. 1981; Liu et al. 1988).
She worked closely with the IVF teams in Taiwan, accompanying
the Joneses on their 1984 visit to Taiwan, giving scientific advice,
and writing a textbook chapter in Chinese together with Taiwanese
doctors.

In addition, young doctors from Taiwan went to the US for hands-
on training in the 1980s. There they attended the ASRM annual
meetings more often than the ESHRE ones. Several doctors met
Min Chueh Chang, the China-born American reproductive biologist

whose study of in vitro fertilization in rabbits and other mammals laid an important foundation for human IVF (Clarke 1988). These Taiwanese doctors called Min Chueh Chang the "true father of IVF," clearly showing their preference for highlighting the contributions of someone of similar ethnic origins. Even though these learning routes extended to France, the UK, and Australia—and though leading experts such as Jacques Testart and Rene Frydman, who succeeded in making the first IVF birth in France, came to Taipei Veterans Hospital for seminars (S.-C. Chen 2020)—the US dominated the map of skill acquisition and also, as we will see, the road map for policy ideas.[3]

"First" discourse helped transform IVF from a possibly controversial technoscience into a glorious one. Like some other Third World countries, Taiwan had started its population control policy in the mid-1960s, so by the early 1980s promoting ART could still be viewed as contrary to the national interest. This was precisely the case in South Korea, where the focus on contraception in the 1970s led Patrick Steptoe and other leading scientists to come there to demonstrate their expertise (Wu, Ha, and Tsuge 2020). Although the aim was birth control, their knowledge of assisted conception inspired doctors in South Korea. Still, leading Korean scientists often claimed that their enthusiasm was due to personal interest in cutting-edge science in order to prevent being criticized as opposing state policy. In contrast, when the superintendent of the government-funded Taipei Veterans Hospital promoted IVF as the organization's ambition, he skipped the issue of population policy and used the rhetoric of "pursuing something number one like National Taiwan University Hospital et al." (Chang and Wu 1999). As a result, doctors on Taipei Veterans Hospital's IVF team, who were paradoxically in the family planning rather than obstetrics-gynecology department, were able to gain generous infrastructural support to begin scientific research and clinical trials. "Something first" became a useful strategy for IVF doctors to use to mobilize expensive hospital resources, from recruiting experts who had trained abroad to funding capital-intensive lab operations (Doctor L, 2011 interview).

"Achieving first" also embodied local competition in terms of expertise. The rivalry among hospitals to achieve the nation's first IVF success was an important part of IVF history in Australia, the US, and Japan. The same was true in Taiwan, but it also involved some local ethnic tension. NTU Hospital—established during the Japanese colonial period (1895–1945) and attracting the cluster of elites of the so-called Taiwanese to work as doctors there—was viewed as the most prestigious medical center. By comparison, Taipei Veterans Hospital, built in 1959, after the Nationalist Party came to Taiwan, provided medical services to veterans—mostly so-called Mainlanders who had migrated to Taiwan with the military from Mainland China after the Chinese civil war.[4] The "Taiwanese" and "Mainlanders" became a new ethnic divide, causing much conflict socially and politically, including in the world of biomedicine.

In terms of research funding for IVF, one senior doctor from NTU Hospital responded after my presentation to their seminar that his research proposal application to the National Science Council had been rejected for not following the national policy (on contraception) (Field note, June 2001). NTU Hospital had great difficulty acquiring sufficient funding to develop IVF, and leadership saw this as the reason it did not achieve the first IVF birth in Taiwan. With the goal of achieving "something first" like the old elite NTU Hospital, Taipei Veterans Hospital received such generous funding from the Veterans Affairs Council that it was able to build a new lab, send young doctors abroad to study, and invite leading scientists to visit for advice and hands-on training. In addition, entrepreneurs in Taiwan started to establish large private hospitals in the late 1970s. Chang-Gung Hospital, founded in 1976 by the leading millionaire of Formosa Plastic Corporation, signaled a new period of commercial competitiveness among hospitals. Competing for "something first" in Taiwan became an important incentive for upgrading IVF.

The two layers of "achieving first"—first in Asia and first in Taiwan—made IVF a medical innovation that was worth pursuing for nationalist glory and local pride. Comparing media reports on the first test-tube baby in Japan and Taiwan shows how the sociotechnical imaginaries of IVF differed greatly among the two East Asian countries. In Japan, as shown in chapter 2, the development of IVF was pervaded by social concerns. When the first test-tube baby was born there, Dr. Masakuni Suzuki showed the media a photo of the delivery, though not focusing on the baby herself (figure 3.1) and creating suspicion that the infant might be deformed. The baby died at one year old, seemingly confirming the rumor (*Yomiuri Shimbun* 12 November 1985: 23). In contrast, the birth of Baby Boy Chang was widely celebrated in Taiwan. All the doctors, nurses, and embryologists were named heroes and heroines by the media. The parents were highly publicized, and the media interviewed them with great joy. A three-layer birthday cake was cut at the press conference that was held when the infant and mother were discharged from the hospital, surrounded by the IVF team (figure

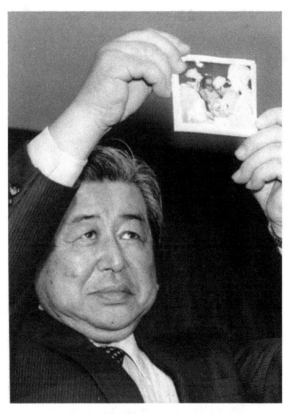

FIGURE 3.1. Dr. Masakuni Suzuki Showing the Photo of Japan's First IVF Baby at Tohoku University Hospital. Source: *Yomiuri Shimbun* 14 October 1983: 15. © Yomiuri News Photo Center (Yomiuri Shimbun), used with permission.

3.2). A survey done one month later showed that over 60.2 percent of the Taiwanese public supported IVF, and 16.2 percent supported it with some conditions (*Ming-Sheng Daily* 7 June 1985: 7). The report compared the result to a survey in Japan at the end of 1982, in which only 18 percent supported IVF. Whereas Japan's first IVF baby died at one year old, which intensified the country's doubts about the technique, Taiwan's media followed Baby Boy Chang for decades, reporting on his academic performance, marriage, and parenthood. Although Taiwan was only "Asia's fourth" in achieving a test-tube baby (after India, Singapore, and Japan), Taipei Veterans Hospital and the media successfully framed the anticipation of IVF as a nationalist glory, which greatly influenced the governance of IVF in seemingly contradictory ways.

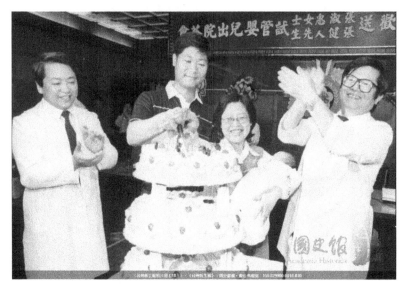

Figure 3.2. The Celebratory Birthday Cake at the Discharge of "Baby Boy Chang," Taiwan's First IVF Baby, at Taipei Veterans Hospital, April 1985. *Left to right* Dr. Hsiang-Da Wu, Mr. Chang, Mrs. Chang, Baby Boy Chang, and Dr. Sheng-Ping Chang. Courtesy of Academia Historica, number 150–029900–0018–030.

Breakthrough or Tragedy?
IVF Twins, Triplets, and Quadruplets

Taiwan's first test-tube baby, Baby Boy Chang, was a singleton. Three eggs were extracted from Mrs. Chang, which developed into two embryos of good quality. Doctors implanted two embryos, leading to the birth of a single child. In the earliest experimental period, doctors in Taiwan, like their international counterparts, tended to implant all available fertilized embryos—generally one or two, since the fertilization rate and the implantation rate were still low and the embryo-freezing technique was not yet available. By the time Taiwan achieved its first IVF birth, clinical data from the international teams were beginning to show that the implantation rate or pregnancy rate increased with the number of embryos transferred (Edwards and Steptoe 1983; Speirs et al. 1983). For the pioneering IVF devotees in Taiwan, the risk of having twins, triplets, or quadruplets was far outweighed by the need to counter the relatively poor results of IVF.

Four months after Baby Boy Chang was born, the second IVF birth was approaching the due date. The mother was expecting twins. Taipei Veterans Hospital revealed the news to the media in April, prompting pages of glorious news (*China Times* 18 April 1985: 3). Unfortunately, early in August, a week before the due date, during their prenatal checkup, doctors detected that the twins would be stillborn. The three major media reported the news, not in the headlines this time but in the corner space of the third or fifth page. *China Times* published a critical comment calling for a medical ethics evaluation to address the possible health risks of IVF (Y.-H. Chang 1985). Taipei Veterans Hospital explained that twins had a higher health risk, and clarified that the stillbirth was not caused by IVF itself (*China Times* 17 August 1985: 3). By the mid-1980s, medical and epidemiological research had documented that the risk of stillbirth for twins was two to three times higher than for singletons (Bleker, Breur, and Huiderkoper 1979; Imaizumi, Asaka, and Inouye 1980). However, none of Taiwan's news reports mentioned that the procedure of multiple embryo transfer (MET) during IVF itself increases the incidence of twins. The next year, another tragedy occurred, with the death of a mother and IVF twins at Taichung Veterans Hospital. The family was angry at the loss of life, and the doctors were frustrated with the incident. Still, the news report emphasized the risk of twin pregnancy rather than of IVF itself (C.-C. Lin 1986).

The fatal events, all caused by multiple pregnancy, did not shadow IVF in Taiwan. The medical breakthrough and the joy about IVF progress still prevailed. The major narrative was focused on achieving more and more "firsts." Every hospital's first IVF birth was reported. Taiwan's first GIFT (gamete intrafallopian transfer) baby, first IVF triplets, first ZIFT (zygote intrafallopian transfer) triplets, and the "world's first IVF case combining the method of zona cutting and cryo-preservation" (S. Y. Chang et al. 1991) were all reported as milestone accomplishments. When parents were portrayed, it was their joy at overcoming infertility that was emphasized—joy that was doubled or tripled for a multiple birth. For example, when the first IVF triplets in Taiwan were born half a year after Baby Boy Chang, even though they were put into incubators for neonatal care, the title of the news report emphasized *yilao yungyi*, meaning "one labor for eternal ease" (*United Daily News* 17 November 1985: 5). When Chang-Gung Hospital delivered its first quadruplet IVF birth, three of the four babies were under fifteen hundred grams, the criterion for "very low birthweight." While showing the scenes

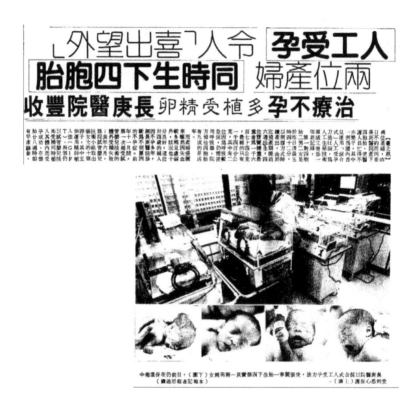

FIGURE 3.3. Report on the Birth of Quadruplets at Chang-Gung Hospital in Taiwan. Source: *Central Daily News* 10 February 1988: 11. Courtesy of Hope Information Technology Co. Ltd.

of four incubators (figure 3.3), the newspaper title emphasized the extreme joy of jumping all at once from barrenness to four babies, phrasing it as *xichu wangwai*, or "joy beyond expectation" (*Central Daily News* 10 February 1988: 11).

Nevertheless, with the quadruplets, the media finally criticized the frequent higher-order multiple birth, highlighting multiple embryo transfer (MET) as the risk factor. Another set of quadruplets, due to the use of an egg stimulation drug, were born on the same day. The very next day, a third set of quadruplets, also by egg stimulation drug, were born, and all died because of premature birth in the twenty-fourth week. The births of three sets of quadruplets within two days at the same hospital created both spectacle and concern. All the major newspapers highlighted the side effects of infertility treatment, calling it a "crisis of multiples" (Tai 1988), and drew attention to MET as problematic. News reports revealed that for the IVF quadruplets, doctors had retrieved ten eggs from the mother, placed five eggs with sperm into the fallopian tube—the so-called GIFT method—and had implanted another two embryos for IVF (*China Times* 10 February 1988: 12). Chang-Gung Hospital emphasized that using the two methods together could enhance the success rate. While some members of the international IVF community began to limit IVF to "three embryos" for transfer, Chang-Gung Hospital "retrieved ten eggs on average, and *implanted only five embryos* ... in order to prevent multiple pregnancy" (*Min Sheng Daily* 11 February 1988: 14, emphasis added). Yet five embryos certainly could not prevent multiple pregnancy, and such practice was not limited to Chang-Gung Hospital. According to the first national statistics report in Taiwan, between 1985 and 1993, 51 percent of IVF cycles were implanted with four or more embryos, which led to one in every four live births being multiples (Yuan 1995).

The risk of multiple pregnancy was presented by doctors as an unavoidable consequence when dealing with the fear of a low pregnancy rate. Dr. Yung-Kuei Soong, the leader of the IVF team at Chang-Gung Hospital, responded to the quadruplet controversy in a newspaper:

> Multiples are the new problem that new reproductive technology brings. Due to the immaturity of current technology, the only way to increase the success rate is to implant more embryos. ... When we found the multiple fetuses on the sixth or seventh week through ultrasound, both the pregnant women and doctors would face a new problem: whether we should reduce some fetuses. (Soong 1988)

As discussed in chapter 1, locating the controversy within the framework of "benefit and risk" appeared early on (e.g., Speirs et al. 1983), although not without contention (e.g., Wagner and St. Clair 1989). In the early emergence of frequent multiple births in Taiwan, doctors maintained that MET was beneficial to patients, focusing on the suffering of repeated IVF failure rather than on the risk of multiple pregnancy.

In addition, Dr. Soong's remark shows that Taiwan had moved from "successful event" to "success rate." While some hospitals were still struggling to achieve a first successful case, some leading centers were beginning to pursue higher success rates. Dr. Soong's comment also reveals that fetal reduction became an option after ultrasound detection of higher-order multiple pregnancies such as the three sets of quadruplets in Chang-Gung Hospital, though it was not practiced by Dr. Soong due to ethical concerns. Instead, he asked for social support, religious understanding, and legal approval of fetal reduction so that women could both achieve pregnancy through MET and have fetal reduction ready in case of multiple pregnancy. In reality, however, Chang-Gung Hospital did not wait for the sociolegal system to be ready to practice fetal reduction in Taiwan. Only two months after the quadruplets event and Dr. Soong's commentary, fetal reduction became another news event, not as a controversy but as a medical accomplishment.

Fetal Reduction as a Technical Solution

Fetal reduction began to become infertility experts' technical solution to multiple pregnancy in Taiwan, and some presented it as another medical breakthrough. Chang-Gung Hospital announced achieving a reduction of four fetuses to three, and calling this four-to-three fetal reduction one of the few successful cases around the world (*Min-Sheng Daily* 25 April 1988: 14). Soon after, some cases that needed fetal reduction included octuplets (eight fetuses) in Taipei Veterans General Hospital (*Min-Sheng Daily* 21 December 1988: 23), nonuplets (nine fetuses) in Hsinchu (*China Times* 27 January 1995: 13), and septuplets (seven fetuses) in Miaoli (*China Times* 12 May 1998, North Taiwan Section: 12). These super-higher-order pregnancy cases were caused by implanting seven embryos or taking egg stimulation drugs, and all planned to reduce to twins with fetal reduction methods. In the early stage of introducing fetal reduction, some IVF experts told the press that the use of fetal reduction was to "keep the remaining babies safe," and they also mentioned the major side effect—namely, that the miscarriage rate of fetal reduction was about 10–15 percent (S.-H. Hung 1995). This statistic was based on the reports in other countries, not the local data in Taiwan. Fetal reduction became the part of the ART network of techniques to handle the risks of multiple pregnancy.

Unlike in Japan and other countries, in Taiwan the practice of fetal reduction was not closely associated with abortion, either technically or legally. As discussed in chapter 1, various methods of fetal reduction were developed in the 1980s in European and North American countries before doctors settled on the method of inserting a needle into the abdomen. Taiwan skipped the transcervical suction aspiration, which was most similar to abortion, occasionally attempted transvaginal reduction, and quickly adopted the transabdominal approach. The earliest published report came from the team at NTU Hospital and shows that nine cases of fetal reduction were performed in 1989–90, and only the first one used the transvaginal route; the other eight cases adopted the injection of KCl into the fetus through the woman's abdomen (Ko et al. 1991).

This was partly because doctors who practiced amniocentesis were soon involved. Amniocentesis requires inserting a needle into a pregnant woman's uterus to remove amniotic fluid for genetic testing. These doctors had the tendency to practice fetal reduction abdominally. I interviewed Doctor Q, the pioneering expert in fetal reduction in Taiwan. He had originally joined the IVF team because of his specialty in chromosomes, and later became one of the leading practitioners to conduct fetal reduction. I asked him whether he still remembered his very first case of fetal reduction:

> Of course I still remember the first case: I had a lot of sweat on my head [*laughs*]. It was actually not difficult. I had practiced amniocentesis since 1982, several years before the first case of fetal reduction [around the late 1980s]. The two procedures were similar. I inserted the needle through the abdominal wall, guided by ultrasound. Other IVF doctors used to retrieve eggs from the vagina, and hence tended to practice fetal reduction from the vagina. However, due to my experience with amniocentesis, I preferred doing it from the abdomen, which could reach a high level of sterility, much better than doing it from the vagina. My way is a much safer method. (Doctor Q, interview 3 August 2017, Taipei)

The early involvement of amniocentesis practitioners such as Dr. Q helped Taiwan move quickly to the transabdominal version of fetal reduction, which later proved to be safer than the transvaginal method in terms of rates of miscarriage and infection (e.g., Timor-Tritsch et al. 2004). Most reports show that IVF teams in other hospitals adopted the transabdominal approach of fetal reduction as well (Hwang et al. 2002; Cheang et al. 2007).

In addition, Taiwan passed the Genetic Health Act in 1984, which legalized intrusive prenatal testing for genetic diseases such as Down syndrome and abortion. The act laid the legal foundation for practicing amniocentesis (F.-J. Hsieh 2014). Doctors I interviewed told me that practicing fetal reduction may have involved some moral uneasiness but never met with any legal problem. In terms of methods, practitioners involved, and legal implications, fetal reduction in Taiwan was associated more with amniocentesis than with abortion.

Overall, without linking it to abortion, as in Germany and the US, or creating intraprofessional conflict, as in Japan, fetal reduction soon became routinized in Taiwan as a way to deal with multiple pregnancy. Some media reports used the term "feticide" to indicate the controversy over the procedure (e.g., Y.-M. Chang 1994b; Hsueh 1994), but without any stakeholders to engage with the issue, the term and the accusation did not last long. A new division of labor in ART gradually emerged: infertility experts to achieve pregnancy, and amniocentesis experts (or general gynecologists) to reduce fetuses when necessary. Some IVF experts in Taiwan who had practiced fetal reduction tended to ask other doctors to do the job (Y.-M. Chang 1994b). A common response to my questions during interviews was that "my work is to create the life, so I do not like to reduce the fetuses." This shows that doctors did face some moral dilemma about fetal reduction, yet they handled it not by reducing cases of multiple pregnancy from the outset but by having someone else later do the job of reduction.

By the late 1990s in Taiwan, the sociotechnical imaginary that pictures IVF as a nationalist glory led an anticipatory framing that focused more on success than on risk. This is not to say that the tragedy of maternal and infant death and the moral discomfort of fetal reduction caused no concern in Taiwan. However, what prevailed in media reports was various successful events: making the first IVF baby in the southern part of Taiwan, achieving the first IVF birth through a frozen embryo, and even the successes of delivering quadruplets and of accomplishing fetal reduction, which were controversial in some other countries. Perhaps most stunning was the case of a pregnancy with ten fetuses in 1997, which Dr. Maw-Sheng Lee claimed might be a national record (Y.-L. Li 1997); the ten fetuses were reduced to two, leading to a twin birth. Facing increasing numbers of multiple pregnancies, IVF specialists in Taiwan began to offer some techniques of risk management, preferring to try new technologies such as cryopreservation and embryo selection methods. These new technologies took time to mature. The need for legal regulation of the number of embryos transferred (NET) began to be voiced, even among the IVF experts themselves. What about government regulation?

Regulatory Agency: Leave Clinical Procedures Alone

Governmental regulation of IVF in Taiwan did start early, but it first focused on the perceived "social issues," rather than clinical practices. The headline news of the first IVF birth also attracted some comments from legal experts (e.g., K.-T. Chen 1985; *United Daily News* 15 October 1985: 3). These legal concerns focused mostly on third-party donation, surrogacy, and associated parent-child relationships, which had either already been practiced in donor insemination since the 1950s or were not the status quo in IVF. The Department of Health established an advisory committee on assisted reproduction to offer advice, composed of eleven members, six of whom were doctors. One senior government official told me that this kind of ad hoc committee followed the pattern used to deal with family planning and the legalization of abortion (Official Q, 2011 interview). Called "Ethical Guidelines for Practicing ARTs," the first official regulation was announced in 1986, one year after the birth of Baby Boy Chang. The guideline specified that ART be made available only to infertile married couples and be operated by qualified medical personnel, and it prohibited the commodification of donated sperm and eggs. This simple statement responded to major concerns in the earliest period.

Two IVF-related medical societies were established in Taiwan in 1990: the Society of Infertility Treatment of the Republic of China, renamed the Taiwanese Society for Reproductive Medicine (TSRM) in 2000, and the Fertility Society of the Republic of China (FSROC). Both societies' presidents routinely became members of consecutive governmental advisory committees. Thus, despite the major role of the government, policy related to the technical aspects of IVF has been dominated by medical professionals.

The official governmental intervention extended to detailed mea- sures, but it still provided no word on number of embryos. In 1994, the new "Regulations Governing ARTs" established an accreditation system to certify IVF centers through governmental evaluation of lab standards, mainly based on the specifications of invited IVF experts. For the first accreditation, forty-eight centers received a formal license to practice IVF and third-party egg and sperm dona- tion. For the lab evaluation, cryopreservation—the preservation of eggs, sperm, and embryos by freezing techniques—counted 3 points in a total possible score of 125, and number of embryos transferred (NET) was not even among the evaluation criteria in the early regulation.

This early absence of multiple embryo transfer regulation in Taiwan shows that the government left the territory of clinical pro- cedure to medical professionals. Some newspaper reports in Taiwan exemplified the British regulation as an ideal from the advanced countries (Y.-M. Chang 1994a; Yuan 1995). When responding to the media's questions about potential regulations such as Britain's 1990 Human Fertilisation and Embryology Act (HFE Act), Taiwan officials emphasized the "fast-changing" character of ART and regarded formal regulation as inflexible for this innovative technology (Y.-M. Chang 1994a). The HFE Act's first edition of its Code of Practice limited NET to three or fewer embryos. One Taiwan official whom I interviewed promoted the self-regulation model:

> The number of embryos transferred is related to doctors' clinical judgment. Cases are diverse, and each judgment differs. Law, such as limiting with a specific number, is rigid; once it is stipulated, if we want to make changes, it has to undergo a lot of procedures. It is better to leave the judgment to doctors themselves. (Official M, 2011 interview)

What Official M argued shows that the Department of Health preferred leaving clinical judgments to the medical community. Compared to statutory regulation, such as what Germany and the UK did in 1990 to legally limit NET to three embryos at most, a voluntary guideline has the advantage of retaining medical professional autonomy while demonstrating professional responsibility.[5]

The medical community in Taiwan preferred no regulation on clinical procedures. It is worth noting that the very existence of statutory regulation on embryo transfer, at least in Britain, inspired a few Taiwanese IVF experts to support regulation. For example, Dr. Tzu-Yao Lee, a pioneering infertility specialist at NTU Hospital, criticized the high incidence of multiple births and asked for standardization (Lee 1995). However, when other leading IVF experts did voice concerns about multiple pregnancy, they favored the technical solutions of perfecting the skills of cryopreservation or improving the quality selection of embryos. They also stressed the limitations of regulation, stating that it could not prevent multiple pregnancy caused by ovulation-induction drugs (Y.-M. Chang 1994b). Their policy suggestions avoided the imposed standardization of clinical procedures found in the British model.

The decision-making structure in Taiwan in this period strengthened medical professionals' autonomy in IVF. The advisory committee in Taiwan, as well as the officials in charge, were all under the Department of Health, in contrast to Britain, where the HFE Authority (HFEA) committee was an independent organization. The HFEA committee was required to include diverse expertise and laypeople (Johnson 1998), whereas in Taiwan medical professionals dominated the committee. Therefore, Taiwan lacked a regulatory regime through which the British model could be executed. Taiwan also lacked most of the policy elements that had forced the British government to regulate. No religious groups or antiabortion

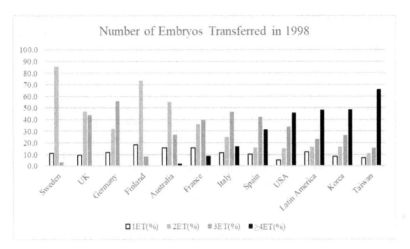

GRAPH 3.1. The Distribution of Number of Embryos Transferred (NET) by Selected Countries in 1998. (1ET = one embryo transferred; 2ET = two embryos; etc.) Source: IWGRAR 2002. © Chia-Ling Wu

groups in Taiwan voiced their concern over the status of embryos (cf. Franklin 1997; Inhorn 2003). Legal experts and social scientists were involved with ART, but they tended to focus on the "social" aspects, leaving the "technical" ones to the medical experts. Overall, in the 1990s, no local stakeholders in Taiwan exerted pressure to regulate the number of embryos transferred.

What about pressure from the international IVF monitoring organizations? Health surveillance through data collecting and reporting has been the common strategy of global governance. The International Working Group for Registers on Assisted Reproduction (IWGRAR 2002) published the data of forty-four countries and found that Taiwan had implanted the highest number of embryos in the world. Taiwan's national registry data started in 1998 so that the national data could be available for the world report. This 1998 global comparison showed that the average NET during IVF was 4.07 in Taiwan, followed by 3.46 in the US and 3.45 in South Korea, while the average NET was less than 2 in Finland and Sweden. Graph 3.1 reveals that 66 percent of IVF cycles in Taiwan involved four or more embryos, while the same column shows zero (no column at all for four or more embryos) for Sweden, the UK, and Germany, where two or three embryos was the maximum number by legal regulation. However, this world's worst ranking was not reported in the Taiwanese media and therefore did not trigger public debate.

I asked several TSRM leaders whether this international comparison was known to the doctors in Taiwan. Dr. S told me how the medical community responded to the international data:

> Right, we did mention the data at our board meeting. Taiwan's statistical result looked bad, and we felt that we needed to improve. However, this kind of pressure did not last long. Most doctors still *cared most about the success rates.* Those centers which did not have a strong lab often depended on implanting more embryos to increase the success rates. And it was also hard to make strict limitations because we [i.e., the TSRM] did not want to make hurdles for some members' running [their] business. It needs the reputation of high success rates to attract clients, so most of them pursue high success rates first, and deal with multiple pregnancy later, with fetal reduction. (Dr. S, 2010 interview, Taipei, emphasis added)

The international report did not create strong pressure. Individual clinics' success rates mattered most. The survival of clinics by keeping high success rates was the main concern. And the medical organization could not easily stand against other members' financial interests in the competitive environment of IVF.

Gathering Test-Tube Babies in the Shape of Taiwan

The health of test-tube babies is conveyed in two types of images: photos of gatherings of IVF children and follow-up statistics. Beginning in the late 1990s, some Taiwanese hospitals and infertility-related organizations would invite all the test-tube babies to get together. For example, the ROC Infertility Foundation, established by the IVF expert Dr. Maw-Sheng Lee, held an event on Children's Day in 1997 that was attended by seven hundred IVF kids, including one hundred twins, fifteen triplets, and three quadruplets, ranging from one to eleven years old. In addition to playing a crawling game and tug of war, two pediatricians offered heart exams by ultrasound on the spot. Dr. Lee claimed that a follow-up survey of twelve hundred IVF children showed that "one-third of test-tube babies were gifted students," possibly due to the selection of sperm during the IVF procedure, as well as to intensive care from their parents (Chao 1997). Combining the survey results and health checkups during the 1997 gathering, the ROC Infertility Foundation announced that "test-tube babies have no problem in IQ and health at all" (C.-H. Chen 1997).

Since then, gatherings of test-tube babies to present the image of happiness and achievement have become a routine event (Ke 2003). Taipei Veterans Hospital held a similar gathering to have "another father" of IVF, Dr. Chang, meet the hospital's IVF children (Wei 2005b). Other clinics used the familial metaphor of "going back to your maternal home" to promote the achievement of the clinic (e.g., C.-L. Li 2006). No IVF entrepreneur could compete with Dr. Maw-Sheng Lee, however, who even applied to break the Guinness World Record of the gathering of 1,180 test-tube babies in Vienna, Austria, in 2007, after 1,232 test-tube babies donned pink hats and gathered in the shape of the island of Taiwan in 2011, the year Taiwan celebrated its centennial (*United Daily News* 17 October 2011). The nationalist glory continues.

In contrast to the joyful and record-breaking gathering, the epidemiology data looked worrisome. From 1987 through 1996, the Taiwan Society of Perinatology had collected data from six hospitals to build the first health patterns of premature babies, finding that the rate of premature birth was 36.9 percent for twins and 75 percent for triplets; the report predicted that premature births would increase with the increasing use of infertility treatments (Y.-F. Shih 1998). Some medical centers had the pediatricians trace the health outcomes of their IVF babies, which revealed that 20 percent had signs of delayed development (S.-H. Hung 2000). The highest-quality data came from Taiwan's ART registry data, built since 1998, which included the health outcomes of the newborns and outshone the data of the voluntary registries in Japan and South Korea (Wu, Ha, and Tsuge 2020). The data revealed that since 1998, more than 40 percent of live births through IVF were of infants weighing less than twenty-five hundred grams, classified as "low birthweight" (ROC Department of Health 2003). This means that nearly half of IVF babies needed extra healthcare after birth. Those who were under fifteen hundred grams, categorized as "very low birthweight," possibly needed long-term care due to disability—an image in stark contrast to the celebratory depictions of test-tube-baby gatherings. A shadow began to fall on the nationalist glory.

Conclusion

This chapter has demonstrated how a nation's sociotechnical imaginaries shape the trajectories and dynamics of anticipatory governance. When IVF debuted as a nationalist glory in Taiwan, the

TABLE 3.1. Anticipatory Governance of In Vitro Fertilization (IVF) in Japan and in Taiwan. (JSOG = Japan Society of Obstetrics and Gynecology.) © Chia-Ling Wu

	Japan	Taiwan
National sociotechnical imaginaries of emerging IVF	Controversy	Glory
Dominant dimension of anticipation	Risk prevention	Pursuing a successful "first"
Framing of fetal reduction	Causing disputes	Medical innovation & routinized technical solution
Anticipatory practices for multiple pregnancy in the 1990s	JSOG's embryo transfer guideline	Professional autonomy

IVF medical community remained the dominant actor to frame the anticipation, primarily in terms of successful events and success rates, and only occasionally in terms of health risk. Even fetal reduction, a controversial procedure in most countries, could be framed as a medical breakthrough and quickly incorporated into the IVF network as the technical solution to the increasing incidence of multiple pregnancy. Facing increasing numbers of cases of quadruplets, maternal and infant death, and worrisome epidemiology of premature babies, the health risks of multiple pregnancy caused by both IVF and egg stimulation drugs attracted debates on regulation. However, the state preferred that IVF professionals self-regulate, leaving much space for practitioners to remain autonomous in their own clinical practices before the 2000s.

The contrast between Japan and Taiwan is revealing (table 3.1). When IVF emerged in East Asia in the early 1980s, it was linked to the management of controversy in Japan and the achievement of nationalist glory in Taiwan. This at least partially explains why Japan governed IVF through strong self-regulation to establish social trust, resulting in the JSOG model to impose a SET guideline to efficiently reduce health risk, which has been far from the case in Taiwan (see table 3.1). More such imaginaries are worth exploring to enrich our understanding of why anticipatory governance takes so many different forms around the world. Even though the medical societies and the state did not actively intervene to change Taiwan's having the world's highest average NET, new voices started to rise in the 2000s: pediatricians, suffering mothers, the Premature Baby Foundation of Taiwan (PBFT), and some reflexive IVF experts all verbalized their concerns on behalf of Taiwan's wordless premature babies. New momentum to anticipate health risk finally started in Taiwan in the 2000s.

Notes

1. Taiwan's media seldom mentioned India's "Baby Durga," born in the same year as Louise Brown (Ferber, Marks, and Mackie 2020).
2. For example, Shirley L. Chang (1992) estimates that in the 1970s nearly half the graduates in engineering and science from National Taiwan University and Tsinghua University, the most prestigious universities in Taiwan, went abroad for graduate study and that 95 percent of them went to the US. Most of them stayed in the US after graduation; the returnee rate was only 5 percent in the 1960s and 15 percent in the 1970s.
3. The trajectory of experimenting with IVF in Taiwan differed greatly from that in China, which involved more of what Fu (2017) calls "*tu* science," a native, local, and Chinese way of doing science. For the making of the first IVF baby in China through *tu* science, see Jiang (2015) and Wahlberg (2016, 2019). I thank one reviewer for pointing out the different beginnings of experimenting with IVF in Taiwan and in China.
4. After defeat by the Communist Party during the 1946–49 civil war in China, the Nationalist Party, led by Chiang Kai-shek, retreated to Taiwan to continue the Republic of China (ROC), while the Communist Party established the People's Republic of China (PRC) on the Mainland. Around 1.2 million Mainlanders migrated to Taiwan and joined the 6 million Taiwanese. The authoritarian rule of the Nationalist Party led to the ethnic tension and inequality between Mainlanders and Taiwanese. For a literature review on this ethnic relationship, see F.-C. Wang 2018.
5. Britain's 1990 Human Fertilisation and Embryology Act (HFE Act) was sometimes mentioned by the media in Taiwan as a policy option, in part because it was the model most widely reported in the English medical journals and mass media (Journalist W, 2011 interview).

Chapter 4

THE MAKING OF THE
WORLD'S MOST LENIENT GUIDELINE

"Unlimited" was a category of the number of embryos to transfer (NET) in the International Federation of Fertility Societies (IFFS) report in 2001 (Jones and Cohen 2001). "Unlimited" indicates the absence of guideline for NET. The IFFS reported that among thirty-nine countries surveyed, more than half had guidelines or statutes to limit NET. Taiwan was included in that report, under the category "unlimited," with "< 6" supplied in parentheses, meaning that the customary NET was fewer than six (ibid.: S12). "Fewer than six" may have looked extreme in comparison with those countries doing double embryo transfer, but it may in fact have been an underestimate in Taiwan, for according to Taiwan's national registry data, in 2000 nearly 20 percent of cycles were implanted with six, seven, eight, or nine embryos (ROC Department of Health 2003). Canada and Greece also reported "unlimited" NET, with "< 6" again supplied in parentheses. In contrast, as chapters 1 and 2 have shown, Sweden, the UK, Belgium, and Japan had moved to a maximum of two or three embryos transferred as early as the 2000s, with enforcement from the state or medical society. Taiwan did not build any guideline on NET until 2005, and it has been revised three times since then. Although Taiwan is no longer listed under the category "unlimited," its NET guidelines have been one of the most lenient in the world.

This chapter analyzes the making of the NET guideline in Taiwan. How did Taiwan start the NET regulation? Who are the key stake-

holders in the process of creating regulation? If doctors have dominated the clinical practices, how could the power dynamics change?
Since NET is a global trend, what kind of available regulatory models
are chosen as the useful reference? What is the contact zone? Most
research discusses ART regulation within the boundaries of a given
nation-state. As the regulation latecomer in the case of NET, Taiwan
can reveal the specificity of interaction between the global and the
local. My analysis begins by identifying the key group of stakeholders who initiated the need to regulate NET. The leverage of the weak
may first come from a sad mother's tears.

"A Sad Mother's True Confession"

In 2000, a story titled "A Sad Mother's True Confession," published
in the newsletter of the Premature Baby Foundation of Taiwan
(PBFT), revealed the suffering of a set of premature triplets and
their whole family. The story began with the implantation of five
embryos, becoming pregnant with quadruplets, reduction to triplets, and birth in the twenty-fifth week. The mother complained
that the doctor in charge gave misleading information:

> The doctor suggested reducing the quadruplets to triplets and gave
> us three factors to consider. First, there are several success stories
> of triplets. Second, parents would have a difficult time. Third, the
> pediatric section in that hospital had a strong team. We came from a
> farmers' family, so we were not afraid of the heavy care burden. ...
> However, what the doctor did not tell us was the health risk of
> triplets. ... I would like to warn future parents that a singleton is what
> you should consider. ... And for doctors, you should bear kindness in
> mind and tell the patients the danger that multiple babies would face.
> (A Sad Mother 2000)

The voices of such "sad mothers" had seldom before been heard.
The PBFT created a platform to reveal the medical misconduct from
the mothers' perspectives, as well as the direction of policy changes,
such as correct information on the health risks of multiple birth.
Some follow-up reports indicated that the sad mother's triplets suffered lingering health problems (Yang 2002), echoing the major
concern of the PBFT, which gradually became the major public
voice for wordless premature babies. The statistics of increasing premature babies caused by IVF looked alarming, but it is the personal
tragedy that often resonated most.

Witnessing the rapid increase in similar cases and the upsetting statistical numbers, the PBFT became a new actor to confront the practices of assisted reproductive technology. The PBFT had been founded in 1992 to provide adequate medical care for premature babies and support for their parents. The main office was in MacKay Memorial Hospital, famous for its pediatric care. In the 2000s, the PBFT began to respond to the increasing multiple births of premature babies, from twins and triplets to quadruplets and even quintuplets. For example, responding to a quintuplet birth, Dr. Kuo-Inn Tsuo, a PBFT board member and the leading pediatrician in the neonatal care unit at NTU Hospital, argued that babies born of IVF overall had poorer health outcomes, mainly due to the prematurity caused by multiple pregnancy (Yang 2000); the response was based on her team's research on the outcomes of one hundred IVF births at NTU Hospital in 1995–96 (Chou et al. 2002). Prevention gradually stood out as a new agenda item for the PBFT, including the misuse of ARTs (Yang 2002). At the PBFT's tenth-anniversary event in 2002, a father of two sets of twins testified how his wife had been pregnant with quadruplets and septuplets, which had been reduced to twins in both cases who had nevertheless been born prematurely. His tearful testimony was widely reported in the media (e.g., C.-C. Chiu 2002).

The PBFT began to pressure the IVF community to act on prevention. In addition to these emotional personal stories, national registry data became a useful force. In 2002, when the PBFT celebrated its tenth anniversary, the premature rate of IVF babies was 43.8 percent, including 6.2 percent weighing less than fifteen hundred grams, categorized as "very low birthweight," the highest percentage ever recorded in Taiwan (ROC Department of Health 2005a). One active member of the PBFT described how she used the data to press the IVF leaders:

> 43 percent of IVF babies were premature. And about 7 percent less than 1,500 grams. This is horrible! These were caused by the 65 IVF centers. I presented the statistics to Dr. Kuo-Kuang Lee and kept asking him what to do. ... He said let's have some education seminars for our members. Since the introduction of National Health Insurance [in 1995], we have traced the health outcomes of premature babies. We have done two white papers on the health outcomes of premature babies. One-fourth to one-fifth of them have some mild or serious neuro and developmental problems. Really sad. I hope they can provide the information well. (PBFT key member, 2002 interview)

Presenting "horrible" numbers and sad stories, the PBFT persuasively asked the IVF community to take action. Thus, unlike the interprofessional conflicts between neonatologists and IVF practitioners that spurred reform in Japan, in Taiwan it was the PBFT that was the main engine of reform. Dr. Kuo-Kuang Lee, who was both the IVF leader at MacKay Memorial Hospital, where the PBFT was based, as well as the president of the Taiwan Society for Reproductive Medicine (TSRM), became the bridge between the PBFT, as the spokesperson for premature babies, and IVF practitioners. The new anticipation of new success—achieving live birth without health risk—finally took off in Taiwan.

The TSRM took two initial steps: education, and informed consent. Seminars and continuing education classes were held to recommend that doctors implant an appropriate number of embryos. This included a 2002 seminar, co-chaired by PBFT director Hui-Chen Lai and TSRM president Kuo-Kuang Lee, titled "Minimizing the Risk of Multiple Pregnancy" that included three speakers who talked about the feasibility of single embryo transfer (SET), fetal reduction, and the relationship between ART and premature babies. The TSRM also offered new information about the increasing risk of multiples and premature babies on the official informed-consent form for ART, adding the sentence, "Assisted reproduction would increase the chances of multiple pregnancy and premature birth." In an interview, Dr. Lee also advocated that doctors follow the guidelines from the American Society for Reproductive Medicine (ASRM) to implant three to five embryos depending on the woman's age (Yang 2002). As chapter 1 has shown, state or medical society guidelines to limit the number of embryos had been practiced by other countries since the late 1980s, and these were deemed the most effective way to change clinical practice. As the president of the TSRM, Dr. Lee obviously knew the importance of guidelines. But why did he advocate the ASRM's guidelines for Taiwan instead of those from the UK, Germany, or Japan?

"American Model Plus One"

By 2002, limiting the number of embryos transferred was the common effort worldwide to reduce the troubling trend of multiple pregnancy. The most lenient guideline came from the US, which showed a NET on the IFFS report of two to five embryos by age group in 1999 (Jones and Cohen 2001: S12), a guideline revised to one to five embryos in 2004. Taiwanese doctors knew well that the trend in European countries and Australia was toward double or single embryo transfer, and some even introduced this trend to Taiwan in popular media articles (C.-H. Lai 1998, 2002; C.-C. Tsai 1999; Chien 1999). Nevertheless, the American guideline became the model to follow.

In 2005, the TSRM announced its own voluntary guidelines for the very first time. At the board meeting in February of that year, Dr. Ying-Ming Lai drafted a qualitative guideline on NET, stating that "if we carefully select *two to three embryos of good quality*, we could reach ideal pregnancy ... if we limit to transferring *two blasto-cysts*, this could both reach a high pregnancy rate and avoid higher-order multiple pregnancy" (Y.-M. Lai 2005: 7, emphasis added). However, in June 2005, the publicized TSRM guideline was much more lenient: two or three embryos for women thirty-five years old or younger; three or four for women thirty-five to forty years of age; and for women forty years old or more, doctors could implant five or more embryos. The guideline followed the recommendations of the revised 2004 ASRM guideline but added one more embryo for each age group (table 4.1). Several doctors termed it the "American model plus one."

Issuing a guideline was an important step, but why did the TSRM move from its original proposal of a two-to-three NET guideline to a two-to-five one? One doctor who became involved with the guidelines explained the result:

> The overall pregnancy rate in Taiwan looked good, but it was uneven: some centers were good, and some were bad. The good pregnancy rate is also made by implanting multiple embryos. Our one- or two-embryo implantation rate was still low. Some members still lacked the skill to get a good pregnancy rate with few embryos. If we gave a strict guideline, we were afraid that it would work against some members' interest. We would be badly complained [about]. (Doctor L, 2011 interview)

Dr. L's response was quite similar to the reasoning in the 1990s for not imposing any guideline—namely, to avoid interfering with other clinicians' business. IVF had moved from a technical competition for "First" status in the 1980s to market rivalry for good business in the 2000s. The number of government-accredited IVF centers rose from twenty-five in 1997 to sixty-five in 2001. IVF

TABLE 4.1. ASRM and TSRM Guidelines in 2004 and 2005. (ASRM = American Society for Reproductive Medicine; TSRM = Taiwanese Society for Reproductive Medicine.) © Chia-Ling Wu

ASRM embryo transfer guidelines			TSRM embryo transfer guidelines		
Publication date	Woman's age	Maximum number of cleavage-stage embryos to transfer	Publication date	Woman's age	Maximum number of embryos to transfer
September 2004	< 35	1–2	April 2005	< 35	2–3
	35–37	2–3		35–40	3–4
	38–40	3–4			
	> 40	4–5		> 40	5

centers expanded from the medical centers in metropolitan Taipei to private clinics in other parts of Taiwan. For newcomers particularly, the risk of IVF failure remained a major concern. Given the need of some IVF centers to raise their success rate through higher numbers of embryos transferred, the TSRM further expanded the lenient American guideline when forming a standard.

Why did the ASRM guidelines appeal to the TSRM? Other medical societies, such as the British Fertility Society and the Japan Society of Obstetrics and Gynecology (JSOG), also offered guidelines, but what the TSRM preferred was the American ones. Doctors whom I interviewed offered the following rationales. First of all, the US is a superpower in terms of technological innovation. Following the American guideline thus "cannot be wrong," as one doctor phrased it. Second, the American guideline adds a variable—the mother's age. Doctors believed that this would increase their autonomy to make clinical decisions. Third, by the mid-2000s, the US guideline was very similar to what most Taiwanese doctors practiced—that is, the US's two-to-five embryos was quite close to Taiwan's (misleading) "< 6"—so most did not have to change their clinical behavior to follow it. Fourth, among all the countries with regulation and guidelines, "Taiwan is most similar to the US" (Doctor N, 2011 interview).

Here "similarity" refers to the two countries' lack of health insurance coverage for IVF and their offers of IVF treatment on the free market. One opinion leader explained:

> Taiwan is much like the US. We are very similar. Both do not offer
> health insurance coverage for IVF. Consumers can choose IVF in the
> market. Those European countries offered health insurance coverage,
> so they could afford to limit the number to one or two. We should
> pick a country that is similar to us to follow. (Dr. N, 2011 interview)

Taiwan and the US may not be that similar, however. Since Taiwan
started its National Health Insurance (NHI) in 1995, assisted reproductive technology—joining cosmetic surgery, sex reassignment
surgery, and other medical treatments—is specified in the statute *not*
to be covered. Even though some infertile couples have requested
NHI coverage through public hearings to relieve their financial
burden, these sporadic efforts have not easily moved to the level of
legal change (Wu et al. 2020). By comparison, some US states, such
as Illinois, require mandated insurance coverage for IVF, mainly due
to the lobby of infertility patient groups (King and Meyer 1997).
And by 2001, three states mandated complete coverage (Illinois,
Massachusetts, Rhode Island), while another five states required
partial coverage (Jain 2002; Reynolds et al. 2003). Therefore, it is
misleading to say that the US is like Taiwan in requiring aspiring
parents to pay for IVF fully out of pocket. Taiwan and the US also
differ in terms of geographical space and degrees of competitiveness—factors that affect clinical decisions on NET, but ones that are
seldom highlighted by policymakers.

It was Taiwanese doctors' affinity for the American model, rather
than the similarity of the two IVF systems, that guided the TSRM
to the ASRM. The familiarity of Taiwanese IVF experts with the
American situation began with their early training in IVF. As mentioned earlier, most pioneering Taiwanese IVF specialists learned
IVF in the hospital labs at the University of Southern California
or the University of Rochester (Doctor L, 2011 interview). In the
initial period, some Taiwanese Americans helped several Taiwanese
hospitals build IVF centers, strengthening the link between Taiwan
and the US. Taiwanese doctors also learned IVF skills from the UK,
Australia, France, Japan, and Singapore and attended conferences
held by the IFFS and the European Society of Human Reproduction
and Embryology (ESHRE). Still, they most regularly attended the
annual meeting of the ASRM, selected a US university lab in which
to learn new skills during their sabbatical years, and reported on
their American experiences in the TSRM newsletter or national
newspapers. Taiwan's affinity for the American IVF model reflects
its continuing dependence on the US since the Cold War period in

terms of knowledge acquisition. This affinity extends to policy travel in the regulation of embryo transfer.

Challenge from a Feminist Legislator

When Taiwan's Department of Health first drafted the Assisted Reproduction Act in the 2000s, regulation of the number of embryos transferred was not included, nor was it contained in two later drafts provided by legislators. It was the legislator Shu-Ying Huang, a feminist activist, who in 2006 proposed adding a regulation that would limit the number of embryos to "no more than four." Taiwan Women's Link (TWL) was established in 2000, the very first women's organization that focused on health issues.[1] From the very beginning, TWL has been devoted to women's access to resources of abortion, including RU486. At the same time, TWL shares similar values with FINRRAGE (Feminist International Network for Resistance to Reproductive and Genetic Engineering) in terms of challenging the use of assisted reproduction technology. Legislator Huang has been the main feminist figure against the legalization of surrogacy in Taiwan. When the Assisted Reproduction Act was discussed in the congress, she also insisted on including a new item on NET in the article that listed prohibited practices such as sex selection of embryos during IVF.

Legislator Huang's written proposal emphasized the risks of the fetal reduction technique to women's health as the primary reason for her insistence on regulating NET. In the parliamentary discussion, she stated that there were cases of women dying from fetal reduction, so "in the interest of protecting women's health," limiting NET was important (Legislative Yuan Gazette 2006: 157). What she was referring to had happened at Taipei Veterans Hospital, where the first IVF baby, Baby Boy Chang, had been delivered by Dr. Sheng-Ping Chang in April 1985. Seventeen years later, Dr. Chang had performed a four-to-two fetal reduction for a woman who subsequently died of a serious infection, together with the remaining two fetuses. Dr. Chang faced a legal suit brought by the family that was not settled for more than a decade. Only one major media outlet reported on the case (C.-S. Chen and Chang 2002). Legislator Huang highlighted the case in her opening statement as the main reason to legally limit the number of embryos transferred in IVF.

Legislator Huang also listed the regulations from Belgium, China, Germany, Japan, Sweden, and Switzerland as examples to regulate

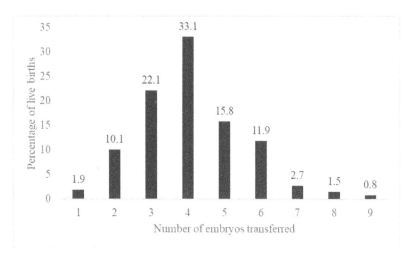

GRAPH 4.1. Taiwanese Government Statistics for 2002 Cited by Legislator Huang. Source: ROC Department of Health 2005a. © Chia-Ling Wu

NET. As a latecomer to legal regulation, Taiwan applied the common strategy of mobilizing an international trend so as to convince others to follow. Legislator Huang further stressed during the congressional meetings that the Nordic countries, Belgium, and the Netherlands had moved to single embryo implantation (Legislative Yuan Gazette 2006: 156). Then she presented the local statistics based on the national registry: the live birth rate for implanting three embryos was 22 percent in 2002, the rate for four was 35 percent, and the rate dropped to 15 percent when five were transferred (graph 4.1). Legislator Huang proposed "no more than four" as a balance between protecting maternal and infant health and maximizing the local success rate of IVF.

Despite the fact that the global trend in IVF was to limit the number of embryos to three or fewer in the 2000s, local practice in terms of pregnancy rate was presented as the most important criterion when considering the extent of limitation. "No more than four" was a compromise for Legislator Huang, considering the dilemma she faced in attempting to protect women's health. That dilemma was to calculate the health risk caused by fetal reduction and repeated IVF. After she learned of the low local success rate using just one or two embryos, she could not just copy the European trend without considering the local situation. Gauging the multiple risks women might face, Legislator Huang chose to limit NET based on the performance of local practice. Dr. Shee-Uan Chen of NTU Hospital, the expert invited to the parliament, admitted that the 3–5 TSRM guideline was more lenient than that of ASRM. He agreed with Legislator Huang that "up to four should be reasonable ... if more than four, it only increases the chances of multiple birth and women's health risk" (Legislative Yuan Gazette 2006). Legislator Huang further echoed Dr. Chen to point out the statistics that "the success rate was 33 percent for four, and dropped to 15 percent [for five embryos], so certainly four was better" (ibid.: 158).

Lack of health insurance was another local practice taken into consideration in the legislature. Asked about the possibility of using single embryo transfer (SET), Dr. Chen responded: "The above-mentioned countries that require one embryo at one time have health insurance coverage, so they can absorb the burden of failure. However, most of the countries in the world do not offer health-insurance coverage" (ibid.: 157). Dr. Chen linked SET to insurance coverage to explain why it wasn't feasible to implant just one embryo at a time in Taiwan. What Dr. Chen described was closer to the Belgian model, or the case in some Nordic countries, as discussed in chapter 2. Still, more countries than Dr. Chen mentioned provide some public financial support of IVF. According to an IFFS survey, half of IFFS-reporting countries offer at least partial insurance coverage (Jones and Cohen 2007). Some countries (such as Israel and France) offer generous coverage without official regulation of NET, while others do not have any national insurance coverage (such as Switzerland and Canada) but nevertheless require that three or fewer embryos be transferred. Although the association between regulation of NET and third-party payment is complicated, a particular image of the global trend was given to justify the permissive regulations in the local proposal before the Taiwanese legislature.

"No more than four" did not encounter any objection in the arena of legislation and soon became part of the drafted Assisted Reproduction Act that was passed by the parliament in 2007. As I investigated this story, I found that the powerful statistics that Legislator Huang relied on were inaccurate, due to badly presented government data. The y-axis on graph 4.1 was mistakenly labeled "Percentage of live births" by the Bureau of Health Promotion; it should be "Percentage of *total* live births," and it would be better presented as a pie chart, since all the percentages would then add up to 100 percent (ROC Department of Health 2005a). If we look

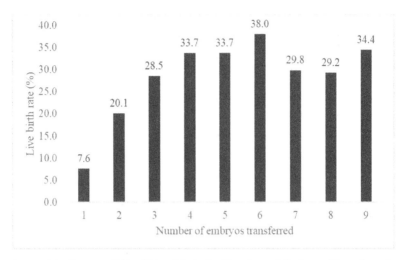

GRAPH 4.2. Percent (%) of Live Births by Number of Embryos Transferred (NET) in Taiwan in 2003. Source: ROC Department of Health 2005b. © Chia-Ling Wu

at the success rate for each number of embryos transferred—the statistics Legislator Huang would have liked to quote—we find that in 2003 the live birth rate was actually highest when six embryos were transferred (graph 4.2), which was also listed in the annual government report of ART practices.

None of the legislators, governmental officials, or IVF experts pointed out Legislator Huang's inadvertent use of misleading government data. This may be because "no more than four" happened to be the best compromise among various stakeholders. For Legislator Huang, a legal enforcement was imposed on doctors. For doctors, "four or fewer" meant a flexible standardization. After all, in 2007, the year the legislation passed, only 13.1 percent of IVF cycles in Taiwan were implantations of five or more embryos (ROC Department of Health 2009). Therefore, despite the fact that the guideline of "no more than four" sprang from a misrepresentation of data, it paradoxically fulfilled the diverse interests of stakeholders and resulted in a consensus on statutory regulation. Feminists such as FINRRAGE members have been the leading actors in selecting multiple pregnancy as the dimension of anticipation of health risk. This also happened in Taiwan. Nevertheless, the newly established regulation of "up to four" embryos transferred in IVF could scarcely reach the goal of reducing the risk of multiple pregnancy.

Voluntary Guidelines: Far from Elective Single Embryo Transfer (eSET)

After the parliament passed the Assisted Reproduction Act in 2007, the TSRM revised its 2005 voluntary guidelines in 2012 and 2016 (table 4.2). In the statement of the 2012 guideline, the TSRM again recognized Taiwan in terms of its world ranking, although this time it was not for a glorious achievement but for a controversial regulation:

> Among all the countries that practiced assisted reproductive tech-
> nologies in the world, for the legal limit on the number of embryos to
> transfer, Taiwan's "up to four" is the highest. ... The goal of ART is to
> help infertile couples have healthy babies. Therefore, while we aim
> to maintain the success rates, we need to reduce the risk of multiple
> pregnancy caused by ART. Our success rates are as good as many
> European and American countries. Based on the trend of developed
> countries, meeting discussions, and surveys of our members, we built
> the following guideline. (TSRM 2012)

The TSRM showed signs of anticipating new success by bringing up the concept of "take a healthy baby home" and working to maintain Taiwan's success rates while reducing the health risk of multiple pregnancy. However, its overall statement leaned toward maintaining Taiwan's high success rates, as contextualized within the global comparison of developed countries. More significantly, the contents of Taiwan's guidelines were far from eSET, which was the most effective way to reduce multiple pregnancy and had been practiced by Sweden, Japan, Belgium, and several other countries for more than a decade by the 2010s.

TABLE 4.2. Taiwan Society for Reproductive Medicine (TSRM) Voluntary Guidelines in 2005, 2012, and 2016. © Chia-Ling Wu

Woman's age	2005	2012	2016
	Maximum number of embryos to transfer		
< 35	2–3	2	1–2
35–37	3–4	2–3	2
38–40		3–4	3
> 41	5	4	4

TABLE 4.3. American Society for Reproductive Medicine (ASRM) 2017 Guideline on the Maximum Number of Embryos to Transfer. Source: Practice Committee of ASRM and Practice Committee of SART 2017: 902. © Chia-Ling Wu

Woman's age	Cleavage-stage embryos			Blastocysts		
	Euploid	Other favorable	All others	Euploid	Other favorable	All others
< 35	1	1	2	1	1	2
35–37	1	1	3	1	1	2
38–40	1	3	4	1	2	3
41–42	1	4	5	1	3	3

Single embryo transfer was not on the TSRM's agenda. The 2012 and 2016 age-specific guidelines did not differ much from the 2005 ones (see table 4.2). They followed the "American model plus one" pattern, with two major differences. First, the TSRM deleted "five" embryos because of the "up to four" rule in Taiwan's 2007 Assisted Reproduction Act, whereas the 2013 ASRM guideline kept "five" for women forty-one to forty-two years old with cleavage-stage embryos (if blastocysts, then three as the maximum) (Practice Committee of ASRM and Practice Committee of SART 2013). Second, the TSRM did not directly follow the ASRM to set up NET according to the prognosis (type of embryos, favorable or not), and hence was more cautious than the ASRM about recommending SET. The 2016 TSRM guideline only asked its members to consider SET for women under the age of thirty-five with a "favorable prognosis," meaning women with (a) excess embryos of quality good enough to warrant cryo-preservation, (b) blastocysts, or (c) previous success with IVF—and for euploid embryos with preimplantation genetic screening (PGS). These conditions showed that the guidelines needed to be updated hand in hand with the advancement of technology for high-quality embryo selection. This is an important part of anticipatory work—abduction—as discussed in chapter 2. When the ASRM announced its 2017 guideline, a lot of "ones" finally appeared in the table (table 4.3), but the TSRM still did not follow the ASRM and revise its own guideline. Overall, both the mandatory restriction (up to four embryos by law) and the voluntary guideline in Taiwan fell far short of encouraging SET.

Disconnected Patchworks of eSET

Other efforts to promote eSET existed but could not be assembled to enact SET. Anticipatory governance requires "ensemblization" (Barben et al. 2008: 990–91)—that is, turning a variety of practices into an ensemble that acts and is viewed as a whole, as a musical or dance ensemble does. I call each such practice a "patchwork" and present the five major types in Taiwan. I then elaborate how the patchworks are disconnected, thereby failing to create a working ensemble.

Patchwork I: Individual exemplar experiments with practicing SET. A few doctors were known to practice eSET and became visible as role models. At the annual meeting of the TSRM in 2010, Dr. Kuo-Kuang Lee, the former TSRM president, gave a keynote speech on higher-order multiple pregnancy since the 2007 regulation. As described earlier, Dr. Lee worked with the Premature Baby Foundation of Taiwan to warn against the health risk of multiple pregnancy, and he also built up some new practices at MacKay Memorial Hospital. In his speech, Dr. Lee did not talk much about the global trend but focused on a sophisticated analysis of local data and evaluation quite unseen in past debates. He then offered the guideline of MacKay Hospital in order to propose a gradual move toward elective single-embryo transfer (eSET) for women under thirty-five years old. This was the most demanding proposal in Taiwan at that time, even stricter than the later 2012 and 2016 TSRM guidelines. The term "SET" was almost synonymous with Dr. Kuo-Kuang Lee and MacKay Hospital whenever multiple pregnancy issues were brought up at annual TSRM meetings. MacKay is the only center that regularly presents a "cumulative pregnancy rate for eSET."[2] However, neither the guideline nor the presentation of eSET results has been followed by other centers.

Patchwork II: Research related to SET. Top IVF experts do publish scientific research related to eSET in both local and international journals. One method is to explore how to improve the selection of embryos by building a score system (Kung et al. 2003; T.-H. Lee et al. 2006) to help assess the possibility of practicing SET in the future. Only a few researchers have really assessed the clinical outcomes of eSET with advanced intervention, including the IVF team from MacKay Memorial Hospital (C.-E. Hsieh et al. 2018) and Dr. Maw-Sheng Lee's team (e.g., P.-Y. Lin et al. 2020). Nevertheless, this shows that a few Taiwanese doctors follow the most advanced scientific breakthroughs, especially the genetic screening of embryos, even though the low percentage of SET from the Taiwan national registry data reveals a gap between research findings and clinical routines.

Patchwork III: An accreditation system to reduce multiple embryo transfer (MET) by encouraging double embryo transfer (DET). In 1998, the government established an accreditation system to issue formal licenses for medical institutions to practice IVF, perform donor insemination, and run sperm and egg banks. Most of the application criteria concern the qualifications of practitioners and the quality of the laboratory. To renew their license, accredited centers must report data to the registry system and reach a certain success rate. In 2014, the government started a new effort to reduce the multiple pregnancy rate—namely, adding a new item about "the percentage of double embryo transfer or less for women under 35 years old" during the accreditation period (usually three years). If a center reaches 55 percent DET or more, it is given the full points for that item—eight points out of one hundred—but if DET is only 30–54 percent, the center gets four points. The threshold was agreed upon by IVF experts before being put into practice. Considering the TSRM guideline, which recommends that women thirty-five or younger be implanted with no more than two embryos, 55 percent DET should not be difficult to reach. Whenever I asked opinion leaders about the policy to reduce multiple birth, the new accreditation rule was brought up as a new limitation.

The accreditation system has therefore become the major force to ask IVF doctors to follow, but its design does not prioritize eSET. First of all, the rule is more about DET than SET. Most importantly, the overall accreditation system still highlights the success rate. Each accredited IVF center needs to reach a cumulative live birth rate of 25 percent for women under thirty-eight years old over the preceding three years to get full points (twenty-six out of one hundred); if the rate is under 15 percent, its license will almost certainly fail to be renewed. Some doctors honestly told me during interviews that they worried that, if they had many difficult cases, they might not reach the required 25 percent rate. Although cumulative live birth rate supports the idea of SET—to transfer embryos one at a time and count the fresh and frozen cycles together—it still means that success rate matters most.

Patchwork IV: Registry data. Taiwan built a mandatory registry data system in 1998, with a 100 percent reporting rate, and collects quite a complete list of indicators, including both clinical practices and health outcomes. However, the registry has not become the resource to reform ART. As discussed earlier, some activists and reflexive doctors did mobilize some descriptive results from the registry data reports to ask for ART reform. Still, much of the hope work and abduction to enact eSET is not carried out in practice, such as aiming for the ideal of "taking a healthy baby home," which would mean increasing the "percentage of cycles/transfers resulting in normal weight & singleton live births"—a number that has been reported in the US in recent years (CDC, ASRM, and SART 2015).

Taiwan has the data available to produce this indicator, yet it has not yet followed the US in this, i.e., in calculating and presenting this percentage in its annual reports. The HFEA in the UK has initiated the "one at a time" SET policy and made a 10 percent rate of multiple birth the target. Taiwan's state bureaucrats have not mobilized the data for a similar policy target. Even though Taiwan began to collect cycle-based data earlier than Japan, since the registry was handled by the state rather than by the medical society, the TSRM never produced an analysis similar to that of the JSOG to determine whether or not the practice of SET could still produce an acceptable success rate. The top-down approach of registry building in Taiwan has yielded complete data but has failed to transform those data into regulations that effectively reduce the health risks involved. In other words, the IVF data registry has not worked as a care infrastructure to strengthen the community's ethical obligations and to inform evidence-based policymaking, and thus it fails to generate better care (Wu, Ha, and Tsuge 2020).

Patchwork V: Public financing requiring SET. Taiwan's subsidy program was proposed several times to boost low birthweights, but it only started in 2015, much later than Japan in 2004 and South Korea in 2006. The three East Asian countries together reached a super-low fertility rate after entering the twenty-first century, but Taiwan did not follow Japan and South Korea in employing subsidies as a pronatalist strategy. Lack of financial resources, concern about a subsidy's effectiveness to increase the population, and criticism from public health experts and feminist scholars vis-à-vis a family policy that was asking for social welfare rather than direct support for IVF all delayed a subsidy program.

Responding to continuous requests from legislators, the government finally built a public financing program in 2015, targeting only low-income households.[3] However, the state required that for those who applied for the subsidy, SET was required for women under thirty-five years old, and a maximum of two embryos for all the others. This restriction is far more demanding than the 2016 TSRM guideline. One governmental official explained the rationale:

> Considering the maternal and infant health risk caused by implanting too many embryos, we require the clinicians to follow our rule if they want to join this game, in order to guarantee the healthcare quality. We the government need to be the gatekeeper, so we impose the SET and DET rule in the subsidy program. (Governmental Official S, July 2019 interview, Taipei)

This became the only mandatory SET requirement in the IVF regime in Taiwan. With the efforts of some governmental officials, a program pressured by pronatalism has turned into one for equal access and health risk prevention.

Unfortunately, the subsidy program for the low-income families did not lead to any change. The eligible users were low-income families, estimated at about 1 percent of total households of married couples. And the applicants have turned out to be fewer than one hundred couples in six years, occupying 0.01 percent of all IVF treatment cycles. In addition, less than one-quarter of IVF centers joined the subsidy program. Some thought that the eligible users would be too few, and others did not want the government to intervene in the IVF market. In September 2020, Legislator Bi-Ling Kuan challenged the policy, claiming that the total expense of the program is about the same as the fireworks budget for the National Birthday. After implementing the policy for five years, only six babies had been born through the subsidy program. It may well be the program with the lowest proportion of eligible users in the world. As a result, its SET guideline for the subsidy program for low-income families has not had any impact.

These diverse anticipatory practices to assess, promote, and impose eSET have not created a working ensemble. The Taiwan Symphony Orchestra of eSET has been disassembled. Using a visual metaphor, the bottom half of figure 4.1 shows that the five patchworks of eSET—the exemplar role model, the academic research published in prestigious journals, the accreditation to give SET some points, the national registry with its 100 percent reporting rate on clinical practices and infant outcomes, and the subsidy requiring SET for young women—do not interact with each other in a way that is effective to enact eSET. In contrast, similar circles of the Belgian Project and the JSOG model, presented in chapter 2, are entangled and thus mutually strengthen each other to create a 60 percent SET rate in Belgium and a rate of over 80 percent in Japan.

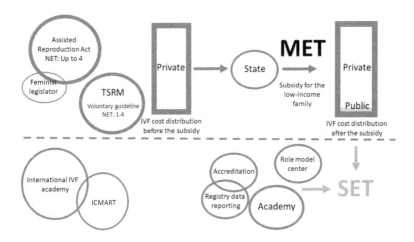

FIGURE 4.1. The Disconnected Patchworks of Single Embryo Transfer (SET) and the Dominance of Multiple Embryo Transfer (MET) in Taiwan, 2005–20. (IVF= in vitro fertilization; NET = number of embryos transferred; TSRM = Taiwan Society for Reproductive Medicine; ICMART = International Committee for Monitoring Assisted Reproductive Technologies.) © Chia-Ling Wu

These trends, as well as warnings from international monitoring organizations such as the ICMART, are cognitively known to the major actors in Taiwan and sometimes serve as the guiding value of each patchwork. However, without integrating the patchwork, the SET rate only reaches 25 percent in Taiwan, one of the lowest percentages in the world.

The ensemble of SET fails, and the MET network remains strong. The upper half of figure 4.1 shows that the permissive legal regulation (up to four embryos to transfer) and the lenient TSRM guideline permit competition among the IVF centers to use MET to meet the promissory capital. The main anticipation still lies in high success rates, and MET is the answer.

Conclusion

Two civic groups in Taiwan, representing the interests of premature babies and mothers, confronted the medical societies and attempted to frame the direction of anticipation on health risk. However, the dilemma of how to balance the success rates against prevention of health risk eventually led to a lenient regulation. IVF doctors managed to build a flexible standardization. Some reflexive IVF practitioners and researchers, engaged governmental officials, and concerned activists have endeavored to promote SET, which is the most effective way to reduce multiple pregnancy/birth. The lack of connected patchworks, which could lead to a SET guideline similar to the ones that Belgium and Japan have established, means that multiple pregnancy remains common in Taiwan.

This chapter also illuminates the specificity of interaction between global and local anticipatory governance. Table 4.4 summarizes the regulatory trajectory of multiple embryo transfer in Taiwan within the analytical framework of global/local dynamics. In different historical periods, the specific Taiwanese stakeholders selected different preferred global forms as a future that Taiwan could follow, such as Britain's code of ethics in the 1990s, the American guideline in the early 2000s, and the European trend in the mid-2000s. The term "global" here is heterogeneous. The configuration of these selected global forms depended on the encountering local network. The British model could serve, at most, as a rhetorical tool for early dissenters in Taiwan because strong pressure had not yet emerged there, as it had in Britain, to limit the number of embryos transferred; moreover, the Taiwanese decision-making structure in IVF regulation favored doctors' autonomy in clinical procedures. When pressure did increase in Taiwan, the American voluntary guideline became a useful policy template for the TSRM to use to balance between the need for self-regulation and market competition. When Taiwanese legislators included number of embryos transferred in the 2007 Assisted Reproduction Act, the international trends acted only to justify legal enforcement, while local statistics became the crucial criterion for specifying "no more than four." The failure to seriously consider adopting the British regulation, the neglect of the JSOG model, the preference for the American guideline (by adding one embryo to its figures), the use of subsidy programs such as that of Belgium as an excuse, and the gap between "no more than four" and the cited European trend all show that Taiwan required a local network as a recontextualized assemblage in order to execute (or not execute) the introduced global model.

The "global" in this case is neither an advanced ideal to copy nor an encompassing force to follow. Due to easy visibility or favored affinity, various stakeholders presented diverse global forms at different stages. The local network further transformed the selected global form, confining it to rhetoric only or tailoring it to local needs. The analytical framework presented here may be most revealing

Table 4.4. The Making of Multiple Embryo Transfer (MET) Regulation in Taiwan, 1980s–2020. (IVF = in vitro fertilization; TSRM = Taiwan Society for Reproductive Medicine; PBFT = Premature Baby Foundation of Taiwan; ASRM = American Society for Reproductive Medicine.) © Chia-Ling Wu

Time period	Key stakeholders	Selected global form	Encountering local network	Recontextualized assemblage
1990s–2000s	Leading IVF experts; the media; TSRM	British model (as a rhetorical tool in addressing the issue of regulating multiple-embryo transfer)	Medical professional dominance; reluctance of the state to intervene in clinical practices	No clinical regulation
2000s–2005	TSRM; PBFT	ASRM guideline (as policy template for guideline formulation)	Professional autonomy & market competition	"American model plus one" (TSRM guideline)
2006–2007	TSRM; feminist legislator; Department of Health	European trends (as justification for legal enforcement); subsidy programs in European countries (as reasons to explain why Taiwan could not practice SET)	Women's health movement & domestic clinical performance	"No more than four" (Assisted Reproduction Act)
2012–2020	TSRM; Ministry of Health	ASRM guidelines	TSRM's preference of flexible standardization	TSRM revised guideline of 1–4 embryos by woman's age

for latecomers, who often turn to international regulatory models for inspiration, but might be useful when analyzing forerunners as well. For example, Franklin (1997: 86–87) argues that the British Parliament limited the use of commercial surrogacy in the 1980s in part because the general public resisted the "Americanisation" of Britain under Thatcher.

The permissive legal regulation and guidelines on the number of embryos to transfer, plus the disconnected patchworks on eSET, mean that multiple embryo transfer (MET) remains a common practice in Taiwan. Graph 4.3 shows that SET increased slowly. Though the graph stops at 2018, in 2019 SET reached 24.9 percent (though some of these are probably compulsory SET rather than eSET); the multiple pregnancy rate declined to 24.1 percent (much higher than the 3 percent in Japan, and the 10 percent goal in UK); and around one-third of test-tube babies were born with low birthweight. Under

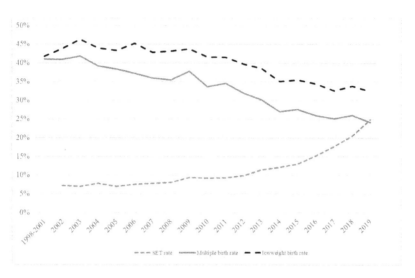

GRAPH 4.3. Trends of Single Embryo Transfer (SET), Multiple Pregnancy, and Low Birthweight Babies in Taiwan, 1998–2019. (ET = embryos transferred.) Source: ROC Ministry of Health and Welfare 2021a. © Chia-Ling Wu

Taiwan's anticipatory governance, "IVF" is almost synonymous with MET and multiple pregnancy in the country. What have women gone through in the IVF regime? Chapters 5, 6, and 7 explore their optimization and "anticipatory labor."

Notes

1. For the history and major contributions of TWL, please see its website: http://twl.ngo.org.tw/about-en (accessed 21 May 2021).
2. MacKay Memorial Hospital's website lists the cumulative pregnancy rate for eSET as 54 percent. See https://ivflab.mmh.org.tw/result (accessed 31 May 2021). However, cumulative live birth rate would be a better indicator.
3. The subsidy is NT 100,000–150,000 dollars (roughly 3,000–5,000 US dollars) for each couple annually. Each IVF cycle costs about NT 120,000–200,000 dollars, so the financial support covers roughly one free cycle.

Chapter 5

OPTIMIZATION WITHIN
DISRUPTED REPRODUCTION

Legislator Lu: "One at a time." Isn't implanting one embryo at a time better than implanting three embryos?

Dr. Chen: The issue is that *patients hope to get pregnant by one time*. The success rate is 20 percent for one-embryo transfer. If one at a time, they would need to come to the hospital many times.

Legislator Lu: You hope that they can achieve success just by one time?

Dr. Chen: Yes. ... Those countries who can have single embryo transfer have insurance coverage, *so that they can endure failure*. However, most countries do not have insurance coverage for IVF.

(Legislative Yuan Gazette 2006: 157, emphasis added)

No laywomen were invited to present their IVF expectations and experiences at the Legislative Yuan during the stipulation of the Assisted Reproduction Act in 2006. Instead, it was left mostly to the legislators, the governmental officials, and the invited doctor to express what women wanted. As shown in chapter 4, the feminist legislator Shu-Ying Huang articulated the various risks that women may meet: failure to become pregnant, fetal reduction, and multiple pregnancy. To balance the needed success rate and the risks to women's health, Legislator Huang proposed four as the maximum number of embryos to transfer, which was supported by Dr. Shee-Uan Chen, chair of the ART center at the prestigious

National Taiwan University Hospital. When another legislator, Mr. Tien-Lin Lu, raised the question of single embryo transfer (SET), Dr. Chen acted as a spokesperson for women and revealed their hope: to get pregnant from their first round of IVF. He also implied that, in the absence of health insurance coverage for the procedure, neither women nor their doctors could afford failure. The issue was quickly settled. Legislator Lu agreed that implanting more embryos to increase the success rate meant fulfilling women's reproductive desire, although he still advised paying attention to the risks of multiple embryo transfer (MET). "No more than four" was written into the law, in the name of women's best interests.

Fast-forward to 2020, and Taiwanese doctors were still voicing women's urgent need to become pregnant the first time they underwent IVF. I interviewed the young Dr. W (at least one generation younger than Dr. Chen) in a café. I asked him why the use of SET remains so low in Taiwan—only around 20 percent of all IVF procedures, possibly the lowest in the world. He cited pressure from patients as the primary reason. He vividly described the suffering that women face: "You know how their hearts break when they see their menstruation has come again." Although he also mentioned the lack of public financial support, and the requirement of reaching certain success rates from the monitoring agency, he saw women's emotional disturbance as the key force that makes doctors reluctant to practice SET. Dr. W reminded me that women request not only quick success but also twins: "People in Taiwan accept 'dragon-phoenix twins' (i.e., one boy and one girl) very much. They do not see twin pregnancy as causing complications, and even praise doctors who can make twins as having superb skills." In Dr. W's words, multiple embryo transfer can "enhance the cp value" (a popular abbreviation for "cost-performance ratio") of IVF.

Women not only want speedy success but also prefer twins? So-called patient demand has been an important angle in figuring out why multiple pregnancy remains popular and whether or not SET works (e.g., Leese and Denton 2010; Adamson and Norman 2020). Dr. Chen and Dr. W implied that women regard multiple embryo transfer as valuable optimization—a way of making their reproductive goal as fully effective as possible. Optimization is an essential part of anticipation work (Adams, Murphy, and Clarke 2009; Clarke 2016). This chapter contextualizes women's optimization within their various experiences of "disrupted reproduction," shaped by medical, social, cultural, legal, and gender politics (Inhorn 2007). Instead of repeating doctors' representations of women's wants and

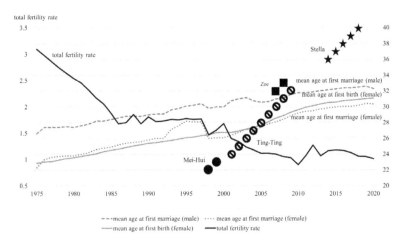

GRAPH 5.1. Changes in Year of First Marriage and Birth in Taiwan, 1975–2020, Showing the Reproductive Trajectories of Four Interviewees (Mei-Hui, Zoe, Ting-Ting, and Stella). Sources: "Demographic Data GIS" 2021; "Population Projection Inquiry System" 2021. © Chia-Ling Wu

needs, I present women's (and a few men's) own voices, focusing on how they seek to achieve their reproductive goals—conflicting and confusing as they may sometimes be—through ART.

The women and men I interviewed anticipated having children at some point in their lives. When they show up at reproductive clinics, they intend to use ART as a tool to solve their perceived reproductive problems. Why do they come to the clinic at this point? What does ART mean to them in terms of achieving their best possible futures? What are their futures? In what follows, I link their personal biographies with the larger social transformation in Taiwan. Only when we understand the different and changing reproductive goals and hurdles these aspiring parents have faced can we know how they view IVF procedures and what the prescribed number of embryos transferred (NET) can mean to them.

Based on interviewing data and participant observation, I present four different anticipatory trajectories of making parents, as well as the optimization to respond to their disrupted reproduction. Graph 5.1 shows the trajectories of Mei-Hui, Zoe, Ting-Ting, and Stella, with Taiwan's dramatic transformation as the backdrop: a declining fertility rate, late marriage, and late birth. Some started their reproductive journey early, and some late. Some took a short period to reach their goal, and others wandered for a longer time. I emphasize that the women's diverse anticipation of becoming parents entailed diverse optimizations of ART, which may differ from what medicine and the media present. Let's meet Mei-Hui first.

"All I Wanted Was to Succeed": Desired Motherhood and Biological Disruption

Mei-Hui became pregnant with triplets by IVF in 1997. Before marrying, she had been pregnant once. It was an ectopic pregnancy, in which the fertilized egg implanted not in the womb but in the fallopian tube. This dangerous situation necessitated termination of the pregnancy and also revealed that her fallopian tube had been damaged. Soon thereafter she married, at twenty-two years old (much sooner than twenty-six, Taiwanese women's average age of first marriage in 1997). At the same time, she quit the job she held as a shop accountant since her high school graduation in order to fully prepare for the couple's fertility plan. She first went to see a doctor of Chinese medicine for about a year. There was no sign of pregnancy, so she went to a medical center for infertility treatment. "We are quite traditional," she told me. "Marriage meant to have children soon." Although Mei-Hui's husband was not the eldest son in his family, her father-in-law emphasized that everyone should have offspring.

Mei-Hui started an IVF cycle immediately because her damaged tube was a clear indication that she should use this advanced infertility treatment. A total of eighteen eggs were retrieved, leading to thirteen embryos in the lab. The doctor transferred eight embryos "to increase the pregnancy rate," Mei-Hui remembered quite clearly. One IVF cycle cost 100,000 NT dollars (roughly 3,000 USD in the late 1990s), and the perseveration of the remaining five embryos cost another 20,000 NT dollars. All the costs were paid by her father-in-law. After the first implantation, there was some sign of pregnancy by testing, but it soon disappeared. Mei-Hui said she was extremely distressed: "The suffering of not getting pregnant was much more serious than the hardship of triplet pregnancy."

In the second attempt, all the remaining five embryos were transferred, leading to triplet pregnancy. All the family were excited. Her mother-in-law joyfully announced: "Triplets are totally fine; we can afford raising three kids altogether." From paying for IVF to paying for childcare, Mei-Hui's in-law family was financially worry free, unlike some other families I met. The doctor did not mention fetal reduction as an option. Mei-Hui, a Christian, said that she would not have opted for fetal reduction in any case due to her religious beliefs. She went through a lot of serious conditions during pregnancy, being hospitalized several times. At one point her father-in-law declared that if Mei-Hui's situation worsened, saving the mother was more important than saving the babies. Mei-Hui gave birth to the triplets around the thirty-fifth week, by cesarean section. All the babies weighed around fifteen hundred grams, the threshold of very low birthweight; two were in incubators for twenty days, and the third for forty days. When I interviewed Mei-Hui at the church she attended, the three teenagers were naughtily playing with each other, waiting for the Sunday school to start.

Mei-Hui's trajectory epitomizes the optimal use of multiple embryo transfer to fix the biological disruption of fertility. For a woman with such a strong desire to bear children, it made sense to pursue methods to increase the success rate of IVF. If multiple embryo transfer (MET) would optimize the chances of becoming pregnant, it was welcomed, not challenged. Mei-Hui was implanted with eight embryos, which was already not permitted in countries such as Sweden, the UK, and Germany in the late 1990s, discussed in chapter 1. However, implanting eight embryos was not rare in Taiwan at that time: according to the registry data, although the mode (the most common value) was four embryos, 5 percent of transfer cycles implanted eight and nine embryos in 1998 (ROC Department of Health 2003). Mei-Hui was in the youngest age group of aspiring mothers, which on average has the highest rate of success; fewer than 2 percent of IVF cycles in the late 1990s were undergone by women who were Mei-Hui's age or younger. Still, the doctor implanted eight embryos on the first round and the remaining five on the second, and Mei-Hui did not object. Not getting pregnant was more torturous than bearing multiple babies. Achieving triplets was a joy that was shared by her family members.

The risks of a multiple birth are not easily registered on the cognitive map of some women's infertility treatment journeys. Some interviewees told me that doctors did tell them that taking fertility drugs and implanting multiple embryos could increase the chances of multiple birth. However, for women who felt frustrated with their failure to conceive even a singleton, the possibility of multiple pregnancy "was for others, [but] impossible for me," as several women told me. As one woman put it, "It is hard to move zero to one, [so] how is it possible to think of two or three?" Instead, it was the failure to conceive that dominated women's minds. When a multiple pregnancy was announced, often after taking an ultrasound image, most women were pleasantly surprised. Gloria, for example, had begun her reproductive journey right after marrying, and when she experienced miscarriage, she told me, "My tears fell like rain." She eventually became pregnant with twins after interuterine insemination (IUI) and compared her excitement to "winning the lottery." This analogy signifies both her perceived low chances of success and a reward beyond all her expectations.

Even though these women show firm determination to become mothers, this does not mean they initially turn to ART. Almost all my interviewees first went through the stage of taking Chinese medicine. As already mentioned, despite Mei-Hui's clear diagnosis of a damaged fallopian tube, she still tried Chinese medicine before moving to IVF. Even women with the strongest desire to bear children tend to first use methods that are perceived as more "natural." Vivian, a customer service staff member at a technology company, got married at twenty-five years old in 1991 and wished to have kids as soon as possible. She said that, because she was a Christian, an "unnatural" method like a test-tube baby was not on the agenda in the beginning. After failure to conceive through sexual intercourse, Vivian took Chinese medicine for a year. Seeing no improvement, she went to see obstetrician-gynecologists and took egg stimulation drugs, but in vain. Then she tried four rounds of IUI, which required her husband to provide sperm that was injected into her womb during her medicated ovulation. IUI failed. Finally, she was persuaded to go to an IVF center where her cousin was working. Due to her preference for naturalness, Vivian had not mobilized her personal network to use the most advanced assisted reproductive technology. The medical center was among the twenty-seven centers in the accredited ART system since 1996. Vivian soon had six embryos ready for use, and the doctor implanted three of them. When I asked whether she was concerned about the possibility of having triplets, she replied:

> Not at all. No such image. *All I wanted was to succeed*, no matter how many fetuses. I tried for so many years, and I felt really bothered. ... I was young, so I did not care much [about the burden of child-raising]. All I wanted was to have a successful pregnancy. (emphasis added)

Vivian became pregnant with twins and went through a very difficult pregnancy (discussed in chapter 7).

Vivian's feeling that "All I wanted was to succeed" was often portrayed in media presentations of the time. In reports seeking legalization of or financial support for surrogacy, for example, the media tended to emphasize how women would take any steps at any cost to achieve their reproductive goals (e.g., Hong 1994), similar to the discourses of desperateness analyzed by Franklin (1990).[1] However, Vivian's case demonstrates the coexistence of strong reproductive desire ("All I wanted was to succeed") with ambivalence toward ART ("It was not natural"). The ideal cultural script was to conceive the natural way: by becoming pregnant through intercourse with one's husband. One woman stressed in her interview with me that although she took a fertility drug to become pregnant, this was much more "natural" than having to go through IUI or IVF. Other things also explained users' hesitancy about IVF. A survey showed that women's top three reasons for not considering IVF were that they thought it was "harmful to health," the "procedures [were] too complicated," and it had a "low success rate"; men's top three were that they thought it was "unnatural," "too expensive," and "against morality" (T.-H. Chen et al. 2009). IVF was not perceived as a magic solution by the general public. The health risk, the financial burden, and the low efficacy were behind this known hesitancy.

Even though my interviewees were concerned about the unnaturalness, intrusiveness, and potential harmful effects of IVF, its leading complication in the medical literature—multiple pregnancy—was scarcely on their mental radar. In Mei-Hui's treatment year (in the late 1990s), although there were some news reports on the controversy of quadruplets, neither a guideline nor informed consent on the risk of multiple birth was in routine practice. In the mid-2000s, the upper limit of number of embryos to transfer was set, and warning signs were listed on the consent form, but the possibility of becoming pregnant with multiples remained hardly a worry during the trajectory to assist conception. Women such as Vivian, who married early and started the reproductive project early, had time to attempt pregnancy using the least intrusive methods first (such as taking Chinese medicine), and gradually moving to fertility drugs, IUI, and finally IVF. Yet these step-by-step strategies were not necessarily appealing to those who began the reproductive project late.

"Take the High-Speed Rail": Rushing toward Delayed Parenthood

Zoe, a middle-tier public servant, used the metaphor of transportation to compare the different methods of infertility treatment she underwent. After failing to become pregnant through a normal sexual life, she went to see a doctor of Chinese medicine but quickly moved to infertility treatment at a medical center, where she began on what she called the "regular train" of taking egg stimulation drugs while having intercourse. After a few cycles, she moved on to what she called the "high-speed rail" (the fastest mode of train travel in Taiwan): IUI, which involved taking egg stimulation drugs and then having washed sperm injected into her womb. She became pregnant with twins after taking her first ride on this "high speed rail."

"We got married late, so we wanted to speed up our schedule to have children," Zoe said in explaining to me why she got off the "slow train." She had married at age thirty-two in 2007, three years older than the mean age of marriage for Taiwanese women in that year. When Zoe stated that she and her husband were a bit behind the ideal schedule, she was referring to the ideal age to become parents, particularly for her husband: "I am already thirty-two, and my husband is three years older than me, so we need to hurry." "Fast" was the keyword for Zoe—and for most of my other interviewees.

Delayed Parenthood

Zoe exemplifies what Lauren Jade Martin (2020) calls "delayers," who want to bear children but start the trajectory late. Much literature has noted that women and men are postponing so-called milestone events, such as marrying and having kids. Taiwan is no exception, and the change there is one of the most drastic in the world. Graph 5.1 (see above) shows that in the last four decades, late marriage, increasing singlehood, and the world's lowest birth rate have become characteristic of Taiwan. Whereas in 1975 the average age at first marriage was twenty-two and twenty-six for women and men, respectively, now it is thirty and thirty-two. For a country with an extremely low rate of births out of wedlock, it is not surprising that, with the postponement of marriage, women are tending to give birth later and later: in 1975 the mean age at which a Taiwanese woman first gave birth was twenty-three, whereas in 2020 it was thirty-one. Moreover, although both Mei-Hui and Zoe planned to have babies, in the 1990s Mei-Hui quit her job early to become a full-time wife/mother, whereas in the 2000s Zoe pursued the goal of becoming a working mother. These two different family/work patterns may partly explain why Mei-Hui began the fertility project early and Zoe began late. In the context of Taiwan today, however, Zoe's approach has become more prevalent than Mei-Hui's.

Studies have shown that many social factors contribute to delayed parenthood in most postindustrial countries, including Taiwan. The subjective evaluation of bodily capacity, the availability of birth control technology, the extension of education duration, the balance of work and family, the worry about inadequate resources for supporting a family, and the changing cultural norms for ideal parenthood—all these lead to late parenthood in many parts of the world today (Sobotka 2010; Brinton 2016; Brinton et al. 2017; Martin 2020). In the specific context of Taiwan, scholars have noted that long working hours, financial instability of the young generation, inadequate family policies, and gender inequality have contributed to late marriage, increasing singlehood, and late parenthood (Raymo et al. 2015; Y.-h. Cheng and Yang 2021). Still, the two-child fertility ideal has persisted in Taiwan (Y.-h. Cheng and Hsu 2020), as it has in Japan, Sweden, Spain, and the US (Brinton et al. 2017). The gap between this ideal and Taiwan's lowest or second lowest fertility rate in the world (less than 1.0 live births per woman over the reproductive years) reflects the struggle and ambivalence of young Taiwanese today.

One consequence for delayers is increasing infertility. Much biomedical literature has emphasized that infertility, miscarriage, maternal complications, and newborns' birth defects increase with women's age (Klein and Sauer 2001). Viewing the trend of increasing numbers of patients in their late thirties and early forties, infertility specialists in Taiwan have warned about starting reproductive action too late. For example, in 2006, the Taiwanese Society for Reproductive Medicine (TSRM) conducted a survey of one thousand men and women aged twenty-five to forty-four to discover their reproductive knowledge and attitudes. The survey found that respondents felt the ideal age to wed is thirty-two years old, and the ideal time to begin a family is two or three years after marriage. When asking, "Compared with 20-year-olds, which age group starts to have decreased fertility capacity?" the TSRM regarded "35-year-olds" as the correct answer but found that about 40 percent of respondents answered "Do not know" or "After 50 years old" (T.-H. Chen et al. 2009). TSRM president Chih-Hong Liu told the press that couples may not be aware that the capacity to conceive declines after age thirty-five, and they may also be misled by some celebrities giving birth in their late forties and early fifties, not realizing that they have done so by using donated eggs (C.-J. Shih 2006).

The TSRM's "deficit model," testing laypeople's knowledge about reproduction, may not be able to fully encompass the complexity of fertility decision-making. Rich social studies of delayed parenthood emphasize a biosocial approach to understanding people's reproductive trajectories (Martin 2017). Whereas Zoe was worried that late parenthood might not be the ideal parenthood, Jane, a PhD student in history, clearly singled out thirty-five (the perceived beginning of "advanced maternal age") as the deadline by which that she wanted to achieve pregnancy. Thinking that "pregnancy should not be a difficult task," she started her pregnancy plan at thirty-four, only to find that she needed to see ob-gyns for medical assistance. Another interviewee, Yi-Fen (details below), insisted that she was voluntarily childless and had even refused parenthood by pursuing graduate study. Facing an intimacy crisis in her eighth year of marriage and passing the age of thirty-five, she finally embarked on a reproductive plan. Various biosocial factors lead people to delay the project—and later speed up the timeline.

The magic number thirty-five was the benchmark among some delayers among my interviewees. Jane, Yi-Fen, and some other women I interviewed used thirty-five as the reference point to calculate the timing of marriage and conception. The deadline for women's fertility plans in Taiwan was quite similar to that in the US (see Martin 2017, 2020). However, as a mark of "advanced maternal age," thirty-five not only denotes declining fertility and increasing health risk for newborns but also exposure to intrusive medical procedures such as amniocentesis. In addition to anticipating infertility (e.g., Martin 2020), women I interviewed attempted to avoid another medical intrusion: amniocentesis. When amniocentesis became available in the early 1980s in Taiwan, it was advised that pregnant women over thirty-five years old undergo the genetic testing. The government offered a subsidy for women above thirty-four, which became a cutoff point for advanced maternal age. Several tragic events happened, such as the harm to the fetus and miscarriage, and were widely reported. This cast a shadow over use of the selective technology. Although advanced maternal age could be associated with infertility and birth defects, avoidance of intrusive risks such as amniocentesis became a matter of women's risk calculation.

The action of "taking the high-speed rail" is not simply one of racing against a woman's biological clock but often a strategy to reassemble various life resources and events. Monica, an elementary school teacher, planned to make full use of the maternity leave resources in Taiwan, for which one must apply within the first three years after the child is born. Therefore, she started her reproductive project when her first child reached one year and seven months, and anxiously calculated whether she could become pregnant and give birth to her second child before her first maternity leave ended. Hsiao-Yen, a lawyer who married at age thirty-eight, started seeing the ob-gyn at a medical center just three months after her wedding, not due to any worry about infertility but because her husband was going to work abroad. And when Yi-Fen began to pursue pregnancy to save her marriage, she made only a two-month attempt to conceive via a regular sexual life before quickly moving on to IVF. As she put it, "I am already at the advanced age. I am thirty-six years old. I did not want to waste time [trying various methods]. *I wanted the fastest one.*" If we use Zoe's transportation metaphor, IVF should be ranked as the *super*-high-speed rail.

Implanting More Embryos with Age

Both delaying parenthood and preferring to speed up the process lead to the increasing use of ART, as well as to increased chances of multiple pregnancy. Taiwan's registry data do not include use of fertility drugs and IUI, so I only discuss IVF here. Taiwan's annual number of IVF cycles performed increased sixfold over twenty years, from around seven thousand cycles in 1998 to forty-four thousand cycles in 2019. In addition, the main users of IVF have become women of advanced reproductive age. In 1998, the median age to undergo an IVF cycle was thirty-two, but by 2019 it had moved up to thirty-eight. The latest data show that 73.3 percent of IVF cycles come from women above thirty-five years old, and, unprecedentedly, more than one-third of the cycles come from women over forty years old (ROC Ministry of Health and Welfare 2021a). If using a woman's own eggs rather than donated eggs, the live birth rate decreases significantly with age after thirty-five. For women above forty years old, the live birth rate per treatment cycle is lower than 10 percent. Therefore, doctors tend to implant more embryos for women over thirty-five as a strategy to prevent the success rate from being too low, often exceeding the TSRM's recommended upper limit, which is already one of most lenient in the world.[2]

The age-specific guideline and practice to implant more embryos for women older than thirty-five increases not only the success rate but also the multiple pregnancy rate. Graph 5.2 shows that among the live birth cycles (except for those using SET, of course), implanting two to four embryos can lead to a multiple birth rate near or over 20 percent, regardless of age group. The highest multiple birth rate is 44 percent, for implanting four embryos for women aged

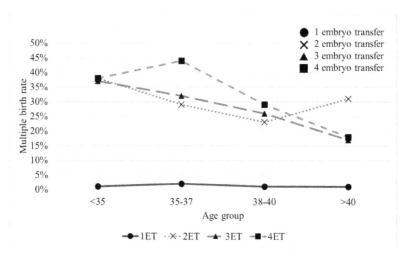

GRAPH 5.2. Multiple Birth Rate of Live Birth Cycles with Number of Embryos Transferred (NET) among Four Age Groups in Taiwan in 2019. Source: ROC Ministry of Health and Welfare 2021a. © Chia-Ling Wu and Wei-Hong Chen

thirty-five to thirty-seven. For those who are more than forty years old, implanting two embryos can lead to a multiple birth rate of 31 percent, possibly due to using donated eggs or taking PGT-A. Viewing the high multiple pregnancy rate for the older women, Doctor Q, an opinion leader of the TSRM, told us in an interview in 2021 that there should be a SET requirement for those who used a donated egg or for taking PGT-A. Such opinions might be discussed informally among medical professionals but are not yet a guideline. Overall, for those who had decided to speed up the timeline, multiple embryo transfer (or a strong dose of fertility drugs) was often viewed as the best strategy for efficiently achieving success. When racing against several biological and social clocks, implanting one embryo at one time did not seem reasonable, and twin births were often welcomed.

Optimization with ART often deals with time too, but in a different way. Like egg freezing, ART is utilized by delayers to optimize their life plan. But unlike egg freezing, using ART is not often in people's original plan. Egg freezing slows down the reproductive clock by "freezing time" (Myers and Martin 2021), whereas ART helps aspiring parents hurtle toward their goal by catching the "superhigh-speed rail." Nevertheless, high-speed rail does not guarantee that people will reach their expected destination. Several countries set the age limit for ART subsidies between forty and forty-three (Keane et al. 2017), indicating the stopping point for pursuing a goal that has a low success rate. However, optimization also offers the promise of some new ART innovations. Donated eggs and PGT-A now mean that people can extend the deadline to a much later age. These new technologies targeting women of advanced reproductive age reveal an important aspect of optimization—namely, that "the pursuit of the 'best possible' is legitimately infinite in its scope and always ongoing" (Adams, Murphy, and Clarke 2009: 256). But what if the best possible future is to remain childless? And how does ART relate to such a future?

Minimizing Compulsory Motherhood

Ting-Ting was one of the few people I interviewed who straightfor-wardly declared she had been forced to undergo ART. I interviewed Ting-Ting in a meeting room of the business building where she worked as an administrative assistant. Ten minutes into the inter-view, in the middle of describing her experience of a clinic visit, she suddenly told me, "I did not tell you in the beginning. In fact, I did not want to have kids in the first place. I was forced to do so." Ting-Ting had polycystic ovary syndrome (PCOS), a hormone disorder that can lead to infrequent menstruation periods. Since girlhood, she had needed to take medicine in order to have regular periods. PCOS is one of the most common factors to cause infertility, so Ting-Ting anticipated this biological barrier to conception, but may have welcomed it. Married at twenty-four years old to a man thirteen years older than she was, she did not plan to have a baby. She explained that this was partly because she did not want to go through the painful infertility treatment: "I hate taking shots and seeing blood." She also regarded taking care of kids as a burden. I am not sure whether this aversion to childcare came from her girlhood or only became clear after she needed to take care of her twins. She stressed that she would have liked to remain voluntarily childless.

"At least I tried," Ting-Ting said, explaining why she had started the infertility treatment after nine years of marriage. The pressure from her parents-in-law had grown over the years. Ting-Ting's husband was the only son in the family. Although he employed the notion of *yuan*—"a cultural idea that congenial and understanding relationships between interdependent people can thrive both within and outside marriage and family" (Huang and Wu 2018: 142)—to support flexibility concerning the couple's reproductive goal, the pressure from his parents became stronger when there were no signs of pregnancy. Ting-Ting's plan of voluntary childlessness was challenged, and she adjusted her strategy:

> I thought that I could just postpone until having kids became impossible [due to biological aging], and then they would understand that nothing can be done. Nevertheless, family members pressured so strongly that I thought, at least I would try once. I thought that I might not succeed the first time anyway.

Ting-Ting delayed the starting time of infertility treatment in order to enhance the chance of *failure*. She expected that ART might not work easily during her early thirties. The doctor implanted four embryos, and Ting-Ting became pregnant with quadruplets. She requested fetal reduction from four to one, but both the doctor and her husband suggested at least keeping two. (Fetal reduction is discussed in detail in chapter 6.) Ting-Ting's twins turned out to have some health problems from birth and needed extra care. Ting-Ting told me that the burden of caring for them exhausted her as well as her husband. She repeatedly lamented that "I did not want to have kids in the first place." Ting-Ting did look tired and depressed to me, but she said that her husband's family was very happy with the twins and that all the in-laws' nagging had finally ended.

Ting-Ting's anticipated voluntary childlessness has become both a practice and a respected choice in twenty-first-century Taiwan. The norm of marriage and parenthood has changed drastically. In 1991, according to the Social Change Survey, around 60 percent of people agreed that married life was not satisfactory without children, and that those who never had their own offspring had empty lives (H.-y. Chiu 1999). However, as table 5.1 shows, support of singlehood, marriage without kids, and same-sex marriage had become majority opinions by 2015. Overwhelmingly, 75 percent agreed that life without marriage can still be fulfilling. Scholars argue that this dramatic change in "family values" not only reflects the preference of the younger generation but also results from the changing values of the older generation, the so-called intracohort effect (Y.-s. Cheng and Yang 2021).

Still, intergenerational conflicts exist. Although Ting-Ting, Hsiao-Yen, and Yi-Fen all welcomed voluntary childlessness, they faced pressure to reproduce from their parents-in-law. ART became

TABLE 5. 1. Changes in Attitude toward Marriage and Parenthood in Taiwan, 1991–2015. Sources: H.-y. Chiu 1999; Fu 2017. © Chia-Ling Wu

Questions (% agree)	1991	2005	2010	2015
People can enjoy a satisfactory and successful life even without getting married	-	63.3%	69.5%	75%
Homosexuals should have the right to get married	11.4%	-	-	54.2%
A marriage without children is not unsatisfactory	27.5%	50.3%	55.7%	59.5%
N	2,488	2,146	1,895	2,034

the concrete recommendation of family members when expressing their concern. The typical advice was, "Why not go to see the doctor?" "If needed, don't hesitate to use ART." The advancement of ART broadens the scope of hope, as if biotechnology can fix any biological problems. Feminists have long argued that ART leads to the medicalization of infertility and also intensifies compulsory motherhood (Corea 1985; Crowe 1987). The availability of new reproductive technologies may lead to a wider range of traps in the name of "choices." Whereas Hsiao-Yen and Yi-Fen changed their reproductive projects and incorporated motherhood into their life agendas, Ting-Ting persisted in her ideal of childlessness and planned to attempt ART only to fulfill her marital and filial duty. New cultural norms could become resources for women such as Ting-Ting in resisting the use of ART against their will.[3]

These "debaters," as Martin (2021) calls those who struggle with the fertility decision, may sometimes withdraw from ART. The changing cultural norms have provided people with more cultural tools for moving away from ART and putting into practice different ideas about what a new kind of future can hold. As early as the 2000s, during my first wave of study on infertile men and women, it was quite frequent to meet working women who wished to withdraw from the treatment journey (Wu 2002b). One approach is to build "social parenthood." After a few failed attempts with ART, one elementary school teacher told me that she wanted to regard her students as her kids; she did not regard biological motherhood as a must. Another approach is to protect loved ones from medical risk. One university professor, who had a low sperm count and witnessed how his wife needed to go through some painful procedures during ART, reflected that "the most rewarding experience was that I witnessed how harmful ARTs are for women … and [that] made me contemplate why I would like to have kids in the first place. If having a kid is at the expense of my wife's health, I would rather not do it." The nationally well-known politician Chien-Shun Wang and his wife Fa-Chao Su went through infertility treatment but failed. In 2011, they started a nonprofit organization for so-called "seedless watermelons" like themselves to collectively arrange life for elders who do not have offspring.[4] ART is not the effective site to relieve people from compulsory biological parenthood; but building more cultural tools might be. However, while heterosexual couples may have created new cultural scripts for being happily married without children, some other groups are excluded from using ART and strive to find access to it so as to fulfill their reproductive goals.

Queer Reproduction and Twin Pregnancy

Stella was pregnant with triplets, conceived in Bangkok. She and her partner (now wife) Jackie were excluded from Taiwan's 2007 Assisted Reproduction Act, which stipulates that only married couples have access to infertility treatments such as IVF and donor insemination.[5] Like some single women and some lesbian and gay couples, Stella and Jackie had achieved their family-building plan abroad. They had a division of reproductive labor: Stella had a problem producing eggs, so she would carry and give birth to the baby, while Jackie contributed her eggs. On their first trip to the clinic in Bangkok in 2014, thirty-five eggs were retrieved from Jackie, leading to twenty-seven day-five blastocysts created with donor sperm. Stella was then implanted with three embryos and became pregnant with a singleton. They stayed in Bangkok for twenty days, and the total cost was about 20,000 US dollars (three or four times the cost if they had been able to access ART in Taiwan). To control the budget, they did not include the preimplantation genetic testing (PGT) to further select the embryos. Stella and Jackie paid the annual fee to freeze the remaining embryos.

When their child reached two years old, in 2017, the Thai government started to tighten its policy on cross-broader use of ART. Thailand had no specific laws to regulate ART (Whittaker 2015).

The change in policy was mainly due to a widely publicized case, dubbed the "'baby factory' mystery" by the BBC (Head 2018): a rich young Japanese man had hired nine women surrogates to bear his children and had been raided by the police in 2014. Stella felt it was urgent to use the couple's remaining embryos because "I was going to be forty years old, and I needed to do it now." Stella and Jackie went to Bangkok again, attempting to best use those frozen embryos and create new family members.

Stella asked the Thai doctor to implant four embryos, the upper limit according to Taiwan's legal regulation. "I had three embryos last time, and only one embryo succeeded. And I am older now, so I should implant more embryos," Stella explained, hoping to maximize her chances of success. The Thai doctor refused and suggested implanting three embryos; plus, he used "embryo glue," a kind of adhesive medium to help the embryo stick to the wall of uterus. The couple only stayed abroad five days this time because the procedure was mainly the embryo transfer. Soon after they went home, they joyfully saw the "positive" sign appear on a pregnancy test kit. In the sixth week of pregnancy, Stella had some bleeding and went to the hospital for care. She found out she was not pregnant with twins, as her earlier ultrasound check had showed, but with triplets.

Stella and Jackie showcase a new wave of queer reproduction in Taiwan.[6] The legal exclusion of unmarried women and men in Taiwan did not prevent them from pursuing ART. To be self-included in the system, the earlier strategy for some lesbians included a marriage of convenience with a gay man to become qualified to use ART in the medical system.[7] Since the early 2000s, some lesbian activists have stopped recommending a marriage of convenience as a way to gain access to ARTs, in view of the unbalanced gender division of labor between the gay father and lesbian mother. Importantly, Taiwan LGBT Family Rights Advocacy (2010) published *When We Build a Family: A Childbearing Guidebook for Lesbians*, the first such book ever to be published in an East Asian country, which warns readers of the troubles that lesbian mothers face in the "heterosexual regime of family" (ibid.: 29).[8] Instead, the guidebook promotes self-insemination: It lists the "Do it ourselves" groups in the US and UK, the successful practices in Taiwan, as well as detailed steps (ibid.: 34–50).[9] It is difficult to know how prevalent this practice was and is, except for a few high-profile cases. Its low success rate and lack of monitoring have caused some concerns within the lesbian community.[10] Cross-border reproductive care has become more visible among the lesbian community in Taiwan since the early 2010s.[11]

The preference for IVF over donor insemination (DI) when lesbians travel abroad leads to higher chances of making multiples. The so-called Tea Tree Moms are often referred to as Taiwan's first lesbian couple to have ART abroad; they have twins. They got married in Canada and gained legal access to use ART there. They shared their reproductive journey in detail in their blog to help other lesbians better understand the situation.[12] Some aspiring parents followed the Tea Tree Moms to Canada, some tried the US, and others built a new network in Thailand, Cambodia, and Japan. Like the Tea Tree Moms, when going abroad, Taiwan's lesbians have preferred IVF to donor insemination. In the beginning, I was puzzled by this preference. IUI has been single women and lesbians' top choice in some Western countries, and I wondered why it wasn't the same for Taiwanese women seeking treatment abroad. Women have their own eggs and womb, so with donated sperm, the simple procedure of IUI—injecting the sperm into the woman's womb during the period of ovulation—can be carried out. Well aware that DI is less intrusive and less expensive than IVF, my interviewees hastened to remind me that its success rate is lower, which matters to them tremendously. I had neglected to consider the constraints that these excluded users have faced, especially the difference between "local use or going abroad."

There are at least three obstacles that women need to face in seeking fertility treatment abroad. First of all, it takes time and courage to build the sense of legitimacy to use a technology that is legally prohibited in one's motherland. These women were moral pioneers to break the norms to fulfill their reproductive desire. Second, traveling abroad takes time, money, and energy. They told me that although IVF costs more, they could not afford to try DI several times first and then move to IVF, like lesbians in Australia, Spain, the US, and the UK who had access to ART locally (Fiske and Weston 2014; Carpinello et al. 2016; Nazem et al. 2019). Third, due to the moral, legal, and financial constraints, by the time Taiwanese lesbians are fully prepared to undergo ART, they tend to be in their thirties, or often in their late thirties, like Stella and Jackie. Hence, like those delayers, they would like to do it fast, with strong measures, such as multiple embryo transfer, with PGT-A, or with the questionable embryo glue that Stella agreed to. These measures tend to enhance chances not only of success but also of multiple pregnancy. Although in Taiwan no systematic data on cross-border ARTs exist, the high prevalence of twin pregnancy is very visible in Taiwan's lesbian and gay community. The Tea Tree Moms have twins—a girl and a boy, often called "dragon and phoenix babies" in Taiwan, indicating the best combination. Chou-Chou and Da Kui, who filed a lawsuit in Taiwan to gain legal parenthood of the nonbirthing partner, also have twins conceived in Canada.[13]

Lesbians' specific practices of Co-IVF also lead to higher chances of making multiples. Taiwan's lesbian couples, such as Stella and Jackie, started to take the "A-egg, B-birth" approach in recent years: A provided the egg, and B carried out the pregnancy. The practice is called ROPA (reception of oocytes from partners) by the Spanish IVF team (Marina et al. 2010), Co-IVF by teams in the US (Yeshua et al. 2015), and "shared motherhood IVF" by British teams (Bodri et al. 2018). In some cases, it is done for medical reasons, such as A not being able to carry the baby to term and B having problems producing eggs. However, many who employ this approach do so to build a biological connection with the children on the part of both parents: A has the genetic linkage through her egg, and B is the birth mother (Machin 2014). In the context of Taiwan, as well as many other countries, "combining gestation and genetics" (Pennings 2016) is also a strategy to maximize the legal rights of the non-birthing partner (Y.-J. Tseng 2013). Taiwan's civil law only recognizes the birth mother as the legal parent, but not the other partner, both before and after the legalization of same-sex marriage in 2019. Recent studies show that shared-motherhood IVF has a higher success rate than autologous IVF and heterosexual couples, possibly due to "the best combination between two oocyte providers and two gestational mothers" (Nunez et al. 2021: 371; also see Hodson, Meads, and Bewley 2017). This is because lesbian couples are "socially infertile," so they often do not have reproductive health problems. The maximization of success by the best combination may also increase the chances of making multiples whenever two or more embryos are chosen to transfer.

Overall, in the face of multiple constraints, lesbian couples may not oppose multiple embryos or strong fertility drugs to reach success quickly, which may increase their multiple pregnancy rate. To reach their goal of having a child, a lesbian couple may need to prepare their reproductive body for IVF by visiting a clinic in Taiwan, order sperm from a commercial bank in Denmark, arrange the medical procedure with a Thai agent, and then take a flight to the IVF destination. After so many troublesome preparations, using Zoe's metaphor of transportation, requesting a supersonic jet—such as the implantation of four embryos in Stella's case—may well be rational thinking.

Surrogacy for gay parents may best illustrate how undergoing hardships to reach a reproductive goal, including high costs, can lead to a preference for multiple embryos. Taiwan's gay men have been traveling abroad to seek parenthood through surrogacy. After Taiwan legalized same-sex marriage in 2019, the international organization Men Having Babies (MHB) came to Taipei to build the link actively. It is estimated to cost 150,000 to 200,000 US dollars for the whole process, and there is no guarantee of taking a baby home. At some point, the elective single-embryo transfer (eSET) policy was brought up during an MHB meeting. One doctor, running an IVF center in California, explained to the aspiring gay parents that with PGT-A, the success rate can be as high as 60 percent, so SET should be fine. The doctor continued to stress that twin pregnancy carries too much health risk for a female surrogate, so it is not encouraged. One Taiwanese gay father offered a recent case of premature twins to support the idea of SET. The babies needed intensive care right after the birth, and medical costs could skyrocket, as in the US. I can easily see that it takes much deliberation to persuade participants to use eSET rather than MET and thus aim for a singleton, not twins. What Dr. W calls the heterosexual couples' "cp value," i.e., getting twins from a single pregnancy, is openly discouraged here. Gays face the most constraints, pay the most money to become parents through ART, and at the same time confront the most demanding requests to practice eSET.

Conclusion

This chapter presents diverse anticipatory trajectories of becoming parents in order to grasp how women and men perceive ART practices and multiple birth. These complex trajectories differ from the simplified representations in the mainstream medicine and media, which tend to highlight those who keep on hoping but may lack knowledge about aging motherhood. Table 5.2 summarizes the major findings. My fieldwork shows that only a small portion of users, such as Mei-Hui, make the reproductive project their life priority. Most interviewees delay, debate, or resist the fertility project or are excluded socially and legally from becoming parents. By the same token, the forms of disrupted reproduction that people face differ greatly, ranging from biological infertility and competing biological and social clocks to social pressure to conceive and legal exclusion from access to ART. As a result, ART is not only a remedy

TABLE 5.2. Anticipation Trajectories with Different Optimizations within Disruptive Reproduction in Taiwan. (ARTs = assisted reproductive technologies.) © Chia-Ling Wu

Type of disruptive reproduction	Exemplar	ARTs as a tool to reach the best possible future	Affective state for multiple pregnancy
Desired motherhood encountering biological obstacles	Reproductive project as main life goal	Fix biological infertility	"Winning the lottery"
Competing biological and social clocks	Delayed parenthood	Speed up the timeline	Efficiency
Pressure against voluntary childlessness	Pressured daughter-in-law	Fulfill the duty	Hesitance
Legal exclusion	Lesbian couples	Remedy for social infertility	Justice

for physical dysfunction but a strategy to speed up an aspiring parent's timeline, fulfill familial duty, and/or fight social discrimination.

When people face the most constraints—such as lack of time and cross-border burdens—they welcome or even require strong measures so as to reach the goal of having a child. Still, what they want most of the time is successful conception, not twins or triplets. "Taking the high-speed rail" means accelerating the timeline, not doubling the results. Aspiring parents' affective states when responding to the announcement of multiple pregnancy range from "winning the lottery" and "efficiency" to "hesitance" and "justice," echoing their anticipatory trajectories. These are mostly responses to surprising pregnancy results, not to their preplanned goal.

While using ART to optimize their reproductive plan, people are aware of various health risks, but not necessarily the risk of making multiple babies. They seek Chinese medicine to find less intrusive treatment. Some withdraw from ART due to its invasiveness. They even worry about the harm caused by amniocentesis. However, the risk of multiple pregnancy is rarely on the list. It is hard for people who are worried about failing to become pregnant to register the possible consequences of bearing twins and triplets who may need ongoing medical care. All the measures to increase the chances of

success—such as strong fertility drugs and multiple embryo transfer—also increase the chance of multiple pregnancy. Therefore, it
should be the task of medical professionals, not their patients, to
initiate the preventive measures required. And conception is only
the first step. When an ultrasound shows triplets or quadruplets,
women face another challenge: how will I bear them? As shown in
chapter 6, their anticipation moves to a new stage: fetal reduction.

Notes

1. In my first wave of interviews in the early 2000s, I found that full-time
   housewives and daughters-in-law in their husband's family business
   felt the strongest pressure to try ART until they experienced success
   (Wu 2002a: 27–28). However, for the second wave of interviewees
   around 2010, the pattern is less clear
2. The latest data show that over one-fourth of the cycles for the thirty-
   five-to-thirty-seven-year-old group exceed the TSRM's recommended
   upper limit of two embryos transferred, and nearly 10 percent are over
   the upper limit of three for the thirty-eight-to-forty-year-old group.
   In addition, SET is not the norm even among the younger group in
   Taiwan, although strong evidence has shown that the cumulative success rate of elective single-embryo transfer (eSET) is as good as that of
   DET (Kamath et al. 2020).
3. Paradox exists. Lack of financial support can create stratified reproduction because only the affluent can afford to pay for IVF out of their own
   pockets, yet when the subsidy is generous, as in the case of Israel, this
   may create new pressure to "keep trying" (Balabanova and Simonstein
   2010: 196).
4. See the official website: http://www.nokids.org.tw/.
5. Legally, from Taiwan's first ethical guidelines in 1986 to the Assisted
   Reproduction Act in 2007, all the ethical and legal regulations continued to prohibit unmarried women and men from using ART. Globally,
   the regulations addressing access to ART are moving toward liber-
   alization, and increasing numbers of countries do not restrict its use
   to married, heterosexual couples alone. However, after the Muslim
   world, (South)East Asia is the second most prominent region where
   ART eligibility criteria are based strictly on marital status. According to
   the latest survey by the International Federation of Fertility Societies
   (IFFS 2019), among the sixty-two countries and regions surveyed,
   only fourteen countries specify married couples as the only eligible
   treatment group by law or guideline, and Taiwan is one of them.
6. ARTs such as IUI, IVF/ICSI, and surrogacy separate heterosexuality
   from reproduction and thus create new opportunities to become par-

ents for single women, lesbians, and gays. However, their utilization depends on complex social, cultural, and legal contexts. In the 1970s, insemination of a friend's sperm or donated sperm to achieve pregnancy, particularly with self-insemination, was a token practice in the women's health movement in the UK and US (Wikler and Wikler 1991). Part of the activist spirit was to reproduce without having sex with men and to stay away from the medical institution. Still, requests to be included in the system of ART increased. By the late 1990s, donor insemination (DI) had become more openly available to single women and lesbians in several Western countries (Moore 2007). By comparison, although DI was equally technically feasible in Taiwan, it was not advocated by feminists there as a way to build an alternative family; instead, fighting against compulsory motherhood by advocating for abortion rights was the main agenda (Wu 2017a).

7. Among my interviewees, Terresa's was the earliest case in which the subject arranged a marriage with a gay man, in the 1990s, to gain legal access to ART, using intrauterine insemination (IUI) to become pregnant. However, the lesbian community gradually found that a marriage of convenience—to secure a marriage license as well as the sperm to conceive through ART—often led to an ongoing burden of care within the patriarchal family, including serving parents-in-law and caring for babies all by oneself. Terresa, for example, got divorced later because she found that the gay father of her child was often absent for childcare. Several interviewees told me a well-circulated story of a mother of triplets to highlight the burden of care: caring for multiple babies intensified the unbalanced gender division of labor between the gay father and lesbian mother. The marriage may have been fake, but the care required was real.

8. Taiwan's gay and lesbian movement had boomed in the early 1990s and soon took on a leading role in Asia (Jackson, Liu, and Woo 2008; Kong 2019). A number of young student activists from the gay and lesbian rights movement initiated the Lesbian Mothers Alliance, which was transformed in 2007 into the Taiwan LGBT Family Rights Advocacy. The organization was intended to offer social support and record the oral histories of lesbian mothers who had mostly become pregnant from previous heterosexual marriage.

9. The activists started to include ART in their agenda of social reform after meeting Vicky, who did DI and self-insemination to have two kids (Wu 2017a).

10. Still, activists' promotion of self-insemination does democratize the use of ART by extending it to these legally excluded persons through sharing simple technology.

11. Scholars prefer to term this "reproductive exile" rather than "reproductive tourism" to emphasize the constraints that force members of the excluded minority to go abroad (Inhorn and Patrizio 2009).

12. When they were invited to write the preface of *When We Build a Family* in 2010, they noted that they wished they had had such guidance at the time, so as to avoid much hesitation and ambivalence. Although cross-border reproduction was not an option listed in the pioneering guidebook, it soon became the most visible strategy.

13. Only a few studies show the multiple pregnancy/birth rate among lesbian couples using IVF or Co-IVF, ranging from 21.3 percent in a medical center in the US (Carpinell et al. 2016) to 14 percent in a British clinic (Bodri et al. 2018).

Chapter 6

WOMEN ENCOUNTER FETAL REDUCTION

"I would reduce only one, and keep two." Stella assertively told me her decision during our lunch, before we headed to the clinic together in the beautiful autumn of 2017. When I had learned several days earlier that she and her partner Jackie planned to travel with their three-year-old daughter on the high-speed rail from southern Taiwan to metropolitan Taipei for fetal reduction, I had volunteered to babysit for them during the procedure, and we all had lunch together after arriving in Taipei. Amid joyfully feeding their toddler in the restaurant, Jackie sighed when Stella raised the topic of how many fetuses to reduce. She believed that a twin pregnancy would be too difficult for Stella, whose previous singleton pregnancy had already been very eventful. "Teacher, please persuade her to keep only one," Jackie implored me, looked more worried than I had ever seen her since first meeting the lovely couple several years earlier. Stella explained her rationale to me: "We did not do PGT [preimplantation genetic testing] for the embryos, so what if only the one [that is not reduced] has something wrong?" Whereas Jackie was concerned that Stella would have to bear the burden of a twin pregnancy, Stella viewed keeping two fetuses as a safe way to guarantee giving birth to at least one healthy baby—or two. As outlined in chapter 5, Stella had already overcome many hurdles in Taiwan and also Thailand to reach the couple's goal of expanding their family, so she viewed conservative fetal reduction as her new task to help ensure the health of the new family member(s).

The doctor at the maternity hospital where Stella received prenatal care had advised Stella, pregnant with triplets, to have fetal reduction, but he would not perform the procedure himself. The maternity hospital, which is also an accredited IVF center, does not offer fetal reduction. The couple researched some options on the internet and quickly found that most women who needed the procedure went to a popular clinic in Taipei that mainly offers genetic testing, including amniocentesis, and fetal reduction.

After lunch, we took the short walk to the clinic. The receptionist first asked Stella to fill out a form, including a consent form to be signed by her spouse. Stella calmly said that she was single, so that there was no spouse to fill out in the form. The staff member empathetically accepted this answer and guided Stella, Jackie, and me to see the doctor. The doctor explained the procedure and pointed out the cross-tabulation of statistics on the desk: it showed the prevalence of cerebral palsy (CP), the most common motor disability for newborns, as 0.23 percent, 1.46 percent, and 4.48 percent for single, twin, and triplet pregnancies, respectively, while neonatal mortality is three to six times higher for twins than for singletons and five to fifteen times higher for triplets. Stella had no qualms about undergoing fetal reduction; instead, the problem was the number of fetuses to reduce. The doctor asked her height, which was less than five feet, so he suggested that reducing to a singleton was better. Stella insisted on keeping two. The negotiation did not last long, and the fetal reduction began in accordance with Stella's stated wishes. The observant staff member soon figured out that Jackie, holding the three-year-old child, was Stella's partner and greeted her in a friendly way, praising her for being a supportive one. This was five months after Taiwan's Constitutional Court ruled in favor of same-sex marriage. The whole island had gone through heated debate about the human rights of gays and lesbians. You could easily tell that the staff were particularly caring toward this couple. On that Monday afternoon, most other clients came to the clinic alone, without any companion.

There were three rooms for the operation. Stella first had an ultrasound examination and then moved to a neighboring room for fetal reduction. While we waited outside, I patted Jackie's shoulder to comfort her, only to find that I myself was almost in tears. I could hear from the lounge that the doctor was telling Stella not to look at the monitor, explaining that he had reduced the smallest fetus. The procedure took only a few minutes. Stella needed to rest for twenty minutes. Then, the doctor confirmed with ultrasonographic imaging that the reduced one was now almost invisible on the monitor and that the remaining twins looked lively. Two ultrasound images of the twins were printed to give to Stella, each one showing one fetus.

Holding the two images, Jackie looked relieved and even excited, cheerfully explaining to their cute toddler that "Mommy is having twin babies."

Fetal reduction has emerged as a new hurdle that women carrying multiples need to jump over, mainly during the first trimester. Its primary purpose is to prevent the health risks of a multiple pregnancy. Cases like Stella's triplet pregnancy are predicted to have preterm labor and various maternal and fetal health risks. Fetal reduction is viewed as a preventive measure by its proponents. In practice, however, to reduce or not to reduce, and how many fetuses to reduce, are not easy questions. Almost all the women I interviewed who had been pregnant with quadruplets, triplets, or even twins had needed to take time, short or long, easy or complicated, to face the option.[1] Even as a companion for a short time on Stella and Jackie's journey of fetal reduction, I felt myself go through some emotional disturbance. Several empirical studies have examined women's fetal reduction experiences, and all recognize the difficulty and complexity of how women go through it in Taiwan (e.g., P.-Y. Chiu 2004; Yu 2015) and in North America (e.g., Britt and Evans 2007a, 2007b; Kelland and Ricciardelli 2015). The repeated keywords are "anxiety" and "ambivalence." Such experiences are shared by other women who use various prenatal testing procedures, such as ultrasound genetic diagnosis to "prevent or allow the birth of certain kinds of children," the main feature of selective reproductive technologies (Gammeltoft and Wahlberg 2014: 201).

Built upon these important research findings, I will discuss the anticipatory labor of women encountering fetal reduction. The essential part of the work at this stage is to collect information on fetal reduction, make sense of the procedure, and come to a decision within a few weeks. The clinic visit, as described above for Stella's family, may only take a couple of hours, during which medical practitioners do most of the work. The decision-making prior to the visit is, however, much more complicated, and it is often women who take up this task. Most research to date has focused on women's "personal value system" and socioeconomic status to understand their experiences. Dimensions such as religious belief, ethical considerations, perceived care responsibility, and estimated financial burden play important roles. Little research has been done, however, about how women evaluate and encounter the medical technology and system itself, which is the ultimate force that initiates the roller-coaster experiences that many women go through. Therefore, in contrast to earlier studies, I focus on (1) how women critically evaluate fetal reduction, and (2) how they navigate the conflicting information about it, including the different opinions among various forms of available guidance. Women in the end sometimes need to rebuild the network of fetal reduction, which is very often disassembled by doctors themselves, in the context of Taiwan.

Detecting the Multiple Fetuses

The early reveal of multiple pregnancy has become possible with the blood test and the routine use of ultrasonography during prenatal care. The level of human chorionic gonadotropin (hCG), or pregnancy hormone, rises quickly from the fourth week from the last menstrual period, or two weeks after the embryo transfer during IVF. A much higher hCG value indicates the possibility of multiple pregnancy, compared with that of a singleton (Chung et al. 2006; Seeber 2012). Doctors tend to follow hCG closely for signs of pregnancy in women who undergo fertility treatment. For example, Yi-Wen, who started IVF at age thirty-one, vividly remembered that she was informed that she might have a twin pregnancy as early as at the fourth week because "the technician told me that the value skyrocketed."

Confirmation of the number of fetuses relies on ultrasound examination as well as on the passage of time. As early as at the fifth postmenstrual week, the number of chorionic sacs can be detected through ultrasound imaging (Timor-Tritsch and Monteagudo 2005). Experts suggest that it is possible to determine the number of fetuses by detecting the number of heartbeats around the sixth week (ibid.: 293). For Yi-Wen, Stella, and some others, a notification of twin pregnancy was later replaced by confirmation of triplets, mainly due to the limitations of the blood test and sonography at the earliest stage. Some opposite situations may happen too. Spontaneous fetal loss, or the so-called vanishing twin or triplet, occurs quite frequently (Landy and Keith 2006). A woman might be informed that she is pregnant with four fetuses in the seventh week but later find out that only one remains. Overall, women who see ultrasound images of more than one sac within the womb have some time to figure out whether or not to undergo fetal reduction around the tenth to fourteenth week.

Never before has it been possible so early in pregnancy for women to view images and hear internal sounds of the multiple fetuses they are carrying. In the millennia before ultrasonography was available, women might not be aware of a twin pregnancy until after the babies were delivered. A woman I interviewed who gave birth in a midwife's clinic in the 1970s recalled that, after the birth of the first twin, the midwife announced that there was another baby about to be born. The mother suddenly realized that it was "no wonder my belly was so large." How large? She described that while she was sitting on a stool, bending over to handwash clothes, her belly was so big that it reached the floor. Still, she and her family members did not suspect a twin pregnancy. In the past, twins might be detected by experienced midwives' delicate hands touching two little baby bottoms under the belly, or with the assistance of a fetoscope and stethoscope that detected two heartbeats. Twins could be detected in the late second trimester at the earliest. The number of fetuses gestating within a woman's womb was simply information to receive, not something about which there was the room for negotiation.

Fetal Reduction as an Option

Today, women may start wondering what to do with multiples as early as the sixth week, before they have any bodily awareness of twins, triplets, or quadruplets. As discussed in earlier chapters, fetal reduction became an option for higher-order pregnancy in the mid-1980s and was steadily practiced in the 1990s in Taiwan. Various studies have compared the outcomes with and without fetal reduction, and these show evidence that the procedure significantly reduces the incidences of spontaneous loss and preterm birth (see review of Evans, Andriole, and Britt 2014). The common tendency is to reduce from triplets or more fetuses to twins. Given that twin pregnancy still carries higher health risks compared with singleton pregnancy, reduction to a singleton has increased and is supported by the medical community, such as the ethical committee of the American College of Obstetricians and Gynecologists (ACOG 2017).

In Taiwan, no guideline has been issued from any medical society. There are no published local data on the outcomes before and after fetal reduction.[2] Taiwanese doctors who practice fetal reduction often suggest reduction to twins (A.-F. Li 2009; Y.-C. Hung 2018). Considering the health issues, such as in Stella's case, reduction to a singleton might be proposed by doctors, or by women and their family members, such as Stella's partner Jackie. In a survey of 112 cases of fetal reduction in a Taipei clinic, nearly half the women said

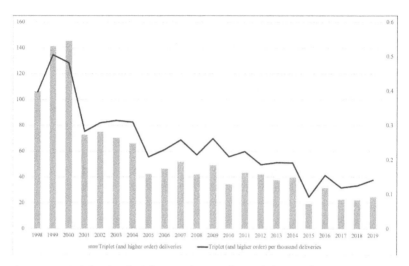

GRAPH 6.1. Triplet (and Higher-Order) Births and the Triplet (and Higher-Order) Birth Rate per Thousand Deliveries in Taiwan, 1998–2019. Source: "Demographic Data GIS" 2021. © Chia-Ling Wu

that they had reduced the multiple fetuses to a singleton, possibly due to the advanced age of the surveyed women, over two-thirds of whom were more than forty years old (Yu 2015).

Taiwan may well have one of the highest rates of fetal reduction in the world. Statistics on the prevalence of fetal reduction are just emerging. The annual report of Taiwan's ART registry disclosed, for the very first time, that out of 11,402 pregnancies in 2019, fetal reduction was practiced in 135 cases (ROC Ministry of Health and Welfare 2021a: 9).[3] The reported number exceeds that in any European country (ESHRE 2020). The UK reported 155 fetal reductions, but its number of IVF cycles is three times greater than that of Taiwan (HFEA 2020). Taiwan's report does not include cases of multiple pregnancy due to spontaneous conception, IUI (interuterine insemination), or IVF done abroad, such as Stella's situation. Most doctors told me that in Taiwan, cases of multiple pregnancy caused by taking fertility drugs outnumber cases resulting from IVF. Probably more than in any other country, women in Taiwan have a higher chance of facing the decision-making process of fetal reduction. At the same time, the very existence of triplet and other higher-order deliveries shows that women do not always use this surgical solution. In 1998, 1999, and 2000, more than one hundred birthing women per year delivered triplets or quadruplets in Taiwan (graph 6.1). Both the number of cases and the triplet birth rate have decreased since then, at least partly due to the increasing acceptance of fetal reduction.

Women Execute Technological Assessment

Some women I interviewed bluntly emphasized the risk that fetal reduction *creates* rather than the risk this intrusive surgery intends to *mitigate*. In their assessment, fetal reduction is an unreliable technology, or even a threat, in three ways: (1) it has the potential to cause miscarriage or total pregnancy loss, (2) it poses a risk to the safety of the remaining fetuses, and (3) doctors don't yet know exactly how to discern and keep the fittest fetuses during the procedure. Therefore, contrary to the medical benefits that proponents would list, some women regard fetal reduction not as a problem-solving technology but as a trouble-making one that needs to be avoided.

The Risk of Miscarriage

The risk of miscarriage after fetal reduction is well known to women facing the option. A study of 112 women undertaking fetal reduction in a clinic showed that 90 percent of them knew the risk (Yu 2015: 33). The possibility of total pregnancy loss makes fetal reduction threatening to women's hard-won achievement. Melody, pregnant with triplets, told me her concerns:

> I did not consider fetal reduction. It has the risk of losing all fetuses, doesn't it? I finally got pregnant, so I'd better not to take the risk. ... I knew it might not be easy to bear triplets, but I had no experience of pregnancy, so I could not imagine how hard it could be.

Especially for women such as Melody, who became pregnant only after a long and difficult journey, the accomplishment needs to be cherished carefully, without introducing a new risky intervention like fetal reduction. Li-Hsueh, who attempted various methods to reach pregnancy, became pregnant with triplets by using fertility drugs. She treasured her first successful pregnancy, and stated that "if fetal reduction led to the loss of all three fetuses, I would go insane." These women are not necessarily unaware of the health risks of triplet pregnancy; carrying triplets itself entails the risk of total pregnancy loss, in addition to other complications. Still, some believe that what they can do to protect the pregnancy is to avoid the new danger created by an intrusive procedure. This uncertainty also looms for women who do choose fetal reduction. In a study of six women undergoing fetal reduction in a medical center, three mentioned the worry of total pregnancy loss (H.-L. Wang and Chao 2006). Such fear of miscarriage also leads to the preference for keeping two fetuses rather than one. As one doctor said when proposing to reduce to twins, "If one is gone, at least another is left" (A.-F. Li 2009). Keeping two thus becomes a safety net to handle the potential disastrous loss that a preventive measure may bring.

The medical community may downplay the risk of fetal reduction. For example, in the American College of Obstetricians and Gynecologists (ACOG) statement on fetal reduction, the "Risks" section only includes the maternal and perinatal mortality and morbidity of multiple pregnancy, as if fetal reduction does not carry any risk.[4] The statement does recognize that fetal reduction "in *rare* cases, may result in the loss of the entire pregnancy" (ACOG 2017: 3, emphasis added). This information appears in the section on "Ethical Considerations," which discusses how women consult their values when deciding between maximizing maternal and fetal health and risking the loss of all fetuses. By comparison, Taiwan's doctors regularly present the loss of all fetuses as the leading complication of fetal reduction. In the 1990s, it was often reported that the rate was 10–15 percent (S.-H. Hung 1995), which has now decreased to 2 percent for twins and 5 percent for triplets, according to a recent media report (Y.-C. Hung 2018).[5] However, doctors tend to present a benefit-and-risk model for evaluation: whereas the miscarriage rate for reduction of triplets is 5 percent, the miscarriage rate is 11.5 percent before the twenty-fourth week if women do not conduct fetal reduction (ibid.). Doctors use statistics to foresee a better future, but pregnant women cannot ignore the near and present threat.

Harm to the fetuses during the procedure is another leading concern. In Yu's study, 87 percent of the surveyed women worried about whether the procedure would harm "the safety of the fetuses" (Yu 2015: 39). Although the main purpose is to "save the lives" of the remaining fetuses, women in my study mentioned concerns about whether the intrusion of the needle, the injection of poison, and the reduced fetuses remaining inside the womb might still hurt the remaining fetuses.

The Selection of Fetuses

Another major uncertainty is the selection of fetuses. Fetal reduction brings with it a new intervention—namely, which fetuses to reduce. Some women do not trust doctors' capacity to select the right ones. For example, Chiu-Yueh was implanted with five embryos, and became pregnant with triplets. The doctor, her husband, and her mother-in-law all suggested that the three be reduced to two, but she cast doubt on the procedure. She wondered whether the fetus selected for reduction might be the best one, not the worst one. Therefore, she decided to keep all three to guarantee that the good ones would remain. Stella had a similar rationale. The main reason that Stella insisted on reduction to two fetuses, not one, was that she had not used PGT-A to select the best embryos. As a result, she worried, "What if the only one [that is not reduced] has something wrong?" For women who go through IVF to become pregnant, the chain of selection extends to the stage of selecting good reproductive cells and embryos. Through donor selection, some traits can be chosen through the commercial gamete banks. PGT-A can help clinicians identify the embryos with the normal number of chromosomes to transfer. After implantation, if pregnancy results, the routine use of prenatal genetic testing can provide further information about the fetuses.

Fetal reduction itself is another selective reproductive technology that brings in a new dimension of selection. Doctors may select the visually worst one, or simply reduce the one(s) whose location lends itself most easily to the procedure. This selectivity is much more inaccurate than that of preimplantation genetic testing such as PGT-A. Stella had not chosen to use PGT-A and felt unsure about the accuracy of selecting fetuses by fetal reduction. Therefore, keeping two became her strategy to help ensure that at least one good fetus would remain.

Incorporating Women's Values into Medicine

Women anticipate the adverse outcomes that fetal reduction may entail and act to handle the new uncertainty. They may reject the technology, do it but keep more fetuses in their wombs, or continue worrying about the adverse outcomes after the operation. These women offer a technology assessment model for evaluating fetal reduction. Such evaluation is seldom presented in the current studies, probably because most research to date has sought samples in the clinics that conduct fetal reduction and hence seldom studies the experiences of women who refuse the procedure.

In addition, current discussion tends to emphasize women's religious beliefs and lifestyle factors to explain why they hesitate, without presenting the so-called women's value system that also involves medicine and technology. Thus, I would like to echo the research on women's refusal of prenatal screening, in which women are found to adopt "the logic of the biomedical paradigm to reject its very offering" (Markens, Browner, and Press 1999: 360). Similarly, in my study, fetal reduction's risk of miscarriage and its inaccuracy of selection are some women's major reasons for their fetal reduction decision. Some new advancements in fetal reduction attempt to reduce such risk by detecting fetal genetic abnormality through chorionic villus sampling (CVS) and other technologies before conducting fetal reduction (Evans, Andriole, and Britt 2014). The chain of selective reproductive technology is thus prolonged, but the issues of inaccuracy remain. Besides, in addition to the technological assessment, women have multiple other dimensions of evaluation to employ on their bumpy road to figuring out what to do with the option of fetal reduction.

The Intensity of Direction Guides

Whereas some women straightforwardly disregard fetal reduction, most women ponder the new option when it pops up unexpectedly during their reproductive journey. When the fetuses become publicly visible in the first trimester, many actors—doctors, family members, bloggers sharing experiences on the internet, and even gods and goddesses—can all get involved in giving women advice about what to do. Yu's survey of 112 women reveals the amazing intensity of their information-seeking behavior after receiving the suggestion of fetal reduction: finding famous doctors (94.6 percent), reading books (94.6 percent), surfing the internet (92 percent), consulting experts on genetics (89.5 percent), looking for cases having similar experiences (77.7 percent), consulting other ob-gyns (75.2 percent), and learning from the experiences of relatives and friends having similar situations (55.4 percent) (Yu 2015: 43).

In my study, most of the women not only searched numerous sources for their decision-making but also found that these sources often conflicted with each other. As earlier research on fetal reduction and other selective reproductive technologies has shown, the diversity of relevant actors may offer the logic of science, the faith of religious orientation, and various cultural conceptions. It takes anxious efforts to navigate divergent information and viewpoints to make the decision. In what follows, I first present Yi-Wen's journey of fetal reduction decision-making. Next, I present the two most conflicting guides that create extra burdens for women to navigate: doctors' contrasting opinions and the related maternal-fetal conflicts.

Yi-Wen's "Most Difficult Time"

Yi-Wen was very excited when she was first informed that she was pregnant with twins after an hCG test at the fourth week. Her fallopian tubes had been damaged when she had an ectopic pregnancy at eighteen years old. Her only option was to undergo IVF for conception. Around her late twenties, she began to consider having a baby. Living in a town that had no accredited IVF center, she had to take a two-hour train ride to Taipei for the fertility treatment. Since her husband, a busy local politician, could not go with her most of the time, she did not persist. Reaching the age of thirty, she resumed IVF treatment when the first accredited IVF center was established in her town. She was implanted with four embryos and became pregnant during the second cycle. The joy of having twins did not last long though, because the ultrasound image conducted at the sixth week showed that she was pregnant with triplets. "Hearing it was triplets, I felt hesitant," Yi-Wen told me during our interview in her husband's office.

The first thing that came to her mind was her eyewitness experience of seriously disabled triplets in the neighborhood of her natal family, two hundred kilometers from where she lived with her husband and in-laws. All the triplets had serious health problems, and one died early. This real case that she had known since childhood gave Yi-Wen firsthand awareness of the hazards triplets faced. She went back to her parents' home and discussed the situation with her natal family members. She also consulted an obstetrician-gynecologist at the nearby medical center. She recounted that the doctor strongly suggested that she undergo fetal reduction, saying that "triplet pregnancy is not for human beings, especially not for Asian people." The doctor's main concern was the maternal health risk to Yi-Wen herself.

Yi-Wen also searched for information online. On the one hand, she read discussions on premature birth caused by triplets, including the high infant mortality rate. These statistics rang a bell for her, as they confirmed what she had witnessed a young girl in her encounters with the triples and their health problems. On the other hand, she learned about the procedure in detail. This disturbed her emotionally, especially the part about the injection of poison into the heart of a fetus, which made Yi-Wen feel "horrible," in her own words. Yi-Wen also wondered whether the reduced fetus, usually remaining in the womb, would influence the other two.

With all these pros and cons, Yi-Wen went back home to consult her IVF doctor, together with her husband. The doctor said that she did not oppose Yi-Wen doing fetal reduction, but she would not do it herself, as the procedure went against the beliefs of the hospital's religious affiliation. When she explained the procedure, highlighting the injection of a needle into the fetus's heart, Yi-Wen felt again how "brutal" the procedure was. The doctor also suggested that Yi-Wen was taller than the average Taiwanese woman, so that she should be able to bear the triplets. Yi-Wen was five feet four inches tall.

Sex preference became another decision criterion. Yi-Wen's husband wanted a baby girl. The ultrasound image showed that two of the fetuses were male and the gender of the third one was uncertain. The doctor asked the "what if" question: What if the reduced one is a baby girl? Yi-Wen's husband nodded positively. The preference of the doctor and the husband not to do fetal reduction became strong guidance. Other family members offered rhetoric such as "following nature," "taking things as they come," and "there must be a reason that these children are following you into the world" to comfort the indecisive Yi-Wen and encourage her to stick with the status quo. Not to act was advised as the best action. Yi-Wen's father-in-law was a Buddhist monk, so Yi-Wen came to believe that he would use religious power to protect her and the fetuses. As time passed, Yi-Wen continued carrying the triplets. "The struggle to decide whether to reduce or not was the most difficult time during the whole pregnancy," Yi-Wen told me as her three children, now healthy toddlers, played around us during the interview.

Doctors with Contrasting Opinions

In a world of evidence-based medicine and standardization, the diverse opinions of healthcare practitioners on the subject of fetal reduction are most striking. Women consult different experts. Yi-Wen consulted her IVF doctor and another ob-gyn for prenatal care. Other women may add a specialist in fetal reduction and genetics to the list, as Stella did. The specialization of doctors in reproductive care has grown over time, especially due to the rise of assisted reproductive technologies to make possible "parceling out the reproductive processes" (Gammeltoft and Wahlberg 2014: 209). As shown in chapter 3, many IVF doctors in Taiwan do not offer prenatal care, and hence women often need to visit other ob-gyns after successful conception. In Yu's study of 112 women undergoing fetal reduction in a specialized clinic, near 70 percent had come to the clinic on the referral of ob-gyns, and 20 percent on referrals from fertility specialists (Yu 2015: 33). Therefore, women carrying multiples due to IVF often need to consult other doctors for guidance and services.

In addition, the easy access to prenatal care in Taiwan's healthcare system makes multiple visits within a short time highly feasible. One dramatic case is Yu-Ping, pregnant with triplets naturally, who visited a total of six doctors to find one who would support her determination not to do fetal reduction. The maternal healthcare program in Taiwan has been promoted since the 1970s and was strengthened after the implementation of National Health Insurance (NHI) in 1995. NHI provides a comprehensive benefit package to all citizens, including 10 prenatal care examinations. Five years before the NHI, women on average already had 10.3 prenatal care visits. After NHI, the average number of visits further increased to 11 (C.-S. Chen, Liu, and L.-M. Chen 2003). People have free choice among providers, easy access to specialists, and short wait times for the services they need (T.-M. Cheng 2015). IVF and fetal reduction have not been covered by NHI, but advice from doctors can be easily accessed. This explains why Yi-Wen could easily reach a doctor working in a medical center for a second opinion, Yu-Ping could visit six ob-gyns during her first trimester, and Stella could easily walk into a clinic specializing in fetal reduction after preregistering online.

Mobilizing Science and Emotion

Doctors are easy to consult in Taiwan, but they offer contrasting judgments. Yi-Wen's body type could be evaluated as *unfit* to carry triplets when the selected reference is Asian versus Western, but change to *possibly capable* when the comparison group is other Taiwanese women. Women's height has been selected by doctors as an indicator for evaluation. Stella's doctor preferred that she reduce to one fetus because she was less than five feet tall. By comparison, Mei-Hsueh, a petite self-employed beauty salon owner, was very much impressed when a doctor asked her, "If you did not try carrying [the triplets], how do you know that you cannot?" The criterion of height seems arbitrary. It demonstrates more about doctors' preference than about scientific evidence.

Doctors' rejection of fetal reduction operates in several ways. They may use some scientific criteria, such as height, to express the possibility of successfully carrying triplets. Alternatively, they may directly present how they dislike fetal reduction by refusing to do it, as Yi-Wen's doctor did. Another common strategy is to describe the procedure in detail to make women feel bad about undergoing it. Some doctors also show couples ultrasound images to persuade them to keep all the fetuses. Allison, a lawyer, could not face her twin pregnancy, caused by taking fertility drugs, because she already had one child to care for and busy working hours. She wished the second fetus to vanish by itself within the next two weeks so that she could only have a singleton. When she asked about the option of fetal reduction, she found that her reticent doctor suddenly became talkative:

> The doctor pointed out the ultrasound images to me: "You see, here is the one. The other is over there." ... He explained that medicine had made great progress. It was not a problem to handle twins. Carrying triplets and quadruplets might not be good for the mother, but carrying twins. ... Then he looked at the monitor, saying, "Look how lovely they are."

This mobilization of ultrasound images successfully elicited Allison's sense of responsibility to cherish the twins' lives and be a good mother. She redirected her worry about her career and financial burdens to the feelings of the fetuses. She stated that "if they felt that I did not welcome them, that might not be good for them." She chose to keep the twins and accepted the situation.

Recruiting Husbands as Allies

Doctors sometimes turn to husbands if women are indecisive. Yi-Wen's husband, who did not accompany her to the IVF procedures, suddenly became the doctor's ally. The husband's preference for a baby girl was identified as another reason not to do fetal reduction. Ting-Ting, who preferred voluntary childlessness and only used ART to fulfill her marital duty, described the scene in the clinic after she had been told she was pregnant with quadruplets:

> I only wanted to have one kid, so I thought I would like to reduce three fetuses. But the doctor suggested twins, and my husband agreed. I considered that one is already a burden, and I did not want to have even one kid. Those who raised kids all told me how exhausting it is. One is tiring, so how would it be with two? I was over thirty, and my husband was over forty. Physically and financially, I did not think we could afford to raise twins. ... My husband and I couldn't agree at the clinic, so the doctor asked us to go back home to discuss it. The doctor also mentioned that due to the risk of miscarriage, it is better to have two. After that, I talked to my parents, and they said they respected my decision. My husband's family preferred to keep two. Thinking about how I would be blamed if I only kept one, especially if something went wrong in the future, ... I eventually had to keep two.

When facing quadruplets, all agreed to conduct fetal reduction. However, everyone had different considerations. Ting-Ting's doctor suggested keeping two as the normal clinical practice, mentioning the risk of miscarriage. When the medical framework did not match the expectant mother's wishes, the doctor brought in her husband. The in-laws' long-standing expectations added further weight to the reasons to have twins. Ting-Ting did not have strong support on her side, so she compromised. No professional counseling was involved, and the doctor failed to take Ting-Ting's strong preference seriously. These various kinds of disagreement, both among doctors and between doctors and their clients, often add further strain to women's navigation of the fetal reduction decision. Also, the possible maternal health risk of carrying multiples was the factor least mentioned during the discussions that led to Ting-Ting's decision.

Maternal-Fetal Conflicts

Although other people's various opinions give pregnant women instruction and inspiration as to what to anticipate, it is important to note that maternal-fetal conflicts also come into play. In theory, maternal *and* fetal health should both be taken into consideration in decision-making. In some cases studied here, maternal health risk was at the center of thought, such as when Jackie worried about her partner Stella's second pregnancy in light of her difficult first one, and when the main concern of the second doctor Yi-Wen consulted was the risk of multiple pregnancy to Yi-Wen herself. However, in most other cases it was fetal health that became the center of discussion. The statistics provided to women in the clinics or on the internet often emphasize the preterm births and prematurity of the infants more than the maternal mortality and morbidity of the women. This focus on fetal health can be deployed in two totally different directions: (1) toward rejecting the fatal harm caused by fetal reduction, or (2) toward employing fetal reduction to help ensure that the remaining fetuses will be healthy. Either way, it is fetal health, not women's health, that is the main theme.[6]

Another feature of maternal-fetal conflict lies in the assumption of fetal personhood. As described above, some doctors use ultrasonic images to highlight the loveliness of the "kids" on the monitor. Or they may describe the procedure in a way that stirs up emotions about "killing someone." Family members often refer to the fetuses as "children" or "kids" as well. They may draw upon some religious or supernatural logic to state that "there must be some reasons that the kids are following you," or they may evoke heaven-given bonding to imply that the woman should keep all the "kids."[7] This makes women feel guilty of bad mothering for not loving their "babies" at this stage. When Wen-Min described to me how she hesitated about what to do with the triple fetuses, she said that "in the beginning, I did not have motherly love, so I intended to reduce one." Family members reminded Yi-Wen of her "motherly love" and suggested that the goddess Mazu wanted her to "follow nature" and accept her assigned job of triplet pregnancy. Such rhetoric is an extra burden on women if they consider accepting fetal reduction.

Exercising Skill-Based Autonomy

Overall, women tend to form a hybrid assessment of the proce-dure, taking into consideration the health, social, emotional, moral, social, and financial aspects. Whether they accepted or declined fetal reduction in the end, I argue that many of them practiced what Meyers (2001) calls the skills-based autonomy. To enact their own desires and goals, these women sought out diverse information to compare and contrast (communication and analytical skills), to reflect upon (introspective skills), to consider in the light of relevant experiences (memory skills), and to evaluate in terms of the future (imaginative skills). They went through very complicated reasoning to make their final decisions.

Women's volitional skills are sometimes endangered. In Taiwan, the conflicting opinions of doctors and the subordination of women's interests to those of the fetuses—or even to those of the women's husbands—often create new barriers to women enacting what they really need. Ting-Ting's preference for reduction to a singleton best illustrates such suppression of women's volitional skills. If they are without other support, women may find it very difficult to confront the authoritative knowledge of doctors in the clinics and/or the dominant status of their husband in the patriarchal family, making it doubly hard to "resist the pressure to capitulate to convention" and "to challenge ... the cultural regimes that pathologize or mar-ginalize their priorities" (Meyers 2001: 741–42).

Some women needed to rebuild the network of fetal reduction that some doctors complicated for them. When these women finally decided to undergo fetal reduction, their doctor would refer them to other doctors. They needed to reschedule and even arrange a long trip to carry out the surgery, as Stella and Jackie did (also see P.-Y. Chiu 2004). Even though fetal reduction is legal, financially feasible, and accessible in Taiwan, reaching the clinic service still meant overcoming an additional hurdle, and often not the last hurdle.

Conclusion

The main anticipatory labor concerning fetal reduction consists of navigating complex information. The core work for women is to seek out and clarify the contrasting opinions, advice, insights, and support offered by doctors, family members, women who share their experiences on the internet, and even the gods and goddesses of religious tradition. Information and suggestions can range from statistics shown on clinicians' desks or the life story of a neighbor to popular wisdom, the moral principles of a certain religion, or the gender preferences of certain family members. This can cause the decision-making process to differ widely from the ACOG guideline's statement that "respect for a patient's autonomy acknowledges an individual's right to hold views, make choices, and take actions based on *her personal values and beliefs*" (ACOG 2017: 3, emphasis added). The so-called *personal* is shaped and built by *collective* consultation, which is often very *political*. An individualized ethics model such as informed consent is not adequate.

Although this chapter recognizes women's great efforts to find their own direction amid these divergent recommendations, a collective effort is nevertheless needed to relieve them of carrying these burdens alone. What is most problematic is that health professionals in Taiwan do not have an official guideline, and individual doctors in different specialties and with different values offer opposing directions. A detailed guideline based on global and local data and evidence should be available for women as one of their resources for enhancing their analytical and reasoning skills.

I also highlight women's capacity to conduct a technological assessment. Most research to date has focused on the decision-making processes, tending to separate medical factors (recognizing the health risk of multiple pregnancy) and nonmedical factors (religious belief and lifestyle) (e.g., H.-L. Wang and Chao 2006; Britt and Evans 2007a; Kelland and Ricciardelli 2015). Many women care most about how medical technology has brought new risks to their cherished pregnancies. Their capacity to assess the medical model should become an important part of consultancy. Ethical guidelines and medical communications should not only focus on women's values or on the social dimensions of decision-making but also recognize women's critical evaluations of medical technology.

On some occasions, feto-centrism and the marginalization of women's health risks and social needs can also prevent women from fully assessing various merits of fetal reduction. When women's concerns about their own health, their care responsibilities, and their career development were put aside in the clinic or the living room, the resulting "decision" was often to keep the triplet or twin pregnancy. As we will see in chapter 7, when women carrying multiples move to the second trimester, they immediately become the risk group, start intensive body work, and bear the sole responsibility for fetal health. These should be anticipated and become an important part of deliberations for navigating the decision on fetal reduction.

Notes

1. One exception is Mei-Hui, who was pregnant with triplets. She was not offered the option of fetal reduction. And she said that this would not have been an option due to her religious beliefs.
2. Several local studies compare the results of twin pregnancies with and without fetal reduction (e.g., Hwang et al. 2002; Cheang et al. 2007).
3. This is partly due to my strong suggestion to the Ministry of Health and Welfare to reveal some reported data openly, such as the number of fetal reductions (Wu et al. 2020).
4. "Obstetrician-gynecologists should be knowledgeable about the *medical risks* of multifetal pregnancy, the potential *medical benefits* of multifetal pregnancy reduction, and the complex *ethical issues inherent in decisions* regarding multifetal pregnancy reduction. They should be prepared to respond in a professional and ethical manner to patients who request or decline to receive information, or intervention, or both" (ACOG 2017: 718, emphasis added).
5. Doctors also claimed that the miscarriage rate after reduction to twin pregnancy was about 4–5 percent, which was similar to, or only slightly higher than, that in twin pregnancy without fetal reduction. In addition, taking into account the baseline, the miscarriage rate directly caused by the fetal reduction might be even lower. The experts would like to start to claim that some of the miscarriages may happen naturally, not due to the intervention of fetal reduction. Dr. Ko, the leading expert in this field, provides information based on his long-term experience. He points out that the miscarriage rate, the leading risk of fetal reduction, is about 3.1 percent in Taiwan, which is lower than most of the published reports in the European and American countries (Ko

2021). He also reminds readers that even without the process of fetal reduction, singleton and twin pregnancy has its "natural miscarriage rate," fetal mortality, and very early prematurity. Overall, he suggests that one in every twenty to twenty-five cases seeking fetal reduction would meet with miscarriage, pretty close to the "natural miscarriage rate."

6. In Yu's study of 112 women undergoing fetal reduction, women's prime consideration was the risk of miscarriage caused by multiple pregnancy, immediately followed by the risk to maternal health (Yu 2015: 37).

7. Rich research has shown how fetal personhood works in the abortion debates, as well as how religious entrepreneurs in Japan (Hardacre 1997) and in Taiwan (Chen 2020) draw selectively upon, and creatively assemble, historical religious tradition to pressure women into practicing some rituals to memorialize the aborted fetuses. Whether or not these newly created rituals have influenced how people perceive fetal reduction needs further research.

Chapter 7

AN-TAI

ACTIVE MATERNAL BODY WORK

Five months after Stella's fetal reduction (from three fetuses to two), I visited her in the maternity hospital. She was practicing *an-tai*, the Chinese term for keeping the fetuses (*tai*) safe/calm (*an*). Twin pregnancy often requires bed rest in hospital to prevent premature birth, the leading complication of multiple pregnancy. Stella had started mild contractions during her thirty-first week of pregnancy. To prolong her pregnancy, she was taking medicine (an *an-tai* drug) as well as maximizing time in bed. "I should hang on until at least the thirty-sixth week," she told me. Premature birth is usually defined as birth before the thirty-seventh week, and Stella wanted to get as close as possible to that threshold. Walking slowly down the hall in her pajamas, she said that members of a lesbian social media group she belonged to discussed how "*raising* twins is like hell," but that the hardship of *carrying* twins was still seldom mentioned. The burden of child-rearing was known, but not that of childbearing.

The determined Stella did not quite reach her goal of the thirty-sixth week; she had a cesarean section in the thirty-fourth week. After the birth, the underweight twins were sent to the neonatal intensive care unit (NICU) at a nearby medical center. The same day, Stella's partner Jackie announced the birth on Facebook, posting photos of Stella and the twins in their separate beds in two different hospitals. Jackie's tagline of "the hardworking mom" for the photo of Stella with her eyes closed won countless heart emojis, including mine. The twins grew well. A couple of years later, when

I saw a video Stella posted of the twins copying their older sister doing exercises during the Covid-19 lockdown in Taiwan, I could not help but smile.

Women carrying twins and triplets undertake differing degrees of *an-tai*, including those who, like Stella adopt fetal reduction to "only" have twins. *An-tai* has a long history. The health practices of *an-tai* have been recorded in the classic Chinese medical books since the fifth century (J.-d. Lee 2008). Some traditional rituals of *an-tai* are still in practice in Taiwan to expel spirits dangerous to pregnancy (Sung 1996, 2000). Today, people still use the traditional phrase "*an-tai*" for the medication (*an-tai* drug and *an-tai* shot) given to expectant mothers who are on bed rest, for maternal or sick leave during an eventful pregnancy (*an-tai* leave), and for various activities to protect fetuses from premature birth. Women who carry multiples, whether due to IVF, IUI, fertility drugs, or spontaneous conception, have a higher chance of preterm labor, so they often need to practice *an-tai*. Since 50–60 percent of twin pregnancies result in preterm birth, Stella's situation was typical. Routine interventions to prevent preterm labor include close monitoring, anticontraction medication (tocolytic therapy) if showing symptoms presaging preterm labor, and recommendations to change the mother's activity level, such as increasing rest (Newman 2005; Medley et al. 2018). Stella went through all these precautions for more than a month.

The *an* in the term *an-tai* is a verb meaning "to remain safe/calm," and women are the subjects enacting it. In order to practice *an-tai*, women in my study took on extra tasks and responsibilities. As Stella indicated when stating her goal of "hanging on until at least the thirty-sixth week," keeping the twin fetuses in utero for a certain length of time was her main task during this stage. Medical practitioners may offer the anticontraction drug, advice, and care, but many of the tasks involved rely heavily on the expectant mothers to execute, experiment with, and then adjust accordingly. What exactly do pregnant women do to practice *an-tai*? Since some common practices, such as bed rest, sound quiet and easy, why did Stella call it a hardship? How does *an-tai* differ from other anticipatory labor decisions and actions described in chapters 5 and 6?

This chapter discusses women's active maternal body work during the *an-tai* period. First, I discuss the medical intervention routinely used during *an-tai*. It is stunning that most of the practices are not supported by evidence-based medicine, yet practitioners continue to prescribe them to pregnant women in many parts of the world, including Taiwan. Second, I delineate three major kinds of maternal body work during *an-tai*: self-palpation for prediction, corporeal adjustment, and emotion work. Though a prescribed intervention such as bed rest may sound easy, I will show why it is a strenuous and disturbing task for women. Third, I present women's negotiation between reproductive labor and productive labor to maximize their efforts to prevent preterm labor. To carry out the heavy responsibility of practicing *an-tai*, some women resign from their paid jobs to become full-time mothers, which they may never have anticipated doing when they embarked upon the reproductive journey.

"No Placement in Incubator"

After the hurdles of reaching conception and deciding on fetal reduction, women carrying multiples move to a new task: prolonging the pregnancy. Stella strove to give birth to the twins as close to the thirty-seventh week as possible because sooner than that is defined as preterm. She was quite reasonable not to expect to be able to carry them to full term (such as the fortieth week). Several of my interviewees referred to their goal as "no placement in incubator" for their anticipated newborns. One concern was financial. Before the National Health Insurance (NHI) was implemented in 1995, parents told me that it cost 10,000 NT dollars a day (roughly 300–400 USD) to use the incubator for a preterm baby. This was not affordable for most of families. As Emily, the manager in a small business company who was pregnant with twins in 1993, stated, "It was impossible to pay 10,000 NT dollars per day with my salary, so I needed to do the *an-tai* well." After NHI relieved families of this financial burden, parents tended to cite the health problems of the newborns as their major concern.[1]

Once women were carrying twins or triplets, their goal of avoiding preterm birth was difficult to reach. Various studies have shown that about 50–60 percent of women carrying twins will have preterm birth. In the US, the 2021 CDC flyer "Having Healthy Babies One at a Time" states that "about 3 out of 5 twin babies are born preterm." The online advice for pregnancy care from the Health Promotion Administration in Taiwan states that while only 10 percent of singleton pregnancies have preterm birth, the rate increases to 50 percent for twins and 90 percent for triplets (M.-H. Hsu 2021; see also Hu et al. 2015). All epidemiological research, from global statistics (World Health Organization 2012) to local data (K.-H. Chen et al. 2019; Y.-K. Chang, Tseng, and Chen 2020), demonstrates that multiple

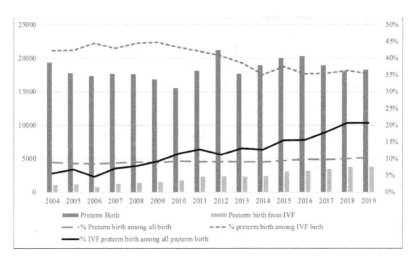

GRAPH 7.1. Trends in Preterm Birth in Taiwan, 2004–19. Sources: ROC Ministry of Health and Welfare 2021a, 2021b. © Chia-Ling Wu

pregnancy is one of the leading causes of preterm birth. As we have seen in chapter 6, for those doctors who advised women to continue twin and even triplet pregnancies, the high prevalence of preterm birth was not a focus of conversation.

Preterm birth has been particularly common for women who have achieved pregnancy through assisted reproductive technology in Taiwan. Graph 7.1 shows that over the fifteen years between 2004 and 2019, about twenty thousand preterm babies were born annually—roughly 10 percent of all newborns. Of these preterm babies, the percentage of IVF babies has increased from 6 percent in 2004 to 21 percent in 2019, shown in the dark horizontal line in graph 7.1. The IVF registry shows that around 35–45 percent of IVF babies are born preterm, mainly due to the high prevalence of multiple pregnancy. There are no data about the relationship between multiple pregnancy or preterm birth and the use of fertility drugs. If such data were included, the rate of ARTs leading to preterm birth would be much higher. Most women who start infertility treatment are seeking to have children through modern technology, and they seldom imagine that their babies from IVF could be preterm babies.

Babies "Born too Soon," as the title of World Health Organization (2012) report summarizes it, have become a global issue that must be tackled. The risks are clear—namely, the high morbidity and mortality of preterm babies and the great care burden this poses for the healthcare system, community, and family. The solutions include preconception prevention of IVF multiples, good maternal care during pregnancy and childbirth, and high-quality infant care after the preterm babies are born. This chapter focuses on the available interventions *during* multiple pregnancy.

Preventing Preterm Labor *during* Multiple Pregnancy

Evidence-based medicine has cast doubt on various commonly practiced interventions during pregnancy to prevent preterm birth. These "pregnancy management" strategies for singleton and multiple pregnancies range from bed rest, home uterine monitoring, and various drug interventions to surgical interventions such as a cervical stitch (cerclage) and good nutrition. Evidence-based medicine shows that almost none of these practices is known to effectively prevent preterm birth. An overview of eighty-three Cochrane systematic reviews of interventions during pregnancy to prevent preterm labor prompted myriad question marks—the icon for "unknown harm or benefit"—on the report (Medley et al. 2018). Please note that this is a review of reviews, so eighty-three systematic reviews mean hundreds of clinical studies. Page after page of question marks are listed in most of the systematic reviews. Among the eighty-three reviews, only one shows "clear evidence of benefit" in lowering perinatal mortality and preventing preterm birth—namely, midwife-led continuity models versus other models of care (Sandall et al. 2016).

The evidence targeting multiple pregnancy specifically for preterm birth prevention is limited. The current evidence shows that "there is no conclusive evidence that any intervention prolongs gestation in multifetal pregnancies" (Biggio and Anderson 2015: 664; see also Jarde et al. 2017). Bed rest stands out as the most dramatic example. Although bed rest is the most frequently prescribed intervention for twin pregnancy, there is no evidence to support its efficacy (Newman 2005; Crowther and Han 2010; Sosa et al. 2015). Due to the lack of evidence on strict bed rest, some experts suggest that "its use to prevent preterm birth cannot be recommended" (Biggio and Anderson 2015: 659). Some doctors emphasize the harm that bed rest can cause pregnant women, from stress to common physical harm, such as a blood clot in a vein or bone demineralization, and therefore even call its prescription "unethical" (McCall et al. 2013).

Intensive Maternal Body Work

Despite the strong evidence that interventions to prevent preterm birth have almost no efficacy for multiple pregnancy, women in my study received a lot of medical advice and prescriptions to keep the fetuses safe. These women carrying twins or triplets, categorized as a high-risk group, often closely followed the advice they received from healthcare providers about ways to prolong their pregnancy. At some point in their pregnancy, most of them felt they needed to practice *an-tai*. In addition to the well-documented statistics of risk, women felt alert to signals from their own changing bodies—especially the "unruly maternal body" (Neiterman and Fox 2017)—such as evidence of bleeding found in the underwear, swelling of the feet, and tightening of the belly. As Vivian described it, the statistics about preterm birth for twin pregnancy did not ring any bells for her until "my belly was so big in the fifth month, as big as if I was close to delivery, that the doctor asked me to stay home to *an-tai* to prevent preterm labor."

The tasks of *an-tai* rely heavily on the expectant mother's body. I borrow and extend the concept "maternal body work" (Gatrell 2011, 2013) to delineate what women do during the *an-tai* period. Most of the literature on body work discusses the paid work undertaken to care for others' bodies (e.g., Wolkowitz 2006). In contrast, a woman's pregnancy is unpaid work, except in cases of commercial surrogacy, and involves practicing on her own body for the sake of another body (or bodies) inside the woman's own body. I present three major forms of maternal body work—self-palpation for prediction, corporeal adjustment, and emotion work—to analyze how women carrying multiples work to avert the threat of preterm birth.

Self-Palpation for Prediction

Predicting the onset of preterm birth is a task that pregnant women often need to share with their medical professionals. If the woman is hospitalized, medical professionals can use devices and vaginal examinations to monitor the pregnancy and make the prediction. However, most women are not hospitalized throughout their pregnancy, so learning to identify the signs of preterm labor becomes part of routine prenatal education for women with multiple pregnancy. The rationale is that if women can detect the early signs of preterm labor, they can ask medical professionals for further assessment and intervention. The signs include tightening of the belly, abdominal cramps, lower backache, bleeding from the vagina, and lack of fetal movement.[2] The umbrella term "home uterine monitoring" includes various elements, ranging from education to the use of monitoring devices at home to detect the early signs of preterm birth. Overall, the women I interviewed were advised to observe their body keenly so as to do self-screening.

Self-palpation of one's uterine contractions and of fetal movement is most challenging. Compared with other signs, such as discharge from the vagina, which can be detected visually, contractions were a new bodily sensation for most women I interviewed. Vivian described the difficulty of identifying contractions as a first-time expectant mother:

> Many twin moms said that by the sixth or seventh month, preterm labor may happen. So I needed to pay attention to the contractions. This was my first pregnancy, so how could I know what contractions were? I asked many of my friends what they were, and they often said it was the tightening of the belly, as hard as a rock. ... During the seventh month, I felt a little bit of pain in the belly, and some funny feeling during the middle of night, so later I went to see the doctor. He said that the contractions had started. Then, I finally knew what contractions meant. I started two months of *an-tai* in the hospital after that.

Monitoring the early signs requires women to observe, feel, record, judge, and then respond by consulting their doctors or midwives. Women enact their new sense of having a pregnant body (Mol and Law 2004). The verbal descriptions of what to watch for may not easily translate into bodily sense, not to mention the fact that there is a wide variation of bodily sensation. Vivian did not experience her belly feeling "hard as a rock," like her friends did, but simply noticed a "funny feeling." Instead, it was menstruation-like cramps in the lower abdomen—another preterm sign—that led Vivian to consult her doctor.

Women sometimes mobilized other resources to practice the palpation. Hsiao-Yen described vividly how feeling the "fetal movement" confused her about her twin pregnancy:

> The doctor advised me to note the fetal movement since the seventh month. He said if one of the twins did not move suddenly, then. ... I felt worried hearing that. How could I know which one was moving? Was it only one moving? Or were both twins moving? I felt the kicking, but was it the two feet of one twin, or two feet from both twins? So I asked help from my sister-in-law (a nurse), and she lent me a stethoscope to figure it out. And then, when she touched my

belly, she said that I had been contracting. I finally got to know, wow, this was a contraction. I was told that contraction meant the tightening of the belly, but I was confused. When the twins kicked, I also felt tightening of the belly. I could not figure out which meant which through the whole pregnancy.

Hsiao-Yen's confusion illustrates the difficulty in distinguishing the normal (fetal movements) from the abnormal (early contractions) and in precisely identifying the sensation (the kicking of just one or of both twins). In some countries, women have easy access to midwives to clarify such kinds of confusion (e.g., Carter et al. 2018). In Taiwan, 99.8 percent of women go to obstetrician-gynecologists for their prenatal visits; although it is free and easy to make appointments in Taiwan's maternity program, women do not regard seeing doctors as a way to seek reassurance or learn how to detect these bodily signals. This explains why Hsiao-Yen mobilized her own social network and asked a relative who was a nurse to bring medical equipment to help her denote the preterm signs more accurately. The task of self-palpation became a new worry for these women. Not only did it consume their attention, but the sensations they were looking for were not easily identified simply by following a book.

What these women never told me is that evidence-based medicine has not firmly supported the efficacy of the home-monitoring program. A systematic review of thirteen randomized trials, involving more than six thousand cases, could not determine whether or not home monitoring is effective in prolonging pregnancy and improving the infants' health outcomes (Urquhart et al. 2017). Nor has evidence-based medicine confirmed the effectiveness of predictive practices, such as cervical-length screening, that only medical professionals can perform (Biggio and Anderson 2015). Still, women often took self-palpation seriously. The self-monitoring can only be done by women themselves. If any suspicious signs appear, women need to decide whether to go to the emergency room or just take more time to rest. Hsiao-Yen, a lawyer, said that after intensive on-site legal investigations and appearances in court, she often found bleeding and needed to go home to rest. However, it is not only such symptoms that can lead to an intervention such as bed rest because carrying multiples itself may require a lot of rest.

Corporeal Adjustment

Twin and triplet pregnancy means a heavy belly—so heavy that women need to develop a lot of strategies to deal with it. When

Neiterman and Fox (2017) investigated how women control the symptoms of their "unruly maternal body," such as morning sickness, nausea, fatigue, shortness of breath, and rapid weight gain, their sample group was women pregnant with a singleton. In my study, most of the women with multiple pregnancy not only shared some typical pregnancy "symptoms" but were also literally carrying a heavier load than they ever had before. It is very common to have a full-term belly by just the fifth month of a twin pregnancy. Gaining twenty kilograms (forty-four pounds) by the eighth month is about the average. In some cases, this prevents women from moving around and doing other things they usually do in daily life. Monica told me that, during the seventh month, she almost never left the house due to her heavy body: "Walking was very tiring. I felt the distance from the living room to the kitchen was very far." She needed to use a wheelchair for her prenatal visits to the hospital. Zoe said that, by the thirty-second week, she was short of breath even when she was sitting: "My boss called me for my latest situation. He wondered whether I had walked from a long distance to pick up the phone because I sounded out of breath. I said I was sitting right next to the telephone. I was out of breath even when I was sitting."

Women needed material support to adjust to this corporeal change and continue the simplest tasks of daily life. Many women mentioned using a maternal support belt to carry the belly. Once walking became difficult, some of them relied on a wheelchair or modified their furniture to help them sit or sleep at home. Almost all mentioned the difficulty of sleeping. Mei-Hui, pregnant with triplets, described vividly how "in the beginning, the right side of the belly was compressed, and then the left side, and later the middle part sprang up." She needed to adjust her sleeping position but eventually could not sleep with the unruly body. Some women had such difficulty lying in bed that they slept in a chair. Yi-Fen, carrying twins, slept in the sitting position for three whole months. Others said that they could not sit because of being afraid their belly would drop to the floor, so they preferred lying on a bed. Women strove hard to figure out how to adjust their body to maintain the basic aspects of daily life, such as moving and sleeping.

"Rest," the common advice given to women carrying multiples, was not easy. In addition to their heavy body that made sleep difficult, some other bodily tasks interfered. During her twentieth week, Zoe started to have contractions every ten minutes, so she was prescribed medicine every two hours, including through the night. By the thirtieth week, frequent urination made Zoe go to the restroom every hour. She often found herself short of breath and woke up gasping for air in the middle of the night, which further deprived her of sleep. Monica described terrible pains during the last few weeks of pregnancy: her belly was pressing on her stomach and sternum so that she even needed a painkiller to reduce the discomfort, but this was often in vain, "so that I could barely rest during the *an-tai* at home." If hospitalized, women were confined to bed. In Mei-Hui's words, "Eating, drinking, and bowel movements were all in bed," which she ranked as the most horrible time during the whole pregnancy. The hospital offered constant monitoring and regular drug taking, and often required strict bed rest. Women described how they endured the side effects of the *an-tai* drugs, as well as their anxiety and impatience. The term "bed rest," either at home or in the hospital, sounds quiet and inactive, but in women's descriptions it was fierce and disturbing.

Again, there is little evidence to support the efficacy of the typical practices to prevent preterm labor in Taiwan, such as taking oral tocolytics, bed rest, and restriction of some strenuous activities (Medley et al. 2018). Women nevertheless try hard to find ways to follow such medical advice, even though it may not work very well. Instead, much research has shown that these so-called prevention measures may cause more anxiety and distress than they assuage, which could increase the chances of preterm birth (MacKinnon 2006; Carter et al. 2018; H.-Y. Hung et al. 2021).

Emotional Work

Despite feeling anxious and stressed, women often engage in emotional work to foster the fetuses. Gatrell (2011: 398) defines "emotion work" as the "emotional energy expended in making decisions about, and implementing, the obligations of pregnancy carework in accordance with medical advice." This is related to how women handle the uncertainty in identifying signs of incipient preterm birth and do their best to adjust their unruly body. Women I interviewed most often used the term *cheng* (hang on) to describe what they did—an action that draws more upon mental strength than physical capacity. Women needed to lift their spirits to foreground the protection of fetuses above their own bodily discomfort. Some described how they imagined the healthy birth of their twins and triplets as powerful motivation for enduring their physical discomfort. After all, in many cases they had achieved the pregnancy only after a long and difficult journey, as described in chapter 5.

Some visualized a better future to further strengthen their determination. For example, Emily stated that "to suffer several months in exchange for healthy twins—it was highly worth doing it, wasn't it?" Hsin-Yu also imagined that child-rearing might be easier as long as she endured all the hardships of the pregnancy.

Such emotion work may intensify for women carrying multiples, due to the increased maternal-fetal conflict. Some honestly expressed how they could not bear it any more at some point in their pregnancy. Yi-Fen kept asking her ob-gyn husband when the earliest time was to deliver the twins, only to hear that she needed to wait until the thirty-sixth week for the cesarean section: "I felt so torn. I felt extremely exhausted, but I also wished they could stay longer to have better lung function." Hsiao-Mei, a cleaner, described the discomfort of the whole twin pregnancy. She recalled the contradiction: "I really wanted to give birth as soon as possible because I felt so uncomfortable. However, doctors told me that the babies were still too small, and their weights too low, so I did my best to eat as much as possible." For Hsiao-Mei, the new task of gaining weight was a way to distract herself from her own suffering. Monica would have liked to give birth to her twins sooner, for relief from various forms of bodily suffering. However, she strongly believed she needed to endure to the thirty-sixth week so that the twins would not have to be placed in incubators, which might prevent her from breastfeeding, her ideal feeding method. Again, her ideals about motherhood enabled her to put her suffering aside. Still, a few days before Monica's scheduled C-section, when she was sent to the emergency room due to contractions, she rejected the ER doctor's advice to practice *an-tai* for a few more days. Monica said that she could not bear the pain of carrying twins, and only wished to give birth as soon as possible. "I just could not hang on anymore," Monica told me. The twins were twenty-three hundred and twenty-five hundred grams when they were born, within the margin of low birthweight.

Although women clearly described how they suffered, I found almost no one who mentioned worrying about their own threatened health. In an important study of women's stress and distress about home rest in Taiwan, the leading worry was "losing baby" and "possible preterm birth" (H.-Y. Hung et al. 2021). That said, the questionnaire that was used included no item about the worry of women losing their own lives, or of possible serious physical and/or psychological harm. Research has shown that, in developed countries, maternal mortality is two to three times higher in twin pregnancy than in singleton pregnancy (Senat et al. 1998; Conde-Agudelo, Belizan, and Lindmark 2000). It is well documented that women carrying multiples have a higher risk of hypertension, anemia, urinary tract infection, and postpartum hemorrhage. However, neither women's narratives nor questionnaire items include the issue of maternal death and health risk. *An-tai* is practiced in anticipation of the better health of fetuses, not mothers.

Negotiating Reproductive and Productive Labor

To execute active maternal body work, women carrying multiples often need to negotiate their reproductive and productive labor. Since bed rest is the key element of *an-tai*, most women need to take leave from their paid jobs. In addition, place matters for *an-tai*. Even for a singleton pregnancy, it is not easy to implement health advice or handle common discomforts such as morning sickness in the workplace (Gatrell 2011, 2013). In the case of multiple pregnancy, where the location of *an-tai* is either the home or a hospital, most women simply cannot practice *an-tai* while continuing to work in an office, shop, or market.

"You want work, or kids?" Emily recalled that her doctor had sharply asked when she was hospitalized for a short time during her second trimester. Emily's doctor created the image of a zero-sum game: women must devote themselves either to *an-tai* or to a job. This narrative places the sole and primary responsibility for the welfare of children at their mother's feet. Some women assumed that their pregnancy care work would not be compatible with their paid work, so quitting their job was part of their maternal body work. Hsiao-Yi was a marketing manager in an international car company when she became pregnant with twins by donor insemination privately arranged by a doctor. A feminist with a strong determination to become a voluntary single mother, she decided to quit her job to focus on "cultivating my belly," in her words. Monica was also reminded by her doctor to rest more and not do strenuous work. For her, "work" meant housework and childcare, so she needed to arrange helpers to take care of her first child. Carrying multiples is itself a full-time job—or more than that, necessitating twenty-four-hour maternal body work in some difficult cases. Sometimes there is no room to manage a second shift.

Maximizing time and energy for *an-tai* means rearranging women's preexisting work. For those who have paid jobs, taking long maternal and sick leaves is most feasible for public servants, teachers, higher-ranked managers, employees of international corporations, and others whose job offers better family policies. Still, it causes much struggle. *An-tai* remained a gray area for any category of leave. In the late 1990s, Mei-Hsiang was working at a national bank that had the most generous paternity leave available at the time in Taiwan. During her *an-tai* period, she combined all her possible leaves—sick leave, annual leave, and maternity leave—to practice *an-tai* at home and in the hospital. Still, after using up all her possible days off, she had no choice but to resign and become a full-time mother and housewife. Hsiao-Yen, a partner at a law firm, used up all her leave and then received support from the firm's other partners to stay home on "special leave." In contrast, part-time workers and private-sector or service-sector employees tend to have to resign in order to practice *an-tai*.

An-tai leaves became part of the Gender Equality in Employment Act in 2010, thanks to the efforts of the feminist legislator Shu-Ying Huang. The revised act specifies that, with their doctor's request and approval, women can follow the regulation of sick leave to practice *an-tai* (Legislative Yuan 2010). If they do not need to be hospitalized, women can have up to thirty days of leave; if hospitalized, following the official rule on sick leave, they can have up to one year. Yet even though women can legally take *an-tai* leave, it can be very stressful to request it. A recent study shows that women who have home rest with threatened preterm labor have higher stress than healthy pregnant women, and "having to ask for leave from work for bed rest" was one of the most stress-inducing items in the survey (H.-Y. Hung et al. 2021). Moreover, legal disputes continue regarding employers' discrimination against women who take *an-tai* leave (e.g., C. Chang 2021).

Conclusion: *An-tai* in Vain?

This chapter reveals women's active maternal body work and reorganization of care to prevent the threat of preterm labor, the leading complication during multiple pregnancy. Unlike most literature that focuses on women's experiences and anxiety surrounding pregnancy and childbirth, this chapter makes women's work visible by highlighting what women do to practice *an-tai*. The women I interviewed were far from being the passive, vulnerable containers of their fetuses. In anticipation of giving birth to healthy newborns, they actively developed various ways to work with the tasks recommended or prescribed for them at this stage.

By the time they practice *an-tai*, women carry the sole responsibility for the welfare of their fetuses. When these women attempted to enhance conception (chapter 5), the major point of contention was optimization of medical intervention, such as determining the best number of embryos to transfer. Here medical professionals bore at least partial responsibility in reaching success. After attaining a multiple pregnancy, fetal reduction (chapter 6) was the major dilemma that women faced, often together with their family members and doctors. In contrast, practicing *an-tai*—to keep the fetuses safe by prolonging their time in the womb—is the embodied responsibility solely of the expectant mother. Over the trajectory of anticipatory labor, from success in conception to stabilizing the pregnancy, the share of responsibility thus gradually increases until it rests on the woman alone.

Most of my interviewees still had preterm births even after all their arduous efforts. This accords with the findings of evidence-based medicine, which show little efficacy for most of the preventive measures encompassed by *an-tai*. Nevertheless, women tend to blame themselves for endangering their children by not being able to further prolong a multiple pregnancy. This sense of guilt may linger. Ya-Wen told me in tears that, "even now, I still blame myself for making him [one of her twins] so small." In contrast, I did not hear anyone mention how fetuses might have harmed their mothers. The closest case was Mei-Hui's father-in-law saying that if the lives of the mother and triplets were endangered, saving the mother's life was more important. Most other cases did not include maternal death as a possible scenario and often positioned fetal health as the priority.

This feto-centrism, as implied in the term *an-tai* ("keep fetus safe/calm") itself, needs to be corrected through policy. First of all, doctors and policymakers need to highlight the maternal health risks of multiple pregnancy rather than focus only on the danger of preterm labor. "Twin pregnancy is risky for baby and mother," as the CDC flyer mentioned earlier emphasizes in bold type. This is even more true of triplet pregnancy. Mothers' health should be part of the prevention agenda, both before and during pregnancy. Second, evidence-based medicine should be followed and become a resource for improving preventive measures. As McCall, Grimes, and Lyerly (2013: 1308) point out, "Findings of fetal harm often lead to immediate prohibitions (such as caffeine or various medication), whereas findings of maternal harm or relative fetal safety are overlooked or slowly integrated into practice." During *an-tai*, women and fetuses are not two different entities, so *an-tai* needs to abandon useless practices that are recommended in the name of protecting fetuses but can harm women's health and/or further burden them.

Finally, the strongest evidence of benefit so far in preventing preterm birth is the midwifery model (Sandall et al. 2016), which has become seriously marginalized in Taiwan (Wu 2017b). This chapter shows that women often either "hang on alone" or have to utilize support by themselves. The midwifery model offers continuity of care, with quick access to advice, judgment, and support. This midwife-led continuity model should be built into *an-tai* as one of the primary ways to safeguard the health of both expectant mothers and their fetuses.

Notes

1. The parents I met at the 2019 triplets gathering told me that they were surprised to find that the expense listed on the bill was more than 2 million NT dollars (roughly 70,000 USD) when their triplets were discharged from the medical center after a two-month stay in the NICU. Taiwan's NHI paid all the fees, and the parents only paid around 50,000 NT dollars (less than 2,000 USD).
2. See the health advice from the National Taiwan University Hospital: https://reurl.cc/o1Qad3 (accessed 8 May 2022).

CONCLUSION

The stories of making multiple babies never stop amazing us. In January 2021 in Texas, in the US, a couple who had struggled with infertility earned 4.3 million hearts on TikTok when they documented how the mother, with an extra-large bump in her thirty-first week of pregnancy, went into the delivery room, where there were forty medical personnel in attendance, for the birth of "surprise pandemic quadruplets" (Dellatto 2021). In May 2021 in Taichung, Taiwan, the most popular IVF center in the country publicly announced the delivery of triplets, under the title "Congratulations," to bring some happy news during Taiwan's so-called level 3 voluntary lockdown (Lee Women's Hospital 2021). In Australia, however, IVF medical societies were celebrating the "world-best twin rate" (Carroll 2021), meaning the world's lowest twin and triplet rate for IVF births, 2.9 percent, along with a record-high success rate for achieving live birth through IVF. And in July 2021, when the UK's Department of Health and Social Care (2021) updated its guidance for the surrogacy process, it assured the populace that "the aim of treatment should be to have a *single* healthy baby, as twins or more carry added risks for mothers and babies" (emphasis added). To avoid having twins, the British government suggested a careful discussion between the intended parents and the surrogates about whether or not double embryo transfer is needed.

These snapshots exhibit again, around the globe and up to the present day, that the making of twins, triplets, and quadruplets provokes strong affect—joy and tears, surprise and concern. Not only aspiring parents and IVF practitioners but also social media followers, medical societies, civic groups, and the state engage in the making or unmaking of multiple babies. Never before in human history has the life and death of twins, triplets, and quadruplets been so salient in the various dimensions of people's social lives.

Thinking with Anticipation

This book invites us to contemplate these palpable stories and events. The foremost task is to understand how people become entangled with the dilemmas that advanced assisted reproductive technologies engender. A clinical practice such as multiple embryo transfer can yield extreme joy or a lifelong nightmare. At one time I focused on the angle of risk involved in ARTs, following those critics who stress how the so-called medical breakthroughs can create serious adverse outcomes. However, both the diversity of governing activities and the narratives of mixed emotions elicited by ARTs soon made it clear that the concept of risk is crucial but inadequate. After all, many of the actions meant to create a bright future from the stakeholders' perspective—whether in terms of a scientific innovation, a medical solution for infertility, a prosperous business, or a new family—are not intended to impose risk. In addition, while the mainstream technological assessment model has put risk in the center, the impact of innovations such as various ARTs is more than risk. Making multiple babies may become an essential part of a nation's pride, of a medical society's development of professionalism, or of a woman's identity, as I have shown. Risk is still largely ignored, and we need a more all-encompassing concept.

Anticipation captures the whole picture, without losing the significance of risk. Anticipation—which juxtaposes hope technology and risky medicine, affection, and knowledge making—helps us better comprehend how making multiple babies emerges and poses problems. In the anticipatory regimes of assisted reproduction, three layers of power dynamics are at work. The first layer consists of how stakeholders frame and act upon their selected dimension of anticipation. Scientists and fertility experts tend to envision and pursue successful events and high success rates. ARTs are the hope technology not only of aspiring parents but also of these professionals. However, the biomedical community of ARTs is not monolithic. Some experts in assisted reproduction join the alert public health sector, societies of pediatricians, and feminist health movements to highlight the risks that ARTs may create. The selected dimension of anticipation for women is particularly revealing. Contrasting images of the future of making multiple babies include highlighting women's strong desire for biological motherhood versus presenting the social options of infertility; showcasing mothers' fulfillment of holding twins versus portraying the burden of care for handicapped triplets; and calculating the live birth rates versus emphasizing women's miscarriage, OHSS, and maternal death caused by carrying multiples. The ways stakeholders negotiate the framing of ARTs and the solutions to settle the contentions surrounding ARTs are the core governing activities.

The second layer consists of the power dynamics among science, state, and society vis-à-vis national sociotechnical imaginaries of assisted conception. The imagined desirable future of ARTs differs from country to country and can range from becoming a world leader in scientific innovation or catching up with forerunners to avoiding harm from the new invention. Every country has had its own first test-tube baby (or babies), usually laden with both positive and negative visions. The main imaginaries still differ, however, as I have argued when examining IVF within the broader historical and political context by contrasting IVF as a nationalist pride in Taiwan but as a troublesome invention in Japan. This accounts for the diverse methods of governing multiple birth ever since the dilemma of balancing ARTs' risk and benefit first arose in the 1980s.

The third layer involves global/local dynamics. IVF as a global technology (Inhorn 2020) has developed at least three mechanisms of global governance: reporting global data through the ICMART; comparing regulations through the IFFS; and evidence-based-medicine debating in academic journals, at conferences, and in systematic reviews such as the Cochrane reports. These global monitoring and recommendation measures sometimes offer strong guidance for state-bound regulations. For example, as shown in chapter 2, Professor Ishihara Osamu, active in both the ICMART and IVF societies in Japan, bridges the global and the local. However, Taiwan shows a different pattern, as analyzed in chapter 3. Although Taiwanese IVF experts actively participate in these international organizations and are aware that single embryo transfer is the trend in Europe and Japan, they tend to select the guidelines of the American Society for Reproductive Medicine and have developed the lenient "American model plus one" criterion in order to build a flexible standardization on the limit of number of embryos to transfer. Feminist legislator Shu-Ying Huang did present the global trend of SET during the stipulation of Taiwan's 2007 Assisted Reproduction Act, but still needed to compromise with the pursuit of a high pregnancy success rate, which was perceived as fulfilling women's most important interests.

I have employed these three layers of analytical framework to explain why Taiwan has the world's highest twin rate after IVF. In Taiwan, the dominance of medical societies in regulating clinical procedures, the perception of IVF as a nationalist pride, and the selection of one global reference point (the US) rather than another (Japan) have created the anticipation of achieving a high success rate while downplaying the urgent need to tackle the health risk of multiple birth. Taiwan's self-congratulatory high pregnancy success rate is achieved at the expense of making too many multiple babies. The analytical framework is also useful for understanding why Japan anticipates risk more than success. This model needs to be further tested in other cases of making multiple babies, such as Australia with its "world-best twin rate" (Carroll 2021) and South Korea with its increasing births of multiples (Kim 2021), as well as in other cases of taking action now for a better future, such as measures to achieve climate security and good death.

Women anticipating having children and carrying multiples are an important part of the anticipatory regimes. This book has coined the term "anticipatory labor" to underscore women's increasingly hard work at different stages of dealing with multiple pregnancy. Women's labor during making multiple babies has been misrepresented and erased in several aspects. First of all, doctors and the media often cite women's requests to achieve success quickly as one of the main reasons that strong measures such as multiple embryo transfer (MET) are favored. This book offers the broader contexts needed to confront these views by delineating the reproductive trajectories of Taiwanese women. Taiwan's low and late marriage trend has led to delayed parenthood. Some gender minorities, such as lesbian couples, must still go abroad to have access to ARTs. Women hesitate to use IVF because they worry about the harm caused by the intrusive infertility treatments; IVF is almost always considered in Taiwan only after the failure of mild interventions such as traditional Chinese medicine. Due to these social and cultural factors, women start IVF late, so implanting more embryos to increase the success rate more quickly turns out to be an option to optimize women's reproductive goal. Women such as Wen-Min (see introduction) may state that they prefer twins to a singleton, but such a preference arises only after long failure and anxious delay in achieving the dream of having kids.

Once a woman becomes pregnant and is carrying multiples, feto-centrism becomes the underlying value of reproductive care. Fetal and infant mortality and morbidity are the risks of multiple pregnancy that are most often stressed in medical textbooks, public health agendas, and medical research. What is less visible is the fact that women carrying multiples face higher chances of dying or suffering physical and/or emotional burnout. Maternal mortality and morbidity are far less likely to become the organizing principle of pregnancy care in Taiwan than are fetal health and survival. In addition, while women's health risks and suffering are marginalized, they also carry almost the sole responsibility for protecting the unborn fetuses. Fetal reduction and preventive measures to prolong multiple pregnancy (which is often preterm) present women with challenging tasks and tremendous burdens. Carrying multiples means that women also face heavy moral struggles and must engage in intensive maternal body work.

Women's anticipatory labor is a continuous process within the changing sociotechnical network of reproductive care. During the stage of achieving conception, successfully becoming pregnant is often attributed primarily to doctors' expertise and high-quality lab facilities, whereas repeated failure to conceive is often attributed to a woman's physical incapacity or advanced maternal age. Moving on to the early confirmation of multiple pregnancy, especially of triplets and quadruplets, the network of fetal reduction emerges as a tough dilemma that most women never thought they would face when they began their reproductive journey. Given that doctors, laypeople, and even the gods offer conflicting evaluation principles and opinions on fetal reduction, women's main task at this stage is to navigate the diverse knowledge and values needed for informed decision-making. If carrying multiples continues, the next sociotechnical network is to prevent preterm labor so as to protect fetal health. It is all up to the woman's maternal body to fulfill the advised tasks—including detecting the early signs of labor, getting sufficient bed rest, and taking some medical drugs—despite most of these measures not being supported by evidence-based medicine. This stage of anticipatory labor is often in vain. Half of the women carrying multiples still have preterm births.

Comparing and contrasting the three networks—achieving conception, fetal reduction, and prolonging pregnancy—reveals that the tasks and responsibility to handle the hurdles gradually rely on women alone. When facing worrisome outcomes, many women feel guilty and blame themselves, even though they have done so much heavy anticipatory labor. Most likely, also, it is women who continue to do the main care work after multiples leave their wombs. Although I do not analyze this aspect in the book, how Ting-Ting cared for her sick twins (chapter 5), how Mei-Hsiang lamented that she had to quit her professional job to become the full-time caregiver of triplets (chapter 7), and how Gloria worried about her early menopause being caused by fertility drugs—all this reminds me that anticipatory labor continues long after multiple birth and needs further investigation. In addition, the extent to which Taiwanese women's anticipatory labor may differ from that of women in other countries will require more studies on women's trajectories of making multiple babies.

Responsible Governance and Solidarity

Collective action is required to relieve individual women of bearing heavy anticipatory labor. Based on the research findings, I propose "responsible anticipatory governance" as the policy recommendation for Taiwan, which would hopefully extend to developing a general framework. Responsible anticipatory governance, following the concept and action of responsible innovation (e.g., Stilgoe, Owen, and Macnaghten 2013), demands the reflexivity of stakeholders and institutions, inclusion of neglected voices—especially those of women carrying heavy anticipatory labor—and responsiveness to changing societal and technical challenges. Through *Making Multiple Babies*, I have shown how, in the world of reproductive medicine, some IVF experts, medical societies, and states reflect upon their own activities, critique themselves, and pay attention to their own biases and limitations. One impressive effort is to invent new concepts for measuring success, such as full-term live singleton births per treatment cycle. Such new indicators may make IVF look less effective than before, but they may also better meet aspiring parents' expectations. Such new calculations of success sometimes become the resources with which to build and evaluate the SET guideline. They can also provide guidance for IVF clinics when reporting their performance on websites for public communication (e.g., in Australia; see Reproductive Technology Accreditation Committee 2017). In the case of Taiwan, where a compulsory registry has been built since the late 1990s, some new concepts of success as well as health outcomes are collected and calculable. However, due in part to the lack of reflexivity among IVF experts and the weak capacity of state bureaucrats to mobilize the data for monitoring, the high quality of data reporting in Taiwan has not yet led to evidence-based policymaking.

Such reflexivity could be enhanced through more public dialogue with diverse groups. I have shown some cases in which feminists, pediatricians, and public health scholars have cast doubt on the practices of the IVF community. Debates and contention need to focus on some mechanisms to make stakeholders work together to increase the momentum of reform. Some effective working examples and mechanisms to date include a special task force with diverse stakeholders (e.g., the UK's Report of the Expert Group on Multiple Birth after IVF; see Braude 2006); inclusive representatives on the official advisory committee to ARTs (e.g., Japan's national ART committee); and the establishment of deliberative forums that encourage the lay public to participate in important ART policymaking (e.g., the deliberative engagement of ART consumers in ART public funding in Australia; see Hodgetts et al. 2014). Women's health organization, feminists, and parents of twins and triplets are often important participants in these committees and meetings. Currently in Taiwan, the state advisory committee of ARTs is mainly composed of IVF experts and scholars; civic groups do not participate regularly. Doctors often act as the spokespersons for their clients, and as I have shown, may sometimes misinterpret women's values and interests.

The integration of efforts to reduce multiple pregnancy is essential to constructing an overarching, consistent, and productive governance approach. In chapter 2, I discussed the Belgian project and the JSOG project, the two exemplars to build the eSET network to effectively reduce multiple pregnancy significantly. The two projects differ in their major movers. The Belgian one was initiated by the state and executed by the medical societies to demand SET with a new public financing program. In contrast, the JSOG led Japan's reform by issuing a voluntary guideline—mainly through mobilization of social responsibility and evidence-based policymaking with new registry data—and by transforming the less generous subsidy from the state as a pronatalist measure. Both projects work well with the alignment of stakeholders' efforts, visually presented by the overlapping circles in figures 2.1 and 2.2. This contrasts with Taiwan's disconnected patchwork (figure 4.1), discussed in chapter 4.

A new opportunity knocks. The Taiwanese state would like to make more babies, which may lead to a decrease in making multiple babies. In April 2021, Taiwan's media widely reported the US

Central Intelligence Agency's latest estimation that Taiwan's total fertility rate would be the lowest in the world in 2021. Although it is not news that the birthrate has been declining for years in Taiwan, the CIA's prediction prompted heated debate in Taiwan's public forums ("Taiwan to Raise Subsidies to Boost Flagging Birthrate" 2021). In response to continuous strong criticism, the government announced some new measures, including a new subsidy program for infertility treatment. The new program no longer targets low-income families only, but grants couples under forty years old six cycles of IVF with subsidies, providing 100,000 NT dollars (roughly 3,500 USD) for the first cycle. For women aged between forty and forty-four, at most three cycles can be subsidized. The new program follows the Belgian project in linking public financing with single embryo transfer. It requires SET for women under thirty-five years old, and a maximum of two embryos for women between thirty-six and forty-four years old. This is by far the most generous subsidy ever offered in Taiwan; the government estimates that the program will benefit 30,000 couples, with a budget of 3 billion NT dollars (roughly 100 million USD).

Can this new subsidy program transform Taiwan from having the world's highest twin rate from IVF? Taiwan's disconnected patch-works of eSET seem to work well with its new subsidy program. The official statement of the new policy lists three goals: (1) to fulfill the reproductive aspirations of the infertile couples, (2) to relieve their financial burdens, and (3) to reduce the multiple birth rate and OHSS caused by ARTs. The TSRM calls this a win-win-win measure: more children may be born to meet Taiwan's societal needs; the health risk of multiple birth can be prevented, to relieve the care burden it places on Taiwan's medical institutions; and couples may have more resources with which to achieve their reproductive goals (Tsui 2021). Instead of calling it win-win-win, however, I would rather bring in the new policy's solidarity in terms of bioethics (Prainsack and Buyx 2012), so as to collectively handle the difficulties of overcoming each hurdle during IVF through redistribution of resources such as money. Still, the new policy is a top-down pronatalist program from the outset, more than being aimed at reducing the multiple pregnancy rate; women's health risk is seldom mentioned. The policymaking process was mainly negotiated between the Ministry of Health and Welfare and the IVF medical societies, without the inclusion of other stakeholders such as pediatricians, health economists, feminists, and lay users. It is predicted that the SET rate will sharply increase and the multiple birth rate will effectively decrease. Yet the new policy is far from responsible anticipatory governance if we look into the pronatalist purpose and top-down policymaking process.

As STS (science, technology, and society) scholarship points out, STS scholars inevitably become part of a country's anticipatory governance (Barben et al. 2008). I did send my published paper on how to design public financing for better healthcare to governmental officials and the opinion leaders of the TSRM on the eve of their finalizing the details of Taiwan's new subsidy program in May 2021. When invited to give talks to IVF practitioners after the program was implemented in summer 2021, I also emphasized the need to reconceptualize the success rate, invite more stakeholders to participate in deliberations, and evaluate the new policy's outcomes not by how many more babies are born but by the extent to which the maternal and infant health risk of making multiple babies has been reduced. Still, I was quite surprised when I heard in July 2021 that the president of the TSRM, Dr. Min-Jer Chen, had announced, "We have lagged behind. Let's have this year as Taiwan's First Year to Promote SET." This happened much earlier than I expected. Who could have guessed that a CIA prediction of Taiwan having the world's lowest 2021 fertility rate would prompt Taiwan to launch a program to lower the world's highest twin rate? Perhaps responsible anticipatory governance is slated to gain momentum. I hope that this book's delineation of making multiple babies since the 1980s will help inspire the building of a solid eSET network in Taiwan. This may demand a new anticipatory regime of assisted reproduction, starting with putting women's anticipatory labor at the forefront.

References

A Sad Mother. 2000. "Mama Xinqing Gushi Laizi Yiwei Beishang Muqin De Zhen qing Gaobai" [Mothers' personal stories: A true confession from a sad mother]. *Taiwan Premature Babies Foundation Newsletter* 35: 22–23.

Abbott, Andrew. 2014. *The System of Professions: An Essay on the Division of Expert Labor.* Chicago: University of Chicago Press.

Aberg, Anders, Felix Mitelman, Michael Cantz, and Jurgen Gehler. 1978. "Cardiac Puncture of Fetus with Hurler's Disease Avoiding Abortion of Unaffected Co-twin." *The Lancet* 312(8097): 990–91.

ACOG (American College of Obstetricians and Gynecologists). 2013. "Multifetal Pregnancy Reduction: Committee Opinion NO. 553." *Obstetrics and Gynecology* 121: 405–10.

———. 2017. "Multifetal Pregnancy Reduction." ACOG Committee Opinion 553. Retrieved 26 October 2021 from https://www.acog.org/clinical/clinical-guidance/committee-opinion.

Adams, Vincanne, Michelle Murphy, and Adele E. Clarke. 2009. "Anticipation: Technoscience, Life, Affect, and Temporality." *Subjectivity* 28: 246–65.

Adamson, G. David. 2009. "Does Self-Regulation Work for Implementation of Single Embryo Transfer?" In *Single Embryo Transfer*, edited by Jan Gerris, G. David Adamson, Petra De Sutter and Catherine Racowsky, 249-267. Cambridge: Cambridge University Press.

Adamson, G. David, Paul Lancaster, Jacques de Mouzon, K. G. Nygren, and Fernando Zegers-Hochschild. 2001a. "A Simple Headstone or Just Eliminate the Chads?" *Fertility and Sterility* 76(6): 1284–85.

Adamson, [G.] D., P. Lancaster, J. de Mouzon, K. G. Nygren, and F. Zegers-Hochschild. International Working Group for Registers on Assisted Reproduction (IWGRAR). 2001b. "World Collaborative Report on Assisted Reproductive Technology, 1998." In *Reproductive Medicine in the*

Twenty-First Century, edited by D. L. Healy, G. T. Kovacs, R. McLachlan, and O. Rodriguez-Armas, 209–19. London: Parthenon Publishing Group.

Adamson, G. David, Jacques de Mouzon, Georgina M. Chambers, Fernando Zegers-Hochschild, Ragaa Mansour, Osaum Ishihara, Manish Banker, and Silke Dyer. 2018a. "International Committee for Monitoring Assisted Reproductive Technology: World Report on Assisted Reproductive Technology, 2011." *Fertility and Sterility* 110(6): 1067–79.

Adamson, G. David, Jacques de Mouzon, Paul Lancaster, Karl-G. Nygren, Elizabeth Sullivan, and Fernando Zegers-Hochschild. International Committee for Monitoring Assisted Reproductive Technologies (ICMART). 2006. "World Collaborative Report on In Vitro Fertilization, 2000." *Fertility and Sterility* 85(6): 1586–622.

Adamson, G. David, and Robert J. Norman. 2020. "Why Are Multiple Pregnancy Rates and Single Embryo Transfer Rates so Different Globally, and What Do We Do about It?" *Fertility and Sterility* 114(3): 680–89.

Adamson, G. D., F. Zegers-Hochschild, S. Dyer, G. Chambers, O. Ishiraha, R. Mansouur, M. Banker, and J. de Mouzon. 2018b. "ICMART World Report." Paper presented at the annual meeting of ESHRE, Barcelona, Spain.

Adrian, Stine Willum. 2010. "Sperm Stories: Policies and Practices of Sperm Banking in Denmark and Sweden." *European Journal of Women's Studies* 17(4): 393–411.

Almeling, Rene. 2015. "Reproduction." *Annual Review of Sociology* 41: 423–42.

American Society for Reproductive Medicine. *See* ASRM.

Andersen, A. N[yboe]. *See under* Nyboe Andersen.

Anonymous. 1969. "What Comes after Fertilization?" *Nature* 221: 613.

Armstrong, Elizabeth M. 1998. *Conceiving Risk, Bearing Responsibility: Fetal Alcohol Syndrome and the Diagnosis of Moral Disorder.* Baltimore, MD: The Johns Hopkins University Press.

Aronowitz, Robert A. 2015. *Risky Medicine: Our Quest to Cure Fear and Uncertainty.* Chicago: University of Chicago Press.

ASRM (American Society for Reproductive Medicine). 1998. "Practice Committee Opinion: Guidelines on Number of Embryos Transferred." Birmingham, AL: American Society for Assisted Reproductive Medicine.

Balabanova, Ekaterina, and Frida Simonstein. 2010. "Assisted Reproduction: A Comparative of IVF Policies in Two Pro-natalist Countries." *Health Care Analysis* 18: 188–202.

Barben, Daniel, Erik Fisher, Cynthia Sellin, and David H. Guston. 2008. "Anticipatory Governance of Nanotechnology: Foresight, Engagement, and Integration." In *The Handbook of Science and Technology Studies*, 3rd ed., edited by Edward J. Hackett, Olga Amsterdamska, Michael Lynch, and Judy Wajcman, 979–1000. Cambridge, MA: MIT Press.

Bardis, Nikolaso, Deivanayagam Maruthini, and Adam H. Balen. 2005. "Mode of Conception and Multiple Pregnancy: A National Survey of

Babies Born during One Week in 2003 in the United Kingdom." *Fertility and Sterility* 84(6): 1727–32.

Barlow, David H. 2004. "A Time for Consensus and Consistency of Reporting in Clinical Studies and the Importance of New Basic Research." *Human Reproduction* 19(1): 1–2.

———. 2005. "The Debate on Single Embryo Transfer in IVF. How Will Today's Arguments Be Viewed from the Perspective of 2020?" *Human Reproduction* 20(1): 1–3.

Bärnreuther, Sandra. 2016. "Innovations 'Out of Place': Controversy over IVF Beginnings in India between 1978 and 2005." *Medical Anthropology* 35(1): 73–89.

Bartels, Ditta. 1993. "The Financial Costs of In Vitro Fertilization: An Example from Australia." In *Tough Choices: In Vitro Fertilization and the Reproductive Technologies*, edited by Patricia Stephenson and Marsden G. Wagner, 73–82. Philadelphia, PA: Temple University Press.

Basu, Narendra Nath, James Hodson, Shaunak Chatterjee, Ashu Gandhi, Julie Wisely, James Harvey, Lyndsey Highton, John Murphy, Nicola Barnes, Richard Jonson, Lester Barr, Cliona C. Kirwan, Sacha Howell, Andrew D. Baildam, Anthony Howell, and D. Gareth Evans. 2021. "The Angelina Jolie Effect: Contralateral Risk-Reducing Mastectomy Trends in Patients at Increased Risk of Breast Cancer." *Scientific Report* 11: 2874. https://doi.org/10.1038/s41598-021-82654-x.

Beresford, David. 1978. "Test Tube Mother Has Girl." *The Guardian*, 26 July: 1.

Bergh, T., A. Ericson, T. Hillensjo, K-G. Nygren, U-B. Wennerholm. 1999. "Deliveries and Children Born after In-Vitro Fertilisation in Sweden 1982–95: A Retrospective Cohort Study." *The Lancet* 354(6): 1579–85.

Berkowitz, Richard L., Lauren Lynch, Joanne Stone, and Manuel Alvarez. 1996. "The Current Status of Multifetal Pregnancy Reduction." *American Journal of Obstetrics and Gynecology* 174(4): 1265–72.

Berkowitz, Richard L., Lauren Lynch, Usha Chitkara, Isabelle A. Wilkins, Karen E. Mehalek, and Emanuel Alvarez. 1988. "Selective Reduction of Multifetal Pregnancies in the First Trimester." *New England Journal of Medicine* 318(16): 1043–47.

Bhalotra, Sonia, Damian Clarke, Hanna Muhlrad, and Marten Palme. 2019. "Multiple Births, Birth Quality and Maternal Labor Supply: Analysis of IVF Reform Sweden." IZA Institute of Labor Economics Discussion Paper Series.

Bharadwaj, Aditya. 2016. "The Indian IVF Saga: A Contested History." *Reproductive BioMedicine and Society Online* 2: 54–61.

Biggio, Joseph R., and Sarah Anderson. 2015. "Spontaneous Preterm Birth in Multiples." *Clinical Obstetrics and Gynecology* 58(3): 654–67.

Birenbaum-Carmeli, Daphna. 1997. "Pioneering Procreation: Israel's First Test-Tube Baby." *Science as Culture* 6(4): 525–40.

———. 2004. "Cheaper than a 'Newcomer': On the Social Production of IVF Policy in Israel." *Sociology of Health and Illness* 26(7): 897–924.

Bleker, O. P., W. Breur, and B. L. Huiderkoper. 1979. "A Study of Birth Weight, Placental Weight and Mortality of Twins as Compared to Singletons." *British Journal of Obstetrics and Gynecology* 86: 111–18.

Bodri, Daniel, Satoshi Kawachiya, Michael De Bruker, Herman Tournaye, Masae Kondo, Ryutaro Kato, and Tsunekazu Matusmoto. 2014. "Cumulative Success Rates Following Mild IVF in Unselected Infertile Patients: A 3-Year Single-Centre Cohort Study." *Reproductive BioMedicine Online* 28: 572–81.

Bodri, D., S. Nair, A. Gill, G. Lamanna, M. Rahmati, M. Arian-Schad, V. Smith, E. Linara, J. Wang, N. Macklon, and K. K. Ahuja. 2018. "Shared Motherhood IVF: High Delivery Rates in a Large Study of Treatments for Lesbian Couples Using Partner-Donated Eggs." *Reproductive Biomedicine Online* 36: 130–36.

Bolton, Virginia N., Christine Leary, Stephen Harbottle, Rachel Cutting, and Joyce Harper. 2015. "How Should We Choose the 'Best' Embryo? A Commentary on Behalf of the British Fertility Society and the Association of Clinical Embryologists." *Human Fertility* 18(3): 156–64.

Bormann, Charles, Prudhvi Thirumalaraju, Manoj Kumar Kanakasabapathy, Hermanth Kandula, Irene Souter, Irene Dimitriadis, Raghav Gupta, Rohan Pooniwala, and Hadi Shafiee. 2020. "Consistency and Objectivity of Automated Embryo Assessments Using Deep Neural Networks." *Fertility and Sterility* 113(4): 781–87.

Botting, Beverley J., Alison J. Macfarlane, and Frances V. Price, eds. 1990. *Three, Four and More: A Study of Triplet and Higher Order Births.* London: HMSO (Her Majesty's Stationery Office).

Brahams, Diana. 1987. "Assisted Reproduction and Selective Reduction of Pregnancy." *The Lancet*, 17 December: 1409–10.

Brandes, Joseph M., Joseph Itskovitz, Ilan E. Timor-Tritsch, Arie Durgan, and Rene Frydman. 1987. "Reduction of the Number of Embryos in a Multiple Pregnancy to Triplets." *Fertility and Sterility* 48(2): 326–27.

Braude, Peter. 2006. *One Child at a Time: Reducing Multiple Births after IVF; Report of the Expert Group on Multiple Birth after IVF.* London: HFEA. Retrieved 14 July 2021 from https://ifqlive.blob.core.windows.net/umbraco-website/1311/one-child-at-a-time-report.pdf.

Brinton, Mary. 2016. "Intentions to Actions: Norms as Mechanism Linking Micro-Macro Levels." *American Behavioral Scientist* 60: 1146–67.

Brinton, Mary, Xiana Bueno, Livia Olah, and Merete Hellum. 2017. "Postindustrial Fertility Ideals, Intentions, and Gender Inequality: A Comparative Qualitative Analysis." *Population and Development Review* 44(2): 281–309.

Britt, David W., and Mark I. Evans. 2007a. "Information-Sharing among Couples Considering Multifetal Pregnancy Reduction." *Fertility and Sterility* 87(3): 490–95.

———. 2007b. "Sometimes Doing the Right Thing Sucks: Frame Combinations and Multi-fetal Pregnancy Reduction Decision Difficult." *Social Science and Medicine* 65: 2342–56.

Bronstein, Janet M. 2016. *Preterm Birth in the United States: A Sociocultural Approach*. New York: Springer International Publishing.

Brown, Eliza, and Mary Patrick. 2018. "Time, Anticipation, and the Life Course: Egg Freezing as Temporarily Disentangling Romance and Reproduction." *American Sociological Review* 83(5): 959–82.

Brown, Nik. 2005. "Shifting Tenses: Reconnecting Regimes of Truth and Hope." *Configuration* 13(3): 331–55.

Brown, Nik, Brian Rappert, and Andrew Webster, eds. 2000. *Contested Futures: A Sociology of Expectations in Science and Technology*. Farnham, Surrey: Ashgate Publishing.

Bryant, Joanne, Elizabeth A. Sullivan, and Jishan H. Dean. 2004. *Assisted Reproductive Technology in Australia and New Zealand 2002*. Australian Institute of Health and Welfare, National Perinatal Statistics Unit.

Callahan, Tamara L., Janet E. Hall, Susan L. Ettner, Cindy L. Christiansen, Michael F. Greene, and William F. Crowley Jr. 1994. "The Economic Impact of Multiple-Gestation Pregnancies and the Contribution of Assisted-Reproduction Techniques to Their Incidence." *New England Journal of Medicine* 331: 244–49.

Campbell, John L. 2002. "Ideas, Politics, and Public Policy." *Annual Review of Sociology* 28: 21–38.

Carpinello, Olivia J., Mary Casey Jacob, John Nulsen, Caludio Benadiva. 2016. "Utilization of Fertility Treatment and Reproductive Choices by Lesbian Couples." *Fertility and Sterility* 106(7): 1709–13.

Carroll, Lucy. 2021. "Unprecedented Rise in IVF Success Rate, but Multiple Births Fall to Record Low." *The Sydney Morning Herald*, 19 September.

Carter, Jenny, Rachel M. Tribe, Andrew H. Shennan, and Jane Sandall. 2018. "Threatened Preterm Labour: Women's Experiences of Risk and Care Management: A Qualitative Study." *Midwifery* 64: 85–92.

Casper, Monica J. 1998. *The Making of the Unborn Patient: A Social Anatomy of Fetal Surgery*. New Brunswick, NJ: Rutgers University Press.

CDC, ASRM, SART, and RESOLVE. 2000. *1998 Assisted Reproductive Technology Success Rates: National Summary and Fertility Clinic Reports*. U.S. Department of Health and Human Services, Centers for Disease Control and Prevention.

———. 2001. *1999 Assisted Reproductive Technology Success Rates: National Summary and Fertility Clinic Reports*. U.S. Department of Health and Human Services, Centers for Disease Control and Prevention.

———. 2002. *2000 Assisted Reproductive Technology Success Rates: National Summary and Fertility Clinic Reports*. U.S. Department of Health and Human Services, Centers for Disease Control and Prevention.

CDC, ASRM, and SART. 2003. *2001 Assisted Reproductive Technology Success Rates: National Summary and Fertility Clinic Reports*. U.S. Department of Health and Human Services, Centers for Disease Control and Prevention.

———. 2004. *2002 Assisted Reproductive Technology Success Rates: National Summary and Fertility Clinic Reports*. U.S. Department of Health and Human Services, Centers for Disease Control and Prevention.

———. 2005. *2003 Assisted Reproductive Technology Success Rates: National Summary and Fertility Clinic Reports.* U.S. Department of Health and Human Services, Centers for Disease Control and Prevention.

———. 2006. *2004 Assisted Reproductive Technology Success Rates: National Summary and Fertility Clinic Reports.* U.S. Department of Health and Human Services, Centers for Disease Control and Prevention.

———. 2007. *2005 Assisted Reproductive Technology Success Rates: National Summary and Fertility Clinic Reports.* U.S. Department of Health and Human Services, Centers for Disease Control and Prevention.

———. 2008. *2006 Assisted Reproductive Technology Success Rates: National Summary and Fertility Clinic Reports.* U.S. Department of Health and Human Services, Centers for Disease Control and Prevention.

———. 2009. *2007 Assisted Reproductive Technology Success Rates: National Summary and Fertility Clinic Reports.* U.S. Department of Health and Human Services, Centers for Disease Control and Prevention.

———. 2010. *2008 Assisted Reproductive Technology Success Rates: National Summary and Fertility Clinic Reports.* U.S. Department of Health and Human Services, Centers for Disease Control and Prevention.

———. 2011. *2009 Assisted Reproductive Technology Success Rates: National Summary and Fertility Clinic Reports.* U.S. Department of Health and Human Services, Centers for Disease Control and Prevention.

———. 2012. *2010 Assisted Reproductive Technology Success Rates: National Summary and Fertility Clinic Reports.* U.S. Department of Health and Human Services, Centers for Disease Control and Prevention.

———. 2013. *2011 Assisted Reproductive Technology Success Rates: National Summary and Fertility Clinic Reports.* U.S. Department of Health and Human Services, Centers for Disease Control and Prevention.

———. 2014. *2012 Assisted Reproductive Technology Success Rates: National Summary and Fertility Clinic Reports.* U.S. Department of Health and Human Services, Centers for Disease Control and Prevention.

———. 2015. *2013 Assisted Reproductive Technology Success Rates: National Summary and Fertility Clinic Reports.* U.S. Department of Health and Human Services, Centers for Disease Control and Prevention.

———. 2016. *2014 Assisted Reproductive Technology Success Rates: National Summary and Fertility Clinic Reports.* U.S. Department of Health and Human Services, Centers for Disease Control and Prevention.

———. 2017. *2015 Assisted Reproductive Technology Success Rates: National Summary and Fertility Clinic Reports.* U.S. Department of Health and Human Services, Centers for Disease Control and Prevention.

———. 2018. *2016 Assisted Reproductive Technology Success Rates: National Summary and Fertility Clinic Reports.* U.S. Department of Health and Human Services, Centers for Disease Control and Prevention.

Centers for Disease Control and Prevention, U.S. Department of Health and Human Services. 2021. "Why Are We Worried about Twin Pregnancies?" Retrieved 28 September 2021 from https://www.cdc.gov/art/pdf/patient-resources/Having-Healthy-Babies-handout-2_508tagged.pdf.

Chambers, G. M., V. P. Hoan, E. A. Sullivan, M. G. Chapman, O. Ishihara, F. Zegers-Hochschild, K. G. Nygren, and G. D. Adamson. 2014. "The Impact of Consumer Affordability on Access to Assisted Reproductive Technologies and Embryo Transfer Practices: An International Analysis." *Fertility and Sterility* 101(1): 191–98.

Chan Chien-Fu. 2005. "Rengong Shengzhi Zhiru Peitai Shumu Ni Shexian" [Assisted reproduction plans to limit the number of embryos transferred]. *Min Sheng Daily*, 6 June: A7.

Chang Chih-Yang. 2004. "Dao Yiwei Weida De Muqin Tan Gaotaishu Duobaotai Renshen De Wenti Yu Chuli" [Mourning for a great mother: On the problems and management of higher-order multiple pregnancy]. *United Daily News*, 6 December: E4.

Chang Chin. 2021. "Qing Wushiqi Tian Antaijia OL Zao Jianxin Ziqian" [Taking 57-day *an-tai* leave, and the office lady had her pay cut and was laid off]. *Apple Daily*, 10 March. Retrieved 26 October 2021 from https://tw.appledaily.com/headline/20210310/6GTRDALDCFEZHLYRCBRBEI VVDQ/.

Chang Sheng-Ping. 1985. "Shiguan Yinger Huiyilu" [Memoir of making a test-tube baby]. *China Times*, 17 April: 5.

Chang, Shirley L. 1992. "Causes of Brain Drain and Solutions: The Taiwan Experiences." *Studies in Comparative International Development* 27(1): 27–43.

Chang, S. Y., Y. K. Soong, M. Y. Chang, P. W. Lin, H. G. Guu, and M. L. Wang. 1991. "A Clinical Pregnancy after a Simple Method of Zona Cutting, Cryopreservation, and Zygote Intrafallopian Transfer." *Fertility and Sterility* 55(2): 420–22.

Chang Yao-Mao. 1994a. "Shatai Rengong Shouyun Duobaotai Zhuochuang Houyizheng Muqin Yisheng Mianlin Shengming Qushe Nanti" [The slow regulation of ART in Taiwan]. *Min-Sheng Daily*, 23 February: 21.

———. 1994b. "Shatai Rengong Shouyun Duobaotai Zhuochuang Houyizheng Muqin Yisheng Mianlin Shengming Qushe Nanti" [Feticide as the complication of multiple implantation by assisted conception: Mothers and doctors faced dilemma of life decision]. *Ming-Sheng Daily*, 1 April: 21.

Chang Yu-Hui. 1985. "Shiguan Yinger Bushi Sushimian" [A test-tube baby is not an instant noodle]. *China Times*, 16 August: 5.

Chang, Yu-Kang, Yuan-Tsung Tseng, and Kow-Tong Chen. 2020. "The Epidemiologic Characteristics and Associated Risk Factors of Preterm Birth from 2004 to 2013 in Taiwan." *BMC Pregnancy and Childbirth* 20: 201.

Chao Hsiao-Ning. 1997. "Xiantian Jingxuan Houtian Zaipei Shiguan Yinger Bijiao Jiechu" [Pre-selection and postnatal care: Test-tube babies are outstanding]. *China Times*, 2 April: 7.

Cheang, Chong-U, Lii-Shung Huang, Tsung-Hsien Lee, Chung-Hsien Liu, Yang-Tse Shih, and Mao-Sheng Lee. 2007. "A Comparison of the Outcomes between Twin and Reduced Twin Pregnancies Produced through Assisted Reproduction." *Fertility and Sterility* 88(1): 47–52.

Chen Cheng-Hsi. 1997. "Cong Yi Sui Dao Shiyi Sui Cong Danbaotai Dao Sibaotai Shiguan Haizi Qibairen Juhui" [From one-year-old to eleven-year-old, from singleton to quadruplets: 700 test-tube kids got together]. *United Daily News*, 5 April: 5.

Chen, Chin-Shyan, Tsai-Ching Liu, and Li-Mei Chen. 2003. "National Health Insurance and the Antenatal Care Use: A Case in Taiwan." *Health Policy* 64: 99–112.

Chen Chong-Sheng and Chang Li-Wen. 2002. "Jiantai Shoushu Yishi San Ming Rongzong Ai Gao" [Fetal reduction caused one dead and three lives: Taipei Veterans Hospital being sued]." *China Times*, 28 December: 9.

Chen Hsuan-Yu. 2020. "Dangdai Taiwan Yingling Xinyang De Fazhan Yu Daojiao Xiehu Chaodu Yishi De Yanyi" [The development of the belief in fetus-ghosts in contemporary Taiwan and how Taoist blood lake rituals have constructed it]. In *Daojiao Fuxing Yu Dangdai Shehui Shenghuo Liuzhiwan Xiansheng Jinian Lunwen Ji* [Taoist revival and contemporary social life: Memorial to Liu Chi-Wan], edited by Jen-Chieh Ting, 309–71. Taipei: Institute of Ethnology, Academic Sinica.

Chen, Kou-Huang, I-Chu Chen, Yi-Chieh Yang, and Kou-Tong Chen. 2019. "The Trends and Associated Factors of Preterm Deliveries from 2001–2011 in Taiwan." *Medicine* 98: 13(e15060).

Chen Kuo-Tzu. 1985. "Shiguan Yinger Dui Falü De Tiaozhan" [The legal challenge of test-tube babies]. *United Daily News*, 17 April: 3.

Chen Shu-Chi. 2020. *Shengming Keji De Qiji Taiwan Shiguan Yinger Fazhan Shi* [Miracle of biotechnology: The development of test-tube babies in Taiwan]. Taipei: uStory.

Chen Tzu-Hui, Hsu Kan-Lin, Wu Meng-Hsing, and Liu Chi-Hong. 2009. "Taiwan Diqu Ershiwu Dao Sishisisui Minzhong De Shengyu Zhishi Yu Taidu Diaocha" [The knowledge of and attitudes toward childbirth among the general public aged 25–44 in Taiwan]. *Taiwan Journal of Public Health* 28(1): 46–52.

Cheng, Tsung-Mei. 2015. "Reflections on the 20th Anniversary of Taiwan's Single Payer National Health Insurance System." *Health Affairs* 34(3): 502–10.

Cheng, Yen-hsin Alice, and Chen-Hao Hsu. 2020. "No More Babies without Help for Whom? Education, Division of Labor, and Fertility Intentions." *Journal of Marriage and Family* 82(4): 1270–85.

Cheng, Yen-hsin Alice, and Chih-lan Winnie Yang. 2021. "Continuity and Changes in Attitudes toward Marriage in Contemporary Taiwan." *Journal of Population Research* 38: 139–67.

Chien Yi-yi. 1999. "Yige Bu Suan Shao!" [One is not too few!]. *United Daily News*, 17 November: 34.

Chiu Chun-Chi. 2002. "Jiayou Si Bazhangxianzi Hongfu Wuweizachen" [Four palm fairies at home, Father Hong: Felt complicated]. *China Times Evening*, 31 January: 6.

Chiu Hei-yuan. 1999. "Taiwan Shehui Bianqian Jiben Diaocha Jihua 1991 Di Er Qi Di Er Ci Jiating Jiao yu Zu" [Taiwan social change survey (round 2, year 2): Family, education (C00003_1) [data file]]." Retrieved 31 July 2021 from Survey Research Data Archive, Academia Sinica. doi:10.6141/TW-SRDA-C00003_1-1.

Chiu Pi-Yu. 2004. "Geshe Yu Weihu Yunyu De Jingyan Licheng Duobaotai Yunfu Jieshou Jiantai Shoushu De Shenghuo Jingyan Yu Yinying Xingwei" [The process of forsaking and maintaining pregnancy-lived experience and coping behaviors of women with multifetal pregnancies and fetal reduction]. Master's thesis, National Taiwan University, Taipei.

Chou, Hung-Chieh, Po-Nien Tsao, Yu-Shih Yang, Jen-Ruey Tang, and Kuo-Inn Tsao. 2002. "Neonatal Outcome of Infants Born after In Vitro Fertilization at National Taiwan University Hospital." *Journal of Formosan Medical Association* 101(3): 203–5.

Chung, Karine, Mary D. Sammel, Christos Coutifaris, Raffi Chalian, Kathleen Llin, Arthur J. Castelbaum, Martin F. Freedman, and Kurt T. Barnhart. 2006. "Defining the Rise of Serum HCG in Viable Pregnancies Achieved through Use of IVF." *Human Reproduction* 21(3): 823–28.

Clarke, Adele E. 1988. *Discipling Reproduction: Modernity, American Life Sciences, and "the Problems of Sex."* Berkeley: University of California Press.

———. 2016. "Anticipation Work: Abduction, Simplification, Hope." In *Boundary Objects and Beyond: Working with Leigh Star*, edited by Geoffrey C. Bowker, Stefan Timmermans, Adele E. Clarke, and Ellen Balka, 85–119. Cambridge, MA: The MIT Press.

Clarke, Adele E., and Joan H. Fujimura, eds. 1992. *The Right Tool for the Job: At Work in Twentieth-Century Life Sciences.* Princeton, NJ: Princeton University Press.

Clarke, Adele E., Laura Mamo, Jennifer R. Fishman, and Janet K. Shim, eds. 2010. *Biomedicalization: Technoscience, Health, and Illness in the U.S.* Durham, NC: Duke University Press.

Coetsier, T., and M. Dhont. 1998. "Avoiding Multiple Pregnancies in In-Vitro Fertilization: Who's Afraid of Single Embryo Transfer?" *Human Reproduction* 13(10): 2663–70.

Cohen, Jean. 1991. "The Efficiency and Efficacy of IVF and GIFT." *Human Reproduction* 6(5): 613–18.

Cohen, Jean, M. J. Mayaux, and M. L. Guihard-Moscato. 1988. "Pregnancy Outcomes after In Vitro Fertilization: A Collaboration Study on 2,342 Pregnancies." *Annals of the New York Academy of Sciences* 541: 1–6.

Cohn, Victor. 1981. "First U.S. Test-Tube Baby Is Born." *Washington Post*, 29 December: 1.

Collopy, Kate Sullivan. 2002. "We Didn't Deserve This: Bereavement Associated with Multifetal Reduction." *Twin Research* 5(3): 231–35.

———. 2004. "'I Couldn't Think That Far': Infertile Women's Decision Making about Multifetal Reduction." *Research in Nursing and Health* 27: 75–86.

Conde-Agudelo, Agustin, Jose M. Belizan, and Gunilla Lindmark. 2000. "Maternal Morbidity and Mortality Associated with Multiple Gestations." *Obstetrics and Gynecology* 95(6): 899–904.

Conrad, Peter, and Miranda R. Waggoner. 2017. "Anticipatory Medicalization: Predisposition, Prediction, and the Expansion of Medicalized Conditions." In *Medical Ethics, Prediction, and Prognosis: Interdisciplinary Perspectives*, edited by M. Gadebusch-Bondio, F. Sporing, and J. S. Gordon, 95–103. London: Routledge.

Corea, Gena. 1985. *The Mother Machine: Reproductive Technologies from Artificial Insemination to Artificial Wombs*. New York: Harper & Row.

———. 1988. "What the King Can Not See." In *Embryos, Ethics, and Women's Rights: Exploring the New Reproductive Technologies*, edited by Elaine Hoffman Baruch, Amadeo F. D'Adamo Jr., and Joni Seager, 77–93. New York: The Haworth Press.

Cowan, Ruth Schwartz. 1993. "Aspects of the History of Prenatal Diagnosis." *Fetal Diagnosis and Therapy* 8, suppl. 1: 10–17.

Crowe, Chirstine. 1987. "Whose Mind over Whose Matter? Women, In Vitro Fertilisation and the Development of Scientific Knowledge." In *Made to Order: The Myth of Reproductive and Genetic Engineering Progress*, edited by Patricia Spallone and Deborah Lynn Steinberg, 27–57. London: Pergamon.

Crowther, Catherine, and Shanshan Han. 2010. "Hospitalisation and Bed Rest for Multiple Pregnancy." *Cochrane Database of Systematic Reviews*, issue 7, art. no. CD000110.

Dancet, E. A. F., T. M. D'Hooghe, C. Spiessens, W. Sermeues, D. De Neubourg, N. Karel, J. A. M. Fremer, and W. L. D. M. Nelen. 2013. "Quality Indicators for all Dimensions of Infertility Care Quality: Consensus between Professionals and Patients." *Human Reproduction* 28(6): 1584–79.

Davis, Owen K. 2004. "Elective Single-Embryo Transfer—Has Its Time Arrived?" *New England Journal of Medicine* 351: 2440–42.

Dean, Jishan H., and Elizabeth A. Sullivan. 2003. *Assisted Conception, Australia and New Zealand, 2000 and 2001*. Australian Institute of Health and Welfare, National Perinatal Statistics Unit.

De Geyter, Christian. 2018. "More than 8 Million Babies Born from IVF Since the World's First in 1978." Press release available at https://www.eshre.eu/Annual-Meeting/Barcelona-2018/ESHRE-2018-Press-releases/De-Geyter.

Dellatto, Marisa. 2021. "TikTokers Fight Texas Winter Storm to See Surprise Quadruplets." *New York Post*, February 23.

"Demographic Data GIS." 2021. Department of Household Registration, Ministry of the Interior, ROC. Retrieved 11 August 2021 from https://gis.ris.gov.tw/dashboard.html?key=D04.

De Neubourg, D., K. Bogaerts, C. Wyns, A. Albert, M. Camus, M. Candeur, M. Degueldre, A. Delbaere, A. Delvigne, P. De Sutter, M. Dhont, D. Dubois, Y. Englert, N. Gillain, S. Gordts, W. Hautecoeur, E. Lesaffre, B. Lejeune, F. Leroy, W. Ombelet, S. Perrier D'Hauterive, F. Vandekerckhove, J. Van der Elst, and T. D'Hooghe. 2013. "The History of Belgian Assisted Reproductive Technology Cycle Registration and Control: A Case Study in Reducing the Incidence of Multiple Pregnancy." *Human Reproduction* 28(10): 2709–19.

Dixon, Jennifer, and H. Gilbert Welch. 1991. "Priority Setting: Lessons from Oregon." *The Lancet* 337(8746): 891–94.

Dumez, Y., and J. F. Oury. 1986. "Method for First Trimester Selective Abortion in Multiple Pregnancy." *Obstetrical & Gynecological Survey* 42(6): 373–74.

Dyer, S., G. M. Chambers, J. de Mouzon, K. G. Nygren, F. Zegers-Hochschild, R. Mansour, O. Ishihara, M. Banker, and G. D. Adamson. 2016. "International Committee for Monitoring Assisted Reproductive Technologies [ICMART] World Report: Assisted Reproductive Technology 2008, 2009 and 2010." *Human Reproduction* 31(7): 1588–609.

Edwards, Robert G. 2001. "The Bumpy Road to Human In Vitro Fertilization." *Nature Medicine* 7(10): 1091–94. doi:10.1038/nm1001-1091.

Edwards, Robert G., B. D. Bavister, and Patrick C. Steptoe. 1969. "Early Stages of Fertilization In Vitro of Human Oocytes Matured In Vitro." *Nature* 221(5181): 632–35. doi:10.1038/221632a0.

Edwards, Robert G., and Patrick C. Steptoe. 1980. *A Matter of Life: The Story of a Medical Breakthrough.* New York: William Morrow and Company.

———. 1983. "Current Status of In-Vitro Fertilisation and Implantation of Human Embryos." *The Lancet* 322(8362): 1265–69. doi: https://doi.org/10.1016/SO140-6736(83)91148-0.

Edwards, Robert G., Patrick C. Steptoe, and J. M. Purdy. 1970. "Fertilization and Cleavage In Vitro of Preovulator Human Oocytes." *Nature* 227(5265): 1307–9. doi:10.1038/2271307a0.

———. 1980. "Establishing Full-Term Human Pregnancies Using Cleaving Embryos Grown In Vitro." *British Journal of Obstetrics and Gynaecology* 87(9): 737–56.

EIM for ESHRE (The European IVF-Monitoring Consortium, for the European Society of Human Reproduction and Embryology). 2016a. M. S. Kupka, T. D'Hooghe, A. P. Ferraretti, J. de Mouzon, K. Erb, J. A. Castilla, C. Calhaz-Jorge, C. De Geyter, and V. Goossens. "Assisted Reproductive Technology in Europe, 2011: Results Generated from European Registers by ESHRE." *Human Reproduction* 31(2): 233–48.

———. 2016b. C. Calhaz-Jorge, C. De Geyter, E. Mocanu, T. Motrenko, G. Scaravelli, C. Wyns, and V. Goossens. "Assisted Reproductive Technology in Europe, 2012: Results Generated from European Registers by ESHRE." *Human Reproduction* 31(8): 1638–52.

———. 2017. C. Calhaz-Jorge, C. De Geyter, M. S. Kupka, J. de Mouzon, K. Erb, T. Motrenko, G. Scaravelli, C. Wyns, and V. Goossens. "Assisted Reproductive Technology in Europe, 2013: Results Generated from European Registers by ESHRE." *Human Reproduction* 32(10): 1957–73.

———. 2018. Ch. De Geyter, C. Calhaz-Jorge, M. S. Kupka, C. Wyns, E. Mocanu, T. Motrenko, G. Scaravelli, J. Smeenk, S. Vidakovic, and V. Goossens. 2018. "Assisted Reproductive Technology in Europe, 2014: Results Generated from European Registers by ESHRE." *Human Reproduction* 33(9): 1586–601.

————. 2020a. "Assisted Reproductive Technology in Europe, 2015: Results Generated from European Registers by ESHRE." *Human Reproduction Open* 2020(3): doi.org/10.1093/hropen/hoaa038.

————. 2020b. C. Wyns, C. Bergh, C. Calhaz-Jorge, Ch. De Geyter, M. S. Kupka, T. Motrenko, I. Rugescu, J. Smeenk, A. Tandler-Schneider, S. Vidakovic, and V. Goossens. "Assisted Reproductive Technology in Europe, 2016. Results Generated from European Registers by ESHRE." *Human Reproduction Open* 2020(3): doi.org/10.1093/hropen/hoaa032.

ESHRE Campus Course Report. 2001. "Prevention of Twin Pregnancies after IVF/ICSI by Single Embryo Transfer." *Human Reproduction* 16(4): 790–800.

ESHRE Task Force on Ethics and Law. 2003. "Ethical Issues Related to Multiple Pregnancies in Medically Assisted Procreation." *Human Reproduction* 18: 1976–79.

Evans, M. I., S. Andriole, and D. W. Britt. 2014. "Fetal Reduction: 25 Years' Experience." *Fetal Diagnosis and Therapy* 35: 69–82.

Evans, Mark I., Doina Ciorica, and David W. Britt. 2004. "Do Reduced Multiples Do Better?" *Best Practice & Research Clinical Obstetrics and Gynaecology* 18(4): 601–12.

Evans, Mark I., Marc Dommergues, Ilan Timor-Tritsch, Ivan E. Zador, Ronald J. Wapner, Lauren Lynch, Yves Dumez, James D. Goldberg, Kypros H. Nicolaides, Mark Paul Johnson, Mitchell S. Golbus, Pierre Boulot, Alain J. Aknin, Ana Monteagudo, and Richard L. Berkowitz. 1994. "Transabdominal versus Transcervical and Transvaginal Multifetal Pregnancy Reduction: International Collaborative Experience of More than One Thousand Cases." 1994. *American Journal of Obstetrics and Gynecology* 170: 902–9.

Evans, Mark I., Marc Dommergues, Ronald J. Wapner, James D. Goldberg, Lauren Lynch, Ivan E. Zador, Robert J. Carpenter Jr., Ilan Timor-Tritsch, Bruno Brambati, Kypros H. Nicolaides, Yves Dumez, Anna Monteagudo, Mark P. Johnson, Mitchell S. Golbus, Lucia Tului, Shawn M. Polak, and Richard L. Berkowitz. 1996. "International, Collaborative Experience of 1,789 Patients Having Multifetal Pregnancy Reduction: A Plateauing of Risks and Outcomes." *Journal of the Society for Gynecologic Investigation* 3: 23–26.

Evans, Mark I., John C. Fletcher, Ivan E. Zador, Burritt W. Newton, Mary Helen Quigg, and Curtis D. Struyk. 1988. "Selective First-Trimester Termination in Octuplet and Quadruplet Pregnancies: Clinical and Ethical Issues." *Obstetrics and Gynecology* 71(3): 289–96.

Evers, Johannes L. H. 2002. "Female Subfertility." *The Lancet* 360: 151–59.

Ezard, John. 1969. "Limitations on Test Tube Babies." *The Guardian*, 15 February: 18.

Ezugwu, E. C., and S. Van der Burg. 2015. "Debating Elective Single Embryo Transfer after In Vitro Fertilization: A Plea for a Context-Sensitive Approach." *Annals of Medical and Health Sciences Research* 5(1): 1–7.

Federal Law Gazette. 1990. *The Embryo Protection Law*. Part I, No. 69. Issued in Bonn, Dec. 19, p. 2746.

Ferber, Sarah, Nicola J. Marks, and Vera Mackie. 2020. *IVF and Assisted Reproduction: A Global History*. Singapore: Palgrave MacMillan.

Ferraretti, A. P., V. Goossens, M. Kupka, S. Bhattacharya, J. de Mouzon, J. A. Castilla, K. Erb, V. Korsak, A. Nyboe Andersen, and the European IVF-Monitoring (EIM) Consortium, for the European Society of Human Reproduction and Embryology (ESHRE). 2013. "Assisted Reproductive Technology in Europe, 2009: Results Generated from European Registers by ESHRE." *Human Reproduction* 28(9): 2318–31.

Ferraretti, A. P., V. Goossens, J. de Mouzon, S. Bhattacharya, J. A. Castilla, V. Korsak, M. Kupka, K. G. Nygren, A. Nyboe Andersen, and the European IVF-Monitoring (EIM) Consortium, for the European Society of Human Reproduction and Embryology (ESHRE). 2012. "Assisted Reproductive Technology in Europe, 2008: Results Generated from European Registers by ESHRE." *Human Reproduction* 27(9): 2571–84.

FINRRAGE no kai. 2000. *New Report on Infertility: The Survey of Real Experiences of Infertility Treatment and Reproductive Technologies*. Tokyo: FINRRAGE no kai.

Fisher, Erik, Roop L. Mahajan, and Carl Mitcham. 2006. "Midstream Modulation of Technology: Governance from Within." *Bulletin of Science, Technology & Society* 26(6): 485–96.

Fiske, Emily, and Gareth Weston. 2014. "Utilization of ART in Single Women and Lesbian Couples since the 2010 Change in Victorian Legislation." *Australian and New Zealand Journal of Obstetrics and Gynaecology* 54: 497–99.

Fitzgerald, Oisín, Katie Harris, Repon C. Paul, and Georgina M. Chambers. 2017. *Assisted Reproductive Technology in Australia and New Zealand 2015*. Sydney, Australia: UNSW (University of New South Wales).

Fitzgerald, Oisín, Repon C. Paul, Katie Harris, and Georgina M. Chambers. 2018. *Assisted Reproductive Technology in Australia and New Zealand 2016*. Sydney, Australia: UNSW (University of New South Wales).

Franklin, Sarah. 1990. "Deconstructing 'Desperateness': The Social Construction of Infertility in Popular Representations of New Reproductive Technologies." In *The New Reproductive Technologies*, edited by Maureen McNeil, Ian Varcoe, and Steven Yearley, 200–229. New York: St. Martin's Press.

———. 1997. *Embodied Progress: A Cultural Account of Assisted Conception*. London: Routledge.

———. 2006. "Origin Stories Revisited: IVF as an Anthropological Project." *Culture, Medicine and Psychiatry* 30: 547–55.

Franklin, Sarah, and Marcia C. Inhorn. 2016. "Introduction." *Reproductive BioMedicine and Society Online* 2: 1–7.

Franklin, Sarah, and Maureen McNeil. 1988. "Reproductive Futures: Recent Literature and Current Feminist Debates on Reproductive Technologies." *Feminist Studies* 14(3): 545–60.

Fu, Jia-Chen. 2015. "Artemsinin and Chinese Medicine as *Tu* Science." *Endeavour* 41(3): 127–35.

Fu, Yang-Chih. 2017. "Taiwan Shehui Bianqian Jiben Diaocha Jihua 2016 Di Qi Qi Di Er Ci Jiating Zu" [2016 Taiwan social change Survey (round 7, year 2): Family (restricted access data) (R090056) [data file]]. Retrieved 15 December 2021 from Survey Research Data Archive, Academia Sinica. doi:10.6141/TW-SRDA-R090056-1.

Gammeltoft, Tine M., and Ayo Wahlberg. 2014. "Selective Reproductive Technologies." *Annual Review of Anthropology* 43: 201–16.

Garcia Jairo E., Georgeanna Seegar Jones, Anibal A. Acosta, and George Wright Jr. 1983. "Human Menopausal Gonadotropin/Human Chorionic Gonadotropin Follicular Maturation for Oocyte Aspiration: Phase I, 1981." *Fertility and Sterility* 39(2): 167–73.

Gatrell, Caroline. 2011. "Putting Pregnancy in Its Place: Conceiving Pregnancy as Carework in the Workplace." *Health & Place* 17(2): 395–402.

———. 2013. "Maternal Body Work: How Women Managers and Professionals Negotiate Pregnancy and New Motherhood at Work." *Human Relations* 66(5): 621–44.

Gerris, Jan, Diane De Neubourg, Kathelijne Mangelschots, Eric Van Royen, Muriel Van de Meerssche, and Marion Valkenburg. 1999. "Prevention of Twin Pregnancy after In-Vitro Fertilization or Intracytoplasmic Sperm Injection Based on Strict Embryo Criteria: A Prospective Randomized Clinical Trial." *Human Reproduction* 14(10): 2581–87.

Gerris, Jan, G. David Adamson, Petra De Sutter, and Catherine Racowsky. 2009. *Single Embryo Transfer*. Cambridge: Cambridge University Press.

Ginsburg, Faye D., and Rayna Rapp. 1995. *Conceiving the New World Order: The Global Politics of Reproduction*. Berkeley: University of California Press.

Glujovsky, Demian, Cindy Farquhar, Andrea Marta Quinteiro Retamar, Cristian Robert Alvarez Sedo, and Deborah Blake. 2016. "Cleavage Stage versus Blastocyst Stage Embryo Transfer in Assisted Reproductive Technology." *Cochrane Database of Systematic Reviews*, issue 6, art. no. CD002118.

Goodman, Lucy Kate, Lucy Rebecca Prentice, Rebecca Chanati, and Cynthia Farquhar. 2020. "Reporting Assisted Reproductive Technology Success Rates on Australia and New Zealand Fertility Clinic Websites." *Australian and New Zealand Journal of Obstetrics and Gynaecology* 60: 135–40.

Gordts, Sylvie. 2005. "Belgian Legislation and the Effect of Elective Single Embryo Transfer on IVF Outcome." *Reproductive BioMedicine Online* 10(4): 436–41.

Grady, Denise. 1988. "The Bitter Cost: Dangers of Multiple Births." *Time*, 2 May. Retrieved 21 June 2021 from http://content.time.com/time/subscriber/article/0,33009,967305,00.html.

Grady, Rosheen, Nika Alavi, Rachel Vale, Mohammad Khandwala, and Sarh D. McDonald. 2012. "Elective Single Embryo Transfer and Perinatal Outcomes: A Systematic Review and Meta-Analysis." *Fertility and Sterility* 97(2): 324–31.

Guston, David H. 2014. "Understanding 'Anticipatory Governance.'" *Social Studies of Science* 44(2): 218–42.

Hammond, Karen R. 1997. "Multifetal Pregnancy Reduction." *Journal of Obstetric, Gynecologic, and Neonatal Nursing (JOGNN)* 27: 338–43.

Harbottle, Stephen, Ciara Hughes, Rachel Cutting, Steven Roberts, and Daniel Brison. 2015. "Elective Single Embryo Transfer: An Update to UK Best Practice Guidelines." *Human Fertility* 18(3): 165–83.

Hardacre, Helen. 1997. *Marketing the Menacing Fetus in Japan.* Berkeley: University of California Press.

Harris, Katie, Oisín Fitzgerald, Repon C. Paul, Alan Macaldowie, Evelyn Lee, and Georgina M. Chambers. 2016. *Assisted Reproductive Technology in Australia and New Zealand 2014.* Sydney, Australia: UNSW (University of New South Wales).

Hazekamp, J., C. Bergh, W. B. Wennerholm, O. Hovatta, P. O. Karlstrom, and A. Selbing. 2000. "Avoiding Multiple Pregnancies in ART: Consideration of New Strategies." *Human Reproduction* 15(6): 1217–19.

Head, Jonathan. 2018. "'Baby Factory' Mystery: Thailand's Surrogacy Saga Reaches Uneasy End." *BBC News*, 26 February 2018. Retrieved 17 December 2021 from https://www.bbc.com/news/world-asia-43169974.

Henahan, John F. 1984. "Fertilization, Embryo Transfer Procedures Raise Many Questions." *Journal of the American Medical Association (JAMA)* 252(7): 877–79 and 882.

Herrero, Javier, and Marcos Mesequer. 2013. "Selection of High Potential Embryos Using Time-Lapse Imaging: The Era of Morphokinetics." *Fertility and Sterility* 99(4): 1030–34.

HFEA (Human Fertilisation and Embryology Authority). 2019. *Fertility Treatment 2017: Trends and Figures.* Retrieved 9 June 2021 from https://www.hfea.gov.uk/media/2894/fertility-treatment-2017-trends-and-figures-may-2019.pdf.

———. 2020. *Fertility Treatment 2018: Trends and Figures.* Retrieved 9 June 2021 from https://www.hfea.gov.uk/media/3158/fertility-treatment-2018-trends-and-figures.pdf.

Hilgartner, Stephen. 2015. "Capturing the Imaginary: Vanguards, Visions, and the Synthetic Biology Revolution." In *Science & Democracy: Making Knowledge and Making Power in Biosciences and Beyond*, edited by Stephen Hilgartner, Clark Miller, and Rob Hagendijk, 33-55. New York: Routledge.

Hodgetts, Katherine, Janet E. Hiller, Jackie M. Street, Drew Carter, Annette J. Braunack-Mayer, Amber M. Watt, John R. Moss, Adam G. Elshaug. 2014. "Disinvestment Policy and the Public Funding of Assisted Reproductive Technologies: Outcomes of Deliberative Engagements with Three Key Stakeholder Groups." *BMC Health Service Research* 14: 204. https://doi.org/10.1186/1472-6963-14-204.

Hodson, K., C. Meads, and S. Bewley. 2017. "Lesbian and Bisexual Women's Likelihood of Becoming Pregnant: A Systematic Review and Meta-Analysis." *BJOG: An International Journal of Obstetrics and Gynecology* 124(3): 393–402.

Hong, Shu-Hui. 1994. "Buyun Yali Funü Zuitong" [The pressure of infertility was most painful for women]. *United Daily News*, 17 December: 03.

Hsieh, Chen-En, Robert Kuo-Kuang Lee, Fang-Ju Sun, Ryh-Sheng Li, Shyr-Yeu Lin, Ming-Huei Lin, and Yuh-Ming Hwu. 2018. "Early Blastublation (EB) of Day 4 Embryo Is Predictive of Outcomes in Single Embryo Transfer (SET) Cycles." *Taiwanese Journal of Obstetrics and Gynecology* 57: 705–8.

Hsieh, Fon-Jou. 2014. "Tangshizheng Zhi Lu Sishi Nian" [A forty-year road to Down's syndrome]." *Jing-Fu Bulletin* 31(11): 58.

Hsieh, Yi-Lien. 1999. "Rengong Shouyun Xinfa Jianshao Duobaotai Changgeng Yiyuan Yi Nangpeiqi Peitai Zhirufa Ke Tigao Shouyunlu Chanfu Qijin Wei Sheng Xia Sanbaotai" [New method of assisted reproduction to lower multiple pregnancy: Chang Gung Hospital uses blastocyst transfer to increase conception rate and no triplets are delivered]. *United Evening News*, 26 May: 6.

Hsu, Chun-Pin. 2005. "Rengong Shou yun Yici Jing Zhi Jiupeitai Zhiliao Buyun Zou Pianfeng Guonei Yuban Zhiru Sange Yishang Peitai Duotai Shengyang Wenti Duo Yixuehui Yu Buzhu Bing Shexian" [Implanting nine embryos for assisted conception: Deviant practice for infertility treatment / Over half cycles implanted more than three embryos / Multiple birth and childcare causing much trouble / Medical society advocates subsidy and limitation]. *United Daily News*, 6 June: A5.

Hsu, Jinn-Yuh, and AnnaLee Saxenian. 2000. "The Limits of Guanxi Capitalism: Transnational Collaboration between Taiwan and the USA." *Environment and Planning* 32: 1991–2005.

Hsu, Ming-Hsin. "Shuang Duo Baotai Zaochan Yufang" [Prevention of preterm birth of twins and triplets]. Retrieved 8 October 2021 from https://mammy.hpa.gov.tw/Home/NewsKBContent?id=1387&type=01.

Hsueh, Kui-Wen. 1994. "Shatai Rengong Shouyun Biyai Zhi E" [Feticide: The necessary evil of assisted conception?]. *Ming-Sheng Daily*, 2 April: 21.

Hu, I-Jan, Chia-Jung Hsieh, Suh-Fang Jeng, Hui-Chen Wu, Chien-Yi Chen, Hung-Chieh Chou, Po-Nien Tsao, Shio-Jean Lin, Pau-Chung Chen, and Wu-Shiun Hsieh. 2015. "Nationwide Twin Birth Weight Percentiles by Gestational Age in Taiwan." *Pediatrics and Neonatology* 56: 294–300.

Huang, Yu-Ling, and Chia-Ling Wu. 2018. "New Feminist Biopolitics in Ultra-low-fertility East Asia." In *Making Kin Not Population: Reconceiving Generations*, edited by Adele Clarke and Donna Haraway, 125–44. Chicago: Prickly Paradigm Press.

Hung, Hsiao-Ying, Pei-Fang Su, Meng-Hsing Wu, and Ying-Ju Chang. 2021. "Status and Related Factors of Depression, Perceived Stress, and Distress of Women at Home Rest with Threatened Preterm Labor and Women with Healthy Pregnancy in Taiwan." *Journal of Affective Disorders* 280: 156–66.

Hung, Shu-Hui. 1995. "Rengong Shengzhi Bu Huai Ze Yi Yi Huai Jing Ren Duobaotai Yao Bu Yao Jiantai" [ART has its surprising outcome: Do we need fetal reduction for multiple pregnancy?]. *United Evening News*, 10 December: 12.

———. 2000. "Shiguaner Zaochan Duo Jiao Ganshou" [Test-tube babies have more premature births and lower birth weights]." *United Evening News*, 12 November: 4.

Hung, Yu-Chun. 2018. "Duobaotai Jiantai Chengjiu Shouzu De Jiankang [Fetal reduction of multiple births to keep the siblings' health]." *Mombaby*, 15 August 2018. https://www.mombaby.com.tw/articles/13526.

Hurst, Tara, and Paul Lancaster. 2001a. *Assisted Conception, Australia and New Zealand, 1998 and 1999*. Australian Institute of Health and Welfare, National Perinatal Statistics Unit.

———. 2001b. *Assisted Conception, Australia and New Zealand, 1999 and 2000*. Australian Institute of Health and Welfare, National Perinatal Statistics Unit.

Hurst, Tara, Esther Shafir, and Paul Lancaster. 1997. *Assisted Conception, Australia and New Zealand, 1996*. Australian Institute of Health and Welfare, National Perinatal Statistics Unit.

———. 1999. *Assisted Conception, Australia and New Zealand, 1997*. Australian Institute of Health and Welfare, National Perinatal Statistics Unit.

Hwang, J. L., H. S. Pan, L. W. Huang, C. Y. Lee, and Y. L. Tsai. 2002. "Comparison of the Outcomes of Primary Twin Pregnancies and Twin Pregnancies Following Fetal Reduction." *Archives of Gynecology and Obstetrics* 267: 60–63.

IFFS (International Federation of Fertility Societies). 2019. "International Federation of Fertility Societies Surveillance 2019: Global Trends in Reproductive Policy and Practice, 8th Edition." *Global Reproductive Health* 4: e29.

Imaizumi, Y. 2005. "Demographic Trends in Japan and Asia." In *Multiple Pregnancy: Epidemiology, Gestation & Perinatal Outcomes*, 2nd ed., edited by Isaac Blickstein and Louis G. Keith, 33–38. Abingdon: Informa.

Imaizumi, Yoko, Akio Asaka, and Eiji Inouye. 1980. "Analysis of Multiple Birth Rates in Japan II: Secular Trend and Effect of Birth Order, Maternal Age, and Gestational Age in Stillbirth Rate of Twins." *Acta Geneticae et Gemellologiae: Twin Research* 29(3): 223–31.

Inhorn, Marcia C. 2003. *Local Babies, Global Science: Gender, Religion, and In Vitro Fertilization in Egypt*. Routledge: New York.

———. 2006. "Making Muslim Babies: IVF and Gamete Donation in Sunni versus Shi'a Islam. *Culture, Medicine and Psychiatry* 30: 427–50.

———. 2020. "Where Has the Quest for Conception Taken Us? Lessons from Anthropology and Sociology." *Reproductive BioMedicine and Society Online* 10: 46–57.

———, ed. 2007. *Reproductive Disruptions: Gender, Technology, and Biopolitics in the New Millennium*. New York: Berghahn Books.

Inhorn, Marcia C., and Daphna Birenbaum-Carmeli. 2008. "Assisted Reproductive Technologies and Cultural Change." *Annual Review of Anthropology* 37: 177–96.

Inhorn, Marcia C., and Pasquale Patrizio. 2009. "Rethinking Reproductive 'Tourism' as Reproductive 'Exile.'" *Fertility and Sterility* 92(3): 904–6.

Irahara, Minoru. 2002. "Funin-chiryo Saizensen: Tatai-ninshin wo yobou suru tameni" [The Frontier of Infertility Treatment: Prevention of multiple pregnancy]. *Nihon sanfujinka gakkai zasshi (Acta Obstetrica et Gynaecologica Japonica)* 54(9): N281–N285.

Irahara, Minoru and Akira Kuwahara. 2003. "ART ni okeru tatai min-shin yobo no tame no kufu" [Prevention of Multiple Pregnancy in Assisted Reproduction]. *Nihon sanfujinka gakkai zasshi (Acta Obstetrica et Gynaecologica Japonica)* 55(8): 1103-12.

Irvin, Alan. 2008. "STS Perspectives on Scientific Governance." In *The Handbook of Science and Technology Studies*, edited by Edward J. Hackett, Olga Amsterdamska, Michael Lynch, and Judy Wajcman, 583–607. Cambridge, MA: The MIT Press.

Ishihara, Osamu, Seung Chik Jwa, Akira Kuwahara, Tomonori Ishikawa, Koji Kugu, Rintaro Sawa, Kouji Banno, Minoru Irahara, and Hidekazu Saito. 2018. "Assisted Reproductive Technology in Japan: A Summary Report for 2016 by the Ethics Committee of the Japan Society of Obstetrics and Gynecology." *Reproductive Medicine and Biology* 18(1): 7–16.

Ishihara, Osamu, Seung Chik Jwa, Akira Kuwahara, Yukiko Katagiri, Yoshimitsu Kuwabara, Toshio Hamatani, Miyuki Harada, and Tomohiko Ichikawa. 2019. "Assisted Reproductive Technology in Japan: A Summary Report for 2017 by the Ethics Committee of the Japan Society of Obstetrics and Gynecology." *Reproductive Medicine and Biology* 19(1): 3–12.

Ishihara, Osamu, Seung Chik Jwa, Akira Kuwahara, Yukiko Katagiri, Yoshimitsu Kuwabara, Toshio Hamatani, Miyuki Harada, and Yutaka Osuga. 2021. "Assisted Reproductive Technology in Japan: A Summary Report for 2018 by the Ethics Committee of the Japan Society of Obstetrics and Gynecology." *Reproductive Medicine and Biology* 20(1): 3–12.

ISLAT Working Group. 1998. "Art into Science: Regulation of Fertility Techniques" *Science* 281(5377): 651–52.

Itskovitz, Joseph, Rafi Boldes, Israel Thaler, Moshe Bronstein, Yohanan Erlik, and Joseph M. Brandes. 1989. "Transvaginal Ultrasonography-Guided Aspiration of Gestational Sacs for Selective Abortion in Multiple Pregnancy." *American Journal of Obstetrics and Gynecology* 160(1): 215–17.

Ivry, Tsipy. 2009. *Embodying Culture: Pregnancy in Japan and Israel.* New Brunswick, NJ: Rutgers University Press.

Iwaki, Akira, Momose Kazuo, Saito Shinichi, and Inshu Yoshitaka. 1979. "Taigai-jusei Ran-ishoku ni taisuru Funin Kanja no Ishiki-chosa" [A survey on awareness of patients in fertility treatments toward IVF-ET]. *Obstetrical and Gynecological Practices* 28(3): 273–78.

Iwaki, Akira, Tachibana Meika, and Ogura Hisao. 1983. "Taigai-jusei Ran-ishoku ni taisuru Funin Kanja no Ishiki-chosa: Dai 2 kai Chosa-seiseki [A survey on awareness of patients in fertility treatments toward IVF-ET: The second survey]. " *Obstetrical and Gynecological Practices* 32(4): 561–67.

IWGRAR (International Working Group for Registers on Assisted Reproduction). 2002. "World Collaborative Report on Assisted Reproductive Technology, 1998." In *Reproductive Medicine in the Twenty-First Century*, edited by D. L. Healy, G. T. Kovacs, R. McLachlan, and O. Rodriguez-Armas, 209–19. London: The Parthenon Publishing Group.

Jackson, Stevi, Jieyu Liu, and Juhyun Woo, eds. 2008. *East Asian Sexualities.* London: Zed Books.

Jain, Tarun, Bernard L. Harlow, and Mark D. Hornstein. 2002. "Insurance Coverage and Outcomes of In Vitro Fertilization." *New England Journal of Medicine* 347(9): 661–66.

Jarde, A., O. Lutsiv, C. K. Park, J. Barrett, J. Beyene, S. Saito, J. M. Dodd, P. S. Shah, J. L. Cook, A. B. Biringer, L. Giglia, Z. Han, K. Staub, W. Mundle, C. Vera, L. Sabatino, S. K. Liyanage, and S. D. McDonald. 2017. "Preterm Birth Prevention in Twin Pregnancies with Progesterone, Pessary, or Cerclage: A Systematic Review and Meta-Analysis." *BJOG: An International Journal of Obstetrics and Gynaecology* 124: 1163–73.

Jasanoff, Sheila. 2005. *Designs on Nature: Science and Democracy in Europe and the United States.* Princeton, NJ: Princeton University Press.

———. 2015. "Future Imperfect: Science, Technology and the Imaginations of Modernity." In *Dreamscapes of Modernity: Sociotechnical Imaginaries and the Fabrication of Power*, edited by Sheila Jasanoff and Sang-Hyun Kim, 1–33. Chicago: University of Chicago Press.

———. 2020. "Virtual, Visible, and Actionable: Data Assemblages and the Sightline of Justice." *Big Data and Society* (July–December): 1–15.

Jasanoff, Sheila, and Sang-Hyun Kim. 2009. "Containing the Atom: Sociotechnical Imaginaries and Nuclear Power in the United States and South Korea." *Minerva* 47: 119–46.

Jiang, Lijing. 2015. "IVF the Chinese Way: Zhang Lizhu and Post-Mao Human In Vitro Fertilization Resarch." *East Asian Science, Technology and Society: An International Journal* 9(1): 23–45.

Johnson, M. H. 1998. "Should the Use of Assisted Reproduction Techniques Be Deregulated? The UK Experience: Options for Change." *Human Reproduction* 13(7): 1769–76.

Johnson, Martin. 2019. "A Short History of *In Vitro* Fertilization (IVF)." *International Journal of Developmental Biology* 63: 83–92.

Johnston, Marie, Robert Shaw, and David Bird. 1987. "'Test-Tube Baby' Procedures: Stress and Judgements under Uncertainty." *Psychology and Health* 1: 25–38.

Jones, Howard W., and Jean Cohen. 1999. "International Federation of Fertility Societies International Conference. IFFS Surveillance 98." *Fertility and Sterility* 71(5), suppl. 2: S1–S34.

———. 2001. "International Federation of Fertility Societies International Conference: IFFS Surveillance 01." *Fertility and Sterility* 76(5), suppl. 2: S1–S36.

Jones, Howard W., et al. 1983. "What Is a Pregnancy? A Question for Programs of In Vitro Fertilization." *Fertility and Sterility* 40(6): 728–33.

Jones, Howard W., Jean Cohen, Ian Cooke, Roger Kempers, Keith Gordon, and Natalia van Houten. 2007. "International Federation of Fertility Societies Surveillance 07." *Fertility and Sterility* 87(4): S1–S67.

JSOG [Japan Society of Obstetrics and Gynecology] Science Committee. 1990. "Seishoku-igaku no Toroku ni kansuru Iinkai Houkoku" [Report on the registry of reproductive medicine]. *Nissanpu-shi (Acta Obstetrica et Gynaecologica Japonica)* 42: 393–97.

———. 2020. "Seishoku-igaku no Toroku ni kansuru Iinkai Houkoku" [Report on the registry of reproductive medicine]. *Nissanpu-shi (Acta Obstetrica et Gynaecologica Japonica)* 72(10): 1229–49.

Kahn, Susan Martha. 2000. *Reproducing Jews: A Cultural Account of Assisted Conception in Israel.* Durham, NC: Duke University Press.

Kamath, M. S., M. Mascarenhas, R. Kirubakaran, and S. Bhattacharya. 2020. "Number of Embryos for Transfer Following In Vitro Fertilisation or Intra-Cytoplasmic Sperm Injection." *Cochrane Database of Systematic Reviews,* issue 8. doi: 10.1002/14651858.CD003416.pub5.

Kanhai, H. H. H., E. J. C. van Rijssel, R. J. Meerman, and J. Bennebroek Gravenhorst. 1986. "Selective Termination in Quintuplet Pregnancy during First Trimester." *The Lancet* 327(8495): 1447.

Katz, Patricia, Robert Nachtigall, and Jonathan Showstack. 2002. "The Economic Impact of the Assisted Reproductive Technologies." *Nature Medicine* 8(10): S29–S32. doi:10.1038/nm-fertilityS29.

Ke, Yung-Hui. 2003. "Sanqianwubai Shiguan Baobao Taizhong Mianduimain" [3,500 test-tube babies gathered together in Taichung]." *United Daily News,* 20 October: A5.

Keane, Martin, Jean Long, Gerald O'Nolan, and Louise Faragher. 2017. *Assisted Reproductive Technologies: International Approaches to Public Funding Mechanisms and Criteria: An Evidence Review.* Dublin: Health Research Board.

Kelland, Jennifer, and Rosemary Ricciardelli. 2015. "Mothers of Multiple Perspectives on Fetal Reduction and Medical Abortion." *Journal of the Motherhood Initiative* 5(2): 123–40.

Kerenyi, Thomas D., and Usha Chitkara. 1981. "Selective Birth in Twin Pregnancy with Discordancy for Down's Syndrome." *New England Journal of Medicine* 304(25): 1525–27.

Kim, Ji-u. 2021. "Increased IVFs, Late Childbearing Lead to Twin-Birth Boom in Korea." *Korea Biomedical Review,* 28 March. Retrieved 17 December 2021 from https://www.koreabiomed.com/news/articleView.html?idxno=10792.

King, Leslie, and Madonna Harrington Meyer. 1997. "The Politics of Reproductive Benefits: US Insurance Coverage of Contraceptive and Infertility Treatments." *Gender and Society* 11(1): 8–30.

Kissin, D. M., A. D. Kulkarni, A. Mneimneh, L. Warner, S. L. Boulet, S. Crawford, and D. J. Jamieson. 2015. "Embryo Transfer Practices and Multiple Births Resulting from Assisted Reproductive Technology: An Opportunity for Prevention." *Fertility and Sterility* 103(4): 954–61.

Klein, Jeffrey, and Mark V. Sauer. 2001. "Assessing Fertility in Women of Advanced Reproductive Age." *American Journal of Obstetrics and Gynecology* 185(3): 758–70.

Ko, Tsang-Ming. 2021. "Duobaotai De Jiantai" [The fetal reduction of the multiple pregnancy]. Ko's Obstetrics & Gynecology Clinic website. Retrieved 30 August from http://www.genephile.com.tw/obs/content/06_02-Multifetal_Reduction.htm.

Ko, Tsang-Ming, Yu-Shih Yang, Fon-Jou Hsieh, Hong-Nerng Ho, Chi-Hong Liu, Li-Hui Tseng, Hsi-Yao Chen, and Tzu-Yao Lee. 1991. "Selective Reduction of Multiple Pregnancies in the First Trimester or Early Second Trimester." *Journal of Formosan Medical Association* 90: 493–97.

Koch, Lene. 1993. "Physiological and Psychosocial Risks of the New Reproductive Technologies." In *Touch Choices: In Vitro Fertilization and the Reproductive Technologies*, edited by Patricia Stephenson and Marsden G. Wagner, 122–34. Philadelphia, PA: Temple University Press.

Kolata, Gina. 1988. "Multiple Fetuses Raise New Issues Tied to Abortion." *New York Times*, 25 January: 1.

Kong, Travis S. K. 2019. "Transnational Queer Sociological Analysis of Sexual Identity and Civic-Political Activism in Hong Kong, Taiwan and Mainland China." *British Journal of Sociology* 70(5): 1904–25.

Krolokke, Charlotte. 2018. *Global Fluids: The Cultural Politics of Reproductive Waste and Value*. New York: Berghahn Books.

Kung, Fu-Tsai, Shiuh-Young Chang, Chun-Yuh Yang, Yi-Chi Lin, Kuo-Chung Lan, Yi-Ying Huang, and Fu-Jen Huang. 2003. "Transfer of Nonselected Transferable Day 3 Embryos in Low Embryo Producers." *Fertility and Sterility* 80(6): 1364–70.

Kupka, M. S., A. P. Ferraretti, J. de Mouzon, K. Erb, T. D'Hooghe, J. A. Castilla, C. Calhaz-Jorge, C. De Geyter, V. Goossens, and the European IVF-Monitoring (EIM) Consortium, for the European Society of Human Reproduction and Embryology (ESHRE). 2014. "Assisted Reproductive Technology in Europe, 2010: Results Generated from European Registers by ESHRE." *Human Reproduction* 29(10): 2099–113.

Laborie, Francoise. 1993. "Social Alternatives to Infertility." In *Touch Choices: In Vitro Fertilization and the Reproductive Technologies*, ed. Patricia Stephenson and Marsden G. Wagner, 37–50. Philadelphia, PA: Temple University Press.

Lachelin, Gillian C. L., H. A. Brant, G. I. M. Swyer, V. Little, and E. O. R. Reynolds. 1972. "Sextuplet Pregnancy." *British Medical Journal* 1: 787–90.

Lai, Chao-Hung. 1998. "Shen Huai Duobaotai Haizi Muti Dou Weixian" [Multiple pregnancy: Children and mothers are all in danger]. *United Daily News*, 15 February: 43.

———. 2002. "Shiguan Yinger Yu Duobaotai" [Test-tube baby and multiple birth]. *United Daily News*, 17 July: 36.

Lai, Ying-Ming. 2005. "Chuli Buyunzheng Zhiliao Bingfazheng Duobaotai Renshen Zhi Zhidao Gangling" [Draft on the guideline to manage the complications of multiple pregnancy]. *Taiwanese Society for Reproductive Medicine Newsletter*, March: 6–8.

Lancaster, Paul, Esther Shafir, and Jishan Huang. 1995. *Assisted Conception, Australia and New Zealand, 1992 and 1993*. Australian Institute of Health and Welfare, National Perinatal Statistics Unit.

Lancaster, Paul, Esther Shafir, Tara Hurst, and Jishan Huang. 1997. *Assisted Conception, Australia and New Zealand, 1994 and 1995.* Australian Institute of Health and Welfare, National Perinatal Statistics Unit.

Landy, H. J., and L. G. Keith. 2006. "The Vanishing Fetus." In *Multiple Pregnancy: Epidemiology, Gestation & Perinatal Outcomes*, 2nd ed., edited by Isaac Blickstein and Louis G. Keith, 108–18. Abington, England: Informa.

Lee, Evelyn, Peter Illingworth, Leeanda Wilton, and Georgina Mary Chambers. 2015. "The Clinical Effectiveness of Preimplantation Genetic Diagnosis for Aneuploidy in All 24 Chromosomes (PGD-A): Systematic Review." *Human Reproduction* 30(2): 473–83.

Lee, Jen-der. 2008. *Nüren De Zhongguo Yiliao Shi Han Tang Zhijian De Jiankang Zhaohu Yu Xingbie* [A women's history of medicine: Gender and health care in early Imperial China]. Taipei: Sanmin Publisher.

Lee, Tsung-Hsien, Chin-Der Chen, Yi-Yi Tsai, Li-Jung Chang, Nong-Nerng Ho, and Yu-Shih Yang. 2006. "Embryo Quality Is More Important for Younger Women whereas Age Is More Important for Older Women with Regard to In Vitro Fertilization Outcome and Multiple Pregnancy." *Fertility and Sterility* 86(1): 64–69.

Lee, Tzu-Yao. 1995. "Guonei Rengong Shengzhi Keji zhi Xiankuang" [The status quo of ART in Taiwan]. *The Taiwanese Law Review* 2: 6–8.

Lee Women's Hospital. 2021. "Gongxi Gongxi Buwei Yiqing Maosheng Yiyuan Kang Yi San Jiemei Chusheng Le" [Congratulations! Not afraid of the pandemic: 'Anti-pandemic triples' have been born]. Lee Women's Hospital website. Retrieved 8 December 2021 from https://www.ivftaiwan.tw/news/?4305.html.

Leese, Brenda, and Jane Denton. 2010. "Attitudes towards Single Embryo Transfer, Twin and Higher Order Pregnancies in Patients undergoing Infertility Treatment: A Review." *Human Fertility* 13(1): 28–34.

Leeton, John. 2004. "The Early History of IVF in Australia and Its Contribution to the World (1970–1990)." *Australian and New Zealand Journal of Obstetrics and Gynaecology* 44: 495–501.

Legislative Yuan Gazette. 2006. "Weiyuanhui Jilu [Committee Records]." *The Legislative Yuan Gazette* 95(33): 143–77.

Li, Ai-Fen. 2009. "Jiantai Shoushu Zhi Duo Shao" [How much do we know about fetal reduction?]. *Mombaby*, 31 July 2009. Retrieved 17 December 2021 from https://www.mombaby.com.tw/articles/1607.

Li, Ching-Lin. 2006. "Guotai Xinzhu Fenyuan Shiguan Baobao Hui Niangjia" [Test-tube babies went back to maternal home at Hsinchu Cathay Hospital]." *United Daily News*, 14 May: C2 Hsinchu edition.

Li, Shih-Cheng. 1982a. "Zhichi Shiguan Yinger" [Support researching test-tube babies]. *Min-Sheng Daily*, 10 October: 4.

———. 1982b. "Shiguan Yinger Daibiao Yiyao Jinbu" [Test-tube babies indicating medical advancement]. *Min-Sheng Daily*, 22 October: 4.

Li, You-Lin. 1997. "Yi Ji Pailuanzhen Shi Mei Luanzi Quan Zhongjiang Jiantai Hou Muqian Zhisheng Shuangbaotai" [One shot of egg stimulation, ten eggs all won the lottery, after fetal reduction, only twins left]." *Ming-Sheng Daily*, 31 August: 29.

Liggins, G. C., and H. K. Ibbertson. 1966. "A Successful Quintuplet Pregnancy Following Treatment with Human Pituitary Gonadotrophin." *The Lancet* 287(7429): 114–17.

Lin, Ching-Ching. 1986. "Sheng Haizi Weixian Guocheng Fuchanke Fengxian Zhiye Shuangsheng Shiguan Yinger Munu Canju Yijie Dazhong Zhide Jiqu Jiaoxun" [Dangerous delivering / Obstetrician is high risk occupation / Test-tube twin tragedy should learn the lesson from this]." *United Daily News*, 26 December: 3.

Lin, Pin-Yao, Chun-I Lee, En-Hui Cheng, Chung-Chia Huang, Tsung-Hsien Lee, Hui-Hsin Shih, Yi-Ping Pai, Yi-Chun Chen, and Maw-Sheng Lee. 2020. "Clinical Outcomes of Single Mosaic Embryo Transfer: High-Level or Low-Level Mosaic Embryo, Does It Matter?" *Journal of Clinical Medicine* 9: 1969. doi:10.3390/jcm9061695.

Liu, Hung-Ching, Georgeanna S. Jones, Howard W. Jones, and Zev Rosenwaks. 1988. "Mechanisms and Factors of Early Pregnancy Wastage in In Vitro Fertilization–Embryo Transfer Patients." *Fertility and Sterility* 50(1): 95–101.

Lopata, Alexander, Ian W. H. Johnston, Ian J. Hoult, and Andrew I. Speirs. 1980. "Pregnancy Following Intrauterine Implantation of an Embryo Obtained by In Vitro Fertilization of a Preovulatory Egg." *Fertility and Sterility* 33(2): 117–20.

Ludwig, M., B. Schopper, A. Katalinic, R. Sturm, S. Al-Hasani, and K. Diedrich. 2000. "Experience with the Elective Transfer of Two Embryos under the Conditions of the German Embryo Protection Law: Results of a Retrospective Data Analysis of 2573 Transfer Cycles." *Human Reproduction* 15(2): 319–24.

Lupton, Deborah, ed. 1999. *Risk and Sociocultural Theory: New Directions and Perspectives.* Cambridge: Cambridge University Press.

Macaldowie, Alan, Yueping A. Wang, Georgina M. Chambers, and Elizabeth A. Sullivan. 2012. *Assisted Reproductive Technology in Australia and New Zealand 2010.* Australian Institute of Health and Welfare.

———. 2013. *Assisted Reproductive Technology in Australia and New Zealand 2011.* Australian Institute of Health and Welfare.

Macaldowie, Alan, Yueping A. Wang, Abrar A. Chughtai, and Georgina M. Chambers. 2014. *Assisted Reproductive Technology in Australia and New Zealand 2012.* Australian Institute of Health and Welfare.

Macaldowie, Evelyn Lee, and Georgina M. Chambers. 2015. *Assisted Reproductive Technology in Australia and New Zealand 2013.* Australian Institute of Health and Welfare.

Macfarlane, A., and B. Blondel. 2005. "Demographic Trends in Western European Countries." In *Multiple Pregnancy: Epidemiology, Gestation and Perinatal Outcomes*, 2nd ed., edited by Isaac Blickstein and Louis G. Keith, 11–21. Abingdon: Informa.

Machin, Rosana. 2014. "Sharing Motherhood in Lesbian Reproductive Practices." *BioSocieties* 9(1): 42–59.

MacKinnon, Karen. 2006. "Living with the Threat of Preterm Labor: Women's Work of Keeping the Baby In." *Journal of Obstetric, Gynecologic, and Neonatal Nursing (JOGNN)* 35: 700–8.

Maeda, Eri. 2019. "How Can We Support Infertile Couples Without Health Insurance: A Public Health Perspective of ART in Japan." Paper presented at the 37th Annual Meeting of Japan Society of Fertilization and Implantation in Tokyo, Japan, August 1.

Maheshwari, Abha, Siriol Griffiths, and Siladitya Bhattacharya. 2011. "Global Variations in the Uptake of Single Embryo Transfer." *Human Reproduction Update* 17(1): 107–20.

Malik, Sonia, and Vinita Sherwal. 2012. "Multifetal Pregnancy Reduction." In *Manual of Assisted Reproductive Technologies and Clinical Embryology*, edited by Lt. Col. Pankaj Talwar, VSM, 125–31. New Delhi: Jaypee Brothers Medical Publishers Pvt. Ltd.

Marina, S., D. Marina, F. Marian, N. Fosas, N. Galiana, and I. Jove. 2010. "Sharing Motherhood: Biological Lesbian Co-others, a New IVF Indication." *Human Reproduction* 25(4): 938–41.

Markens, Susan, C. H. Browner, and Nancy Press. 1999. "'Because of the Risks': How US Pregnant Women Account for Refusing Prenatal Screening." *Social Science and Medicine* 49: 359–69.

Martin, Lauren Jade. 2010. "Anticipating Infertility: Egg Freezing, Genetic Preservation, and Risk." *Gender and Society* 24(4): 526–45.

———. 2017. "Pushing for the Perfect Time: Social and Biological Fertility." *Women's Studies International Forum* 62: 91–98.

———. 2020. "Delaying, Debating and Declining Motherhood." *Culture, Health and Sexuality* 23(8): 1034–49.

Martin, Paul, Nik Brown, and Andrew Turner. 2008. "Capitalizing Hope: The Commercial Development of Umbilical Cord Blood Stem Cell Banking." *New Genetics and Society* 27(2): 127–43.

McCall, Christina A., David A. Grimes, and Anne Drapkin Lyerly. 2013. "'Therapeutic' Bed Rest in Pregnancy: Unethical and Unsupported by Data." *Obstetrics & Gynecology* 121(6): 1305–8.

McKibben, Bill. 2007. *Fight Global Warming Now: The Handbook for Taking Action in Your Community*. New York: St. Martin's Griffin.

Medical Research International and the American Fertility Social Interest Group. 1988. "In Vitro Fertilization/Embryo Transfer in the United States: 1985 and 1986 Results from the National IVF/ET Registry." *Fertility and Sterility* 49(2): 212–15.

Medical Research International and the Society for Assisted Reproductive Technology [SART] of the American Fertility Society. 1989. "In Vitro Fertilization/Embryo Transfer in the United States: 1987 Results from the National VIF-ET Registry." *Fertility and Sterility* 51: 14–19.

Medley, N., J. P. Vogel, A. Care, and Z. Alfirevic. 2018. "Interventions during Pregnancy to Prevent Preterm Birth: An Overview of Cochrane Systematic Reviews." *Cochrane Database of Systematic Reviews* 11. Art. No.: CD012505.

Meyers, Diana Tietjens. 2001. "The Rush to Motherhood: Pronatalist Discourse and Women's Autonomy." *Signs: Journal of Women in Culture and Society* 26(3): 735–73.

Min, Jason K., Sue A. Breheny, Vivien MacLachlan, and David L. Healy. 2004. "What Is the Most Relevant Standard of Success in Assisted

Reproduction? The Singleton, Term Gestation, Live Birth Rate per Cycle Initiated: The BESST [Birth Emphasizing a Successful Singleton at Term] Endpoint for Assisted Reproduction." *Human Reproduction* 19(1): 3.

Mladovsky, Philipa, and Corinna Sorenson. 2010. "Public Financing of IVF: A Review of Policy Rationales." *Health Care Analysis* 18(2): 113–28.

Mol, Annemarie, and John Law. 2004. "Embodied Action, Enacted Bodies: The Example of Hypoglycaemia." *Body & Society* 10(2–3): 43–62.

Monden, Christiaan, Gilles Pison, and Jeroen Smits. 2021. "Twin Peaks: More Twinning in Humans than Ever Before." *Human Reproduction* 36(6): 1666–73.

Moore, Lisa Jean. 2007. *Sperm Counts: Overcome by Man's Most Precious Fluid.* New York: New York University Press.

Moreira, Riago, and Paolo Palladino. 2005. "Between Truth and Hope: On Parkinson's Disease, Neurotransplantation and the Production of the 'Self.'" *History of the Human Sciences* 18: 55–82.

Morgan, Lynn M., and Elizabeth F. S. Roberts. 2012. "Reproductive Governance in Latin America." *Anthropology & Medicine* 19(2): 241–54.

Mori, Takahide. 2010. *Seishoku, Hassei no Igaku to Rinri: Taigai-jusei no Genryu kara iPS Jidai e* [Reproduction, regenerative medicine, and ethics: From the origin of IVF to the era of iPS]. Kyoto: Kyoto University Press.

Mottier, Veronique. 2013. "Reproductive Rights." In *The Oxford Handbook of Gender and Politics*, edited by Georgina Waylen, Karen Celis, Johanna Kantola, and S. Laurel Weldon, 214–35. Oxford: Oxford University Press.

Mouzon, J. de, V. Goossens, S. Bhattacharya, J. A. Castilla, A. P. Ferraretti, V. Korsak, M. Kupka, K. G. Nygren, A. Nyboe Andersen, and the European IVF-Monitoring (EIM) Consortium, for the European Society of Human Reproduction and Embryology (ESHRE). 2010. "Assisted Reproductive Technology in Europe, 2006: Results Generated from European Registers by ESHRE." *Human Reproduction* 25(8): 1851–62.

———. 2012. "Assisted Reproductive Technology in Europe, 2007: Results Generated from European Registers by ESHRE." *Human Reproduction* 27(4): 954–66.

Mugford, Miranda. 1990. "The Cost of a Multiple Birth." In *Three, Four and More: A Study of Triplet and Higher Order Births*, edited by Beverley J. Botting, Alison J. Macfarlane, and Frances V. Price, 205–17. London: HMSO (Her Majesty's Stationery Office).

Mulkay, Michael. 1997. *The Embryo Research Debate: Science and the Politics of Reproduction.* Cambridge: Cambridge University Press.

Munne, Santiago, James Grifo, and Dagan Wells. 2016. "Mosaicism: 'Survival of the Fittest' versus 'No Embryo Left Behind.'" *Fertility and Sterility* 105(5): 1146–49.

Munne, Santiago, Brian Kaplan, John L. Frattarelli, Tim Child, Gary Nakhuda, F. Nicholas Shamma, Kaylen Silverberg, Tasha Kalista, Alan H. Handyside, Mandy Katz-Jaffe, Dagan Wells, Tony Gordon, Sharyn Stock-Myer, and Susan Willman. 2019. "Preimplantation Genetic Testing for

Aneuploidy versus Morphology as Selection Criteria for Single Frozen-Thawed Embryo Transfer in Good-Prognosis Patients: A Multicenter Randomized Clinical Trial." *Fertility and Sterility* 112(6): 1071–79.

Murdoch, Alison P. 1998. "How Many Embryos Should Be Transferred?" *Human Reproduction* 13(10): 2666–70.

Myers, Kit C., and Lauren Jade Martin. 2021. "Freezing Time? The Sociology of Egg Freezing." *Sociology Compass* 15(4). https://doi.org/10.1111/soc4.12850.

Nazem, Taraneh Gharib, Sydney Chang, Joseph A. Lee, Chirstine Briton-Jones, Alan B. Copperman, and Beth McAvey. 2019. "Understanding the Reproductive Experience and Pregnancy Outcomes of Lesbian Women Undergoing Donor Intrauterine Insemination." *LGBT Health* 6(2): 62–67.

Neiterman, Elena, and Bonnie Fox. 2017. "Controlling the Unruly Maternal Body: Losing and Gaining Control over the Body during Pregnancy and the Postpartum Period." *Social Science and Medicine* 174: 142–48.

Netsu, Yahiro. 1998. *Gentai shujutsu no jissai: Sono toikakeru mono; Funin chiryō no fukusanbutsu* [The actual conditions of multifetal pregnancy reduction: The byproduct of infertility treatment; Things it questions]. Tokyo: Kindai bungei-sha.

———. 2015. *Tatai ichibu kyūtai shujutsu: gensū gentai shujutsu* [Multifetal pregnancy reduction]. Nagano: Karamatsushobō.

Neumann, Peter J. 1997. "Should Health Insurance Cover IVF? Issues and Options." *Journal of Health Politics, Policy and Law* 22(5): 1215–39.

Neumann, Peter J., S. D. Gharib, and M. C. Weinstein. 1994. "The Cost of a Successful Delivery with In Vitro Fertilization." *New England Journal of Medicine* 331(4): 239–43.

Newman, J. E., Oisín Fitzgerald, Repon C. Paul, and G. M. Chambers. 2019. *Assisted Reproductive Technology in Australia and New Zealand 2017*. Sydney: UNSW (University of New South Wales).

Newman, J. E., R. C. Paul, and G. M. Chambers. 2020. *Assisted Reproductive Technology in Australia and New Zealand 2018*. Sydney: National Perinatal Epidemiology and Statistics Unit, the University of New South Wales.

Newman, R. B. 2005. "Routine Antepartum Care of Twins." In *Multiple Pregnancy: Epidemiology, Gestation and Perinatal Outcomes*, 2nd ed., edited by Isaac Blickstein and Louis G. Keith, 405–19. Abingdon: Informa.

Ng, Franklin. 1998. *The Taiwanese Americans*. Westport, CT: Greenwood Press.

Noah, Lars. 2003. "Assisted Reproductive Technologies and the Pitfalls of Unregulated Biomedical Innovation." *Florida Law Review* 55(2): 603–66.

Nunez, Anna, Desiree Garcia, Pepita Gimenez-Bonafe, Rita Vassena, and Amelia Rodriguez. 2021. "Reproductive Outcomes in Lesbian Couples Undergoing Reception of Oocytes from Partner versus Autologous In Vitro Fertilization/Intracytoplasmic Sperm Injection." *LGBT Health* 8(5): 367–71.

Nyboe Andersen, A., L. Gianaroli, R. Felberbaum, J. de Mouzon, and K. G. Nygren. The European IVF-Monitoring Programme (EIM) for the European Society of Human Reproduction and Embryology (ESHRE).

2005. "Assisted Reproductive Technology in Europe, 2001: Results Generated from European Registries by ESHRE." *Human Reproduction* 20(5): 1158–76.

———. 2006. "Assisted Reproductive Technology in Europe, 2002: Results Generated from European Registers by ESHRE." *Human Reproduction* 21(7): 1680–97.

Nyboe Andersen, A., L. Gianaroli, and K. G. Nygren. The European IVF-Monitoring Programme (EIM) for the European Society of Human Reproduction and Embryology (ESHRE). 2004. "Assisted Reproductive Technology in Europe, 2000: Results Generated from European Registers by ESHRE." *Human Reproduction* 19(3): 490–503.

Nyboe Andersen, A., V. Goossens, S. Bhattacharya, A. P. Ferraretti, M. S. Kupka, J. de Mouzon, K. G. Nygren, and the European IVF-Monitoring (EIM) Consortium, for the European Society of Human Reproduction and Embryology (ESHRE). 2009. "Assisted Reproductive Technology and Intrauterine inseminations in Europe, 2005: Results Generated from European Registers by ESHRE." *Human Reproduction* 24(6): 1267–87.

Nyboe Andersen, A., V. Goossens, A. P. Ferraretti, S. Bhattacharya, R. Felberbaum, J. de Mouzon, K. G. Nygren, and the European IVF-Monitoring (EIM) Consortium, for the European Society of Human Reproduction and Embryology (ESHRE). 2008. "Assisted Reproductive Technology in Europe, 2004: Results Generated from European Registers by ESHRE." *Human Reproduction* 23(4): 756–71.

Nyboe Andersen, A., V. Goossens, L. Gianaroli, R. Felberbaum, J. de Mouzon, and K. G. Nygren. 2007. "Assisted Reproductive Technology in Europe, 2003: Results Generated from European Registers by ESHRE." *Human Reproduction* 22(6): 1513–25.

Nygren, K. G., and A. Nyboe Andersen. 2001. "Assisted Reproductive Technology in Europe, 1997: Results Generated from European Registers by ESHRE; European IVF-Monitoring Programme (EIM) for the European Society of Human Reproduction and Embryology (ESHRE)." *Human Reproduction* 16(2): 384–97.

Nygren, K. G., A. Nyboe Andersen, and European IVF-Monitoring Programme (EIM). 2001. "Assisted Reproductive Technology in Europe, 1998: Results Generated from European Registers by ESHRE; European Society of Human Reproduction and Embryology (ESHRE)." *Human Reproduction* 16(11): 2459–71.

———. 2002. "Assisted Reproductive Technology in Europe, 1999: Results Generated from European Registers by ESHRE." *Human Reproduction* 17(12): 3260–74.

Ombelet, Willem. 2016. "The Twin Epidemic in Infertility Care—Why Do We Persist in Transferring Too Many Embryos?" *Facts, Views and Vision in Obstetrics and Gynecology* 8(4): 189–91.

Ombelet, Willem, et al. 2005. "Multiple Gestation and Infertility Treatment: Registration, Reflection and Reaction—the Belgian Project." *Human Reproduction Update* 11(1): 3–14.

Overall, Christine. 1990. "Selective Termination of Pregnancy and Women's Reproductive Autonomy." *The Hastings Center Report* 20(3): 6–11.

Ozturk, O., and A. Templeton. 2002. "In-Vitro Fertilisation and Risk of Multiple Pregnancy." *The Lancet* 359(9302): 232.

Pandian, Zabeena, Allan Templeton, Gamal Serour, and Siladitya Bhattacharya. 2005. "Number of Embryo for Transfer after IVF and ICSI: A Cochrane Review." *Human Reproduction* 20(10): 2681–87.

Peeraer, Karen, et al. 2017. "A 50 percent Reduction in Multiple Live Birth Rate Is Associated with a 13 percent Cost Saving: A Real-Life Retrospective Cost Analysis." *Reproductive Biomedicine Online* 35(3): 279–86.

Pennings, Guido. 2000. "Avoiding Multiple Pregnancies in ART: Multiple Pregnancies; A Test Case for Moral Quality of Medically Assisted Reproduction." *Human Reproduction* 15(12): 2466–69.

———. 2009. "International Evolution of Legislation and Guidelines in Medically Assisted Reproduction." *Reproductive BioMedicine Online* 19, suppl. 2: 15–18.

———. 2016. "Having a Child Together in Lesbian Families: Combining Gestation and Genetics." *Journal of Medical Ethics* 42(4): 253–55.

Perrotta, Manuela, and Alina Geampana. 2021. "Enacting Evidence-Based Medicine in Fertility Care: Tensions between Commercialisation and Knowledge Standardization." *Sociology of Health & Illness* 43: 2015–30.

Petersen, Alan, and Ivan Krisjansen. 2015. "Assembling 'Bioeconomy': Exploiting the Power of the Promissory Life Science." *Journal of Sociology* 51(1): 28-46.

Pinchuk, Stacey. 2000. "A Difficult Choice in a Different Voice: Multiple Births, Selective Reduction and Abortion." *Duke Journal of Gender Law and Policy* 7 (Spring): 29–56.

Pharoah, P. O. D. 2005. "Cerebral Palsy and Multiple Births." In *Multiple Pregnancy: Epidemiology, Gestation & Perinatal Outcomes*, 2nd ed., edited by Isaac Blickstein and Louis G. Keith, 807–16. Abingdon: Informa.

"Population Projection Inquiry System." 2021. *National Development Council, R.O.C.* Retrieved 11 August 2021 from https://pop-proj.ndc.gov.tw/dataSearch2.aspx?r=2&uid=2104&pid=59.

Practice Committee and Genetic Counseling Professional Group [GCPG] of ASRM. 2020. "Clinical Management of Mosaic Results from Preimplantation Genetic Testing for Aneuploidy (PGT-A) of Blastocysts: A Committee Opinion." *Fertility and Sterility* 114(2): 246–54.

Practice Committee of ASRM [American Society for Reproductive Medicine] and the Practice Committee of SART [Society for Assisted Reproductive Technology]. 2013. "Criteria for Number of Embryos to Transfer: A Committee Opinion." *Fertility and Sterility* 99(1): 44–46.

———. 2017. "Guidance on the Limit to the Number of Embryos to Transfer: A Committee Opinion." *Fertility and Sterility* 107(4): 901–3.

———. 2018. "The Use of Preimplantation Genetic Testing for Aneuploidy (PGT-AP): A Committee Opinion." *Fertility and Sterility* 109(3): 429–36.

Practice Committee of SART [Society for Assisted Reproductive Technology] and Practice Committee of ASRM [American Society for Reproductive Medicine]. 2004. "Guidelines on the Number of Embryos Transferred." *Fertility and Sterility* 82(3): 773–74.

———. 2018. "Elective Single-Embryo Transfer" *Fertility and Sterility* 97(4): 835-42.

Prainsack, Barbara, and Alena Buyx. 2012. "Solidarity in Contemporary Bioethics—Towards a New Approach." *Bioethics* 26(7): 343–50.

Price, Frances V. 1988. "The Risk of High Multiparity with IVF/ET." *Birth* 15(3): 157–63.

———. 1990. "The Management of Uncertainty in Obstetric Practice: Ultrasonography; *In Vitro* Fertilisation and Embryo Transfer." In *The New Reproductive Technologies*, edited by Maureen McNeil, Ian Varcoe, and Steven Yearley, 123–53. New York: St. Martin's Press.

Rajah, Shantal. 2009. "Elective Single Embryo Transfer (eSET) Policy Implementation to All UK IVF Centers from 2009: Reality or Myth?" 26 January. *BioNews* 492. Retrieved 10 March 2021 from https://www.bionews.org.uk/page_91673.

Raymo, James, Hyunjoon Park, Yu Xie, and Wei-jun Jean Yeung. 2015. "Marriages and Family in East Asia: Continuity and Change." *Annual Review of Sociology* 41: 471–92.

Raymond, Janice G. 1993. *Women as Wombs: Reproductive Technologies and the Battle over Women's Freedom.* San Francisco: HarperCollins.

Redwine, F. O., and R. E. Petres. 1984. "Selective Birth in a Case of Twins Discordant for Tay Sachs Disease." *Acta Genet Med Gemellol* 33: 35–38.

Relier, Jean-Pierre, Michele Couchard, and Catherine Huon. 1993. "The Neonatologist's Experience of In Vitro Fertilization Risks." In *Touch Choices: In Vitro Fertilization and the Reproductive Technologies*, edited by Patricia Stephenson and Marsden G. Wagner, 135–43. Philadelphia: Temple University Press.

Reproductive Technology Accreditation Committee. 2017. "Public Information, Communication and Advertising Australian Clinics." Technical Bulletin 7.

Reynolds, M., L. A. Schieve, G. Jeng, and H. B. Peterson. 2003. "Does Insurance Coverage Decrease the Risk for Multiple Births Associated with Assisted Reproductive Technology?" *Fertility and Sterility* 80(1): 16–23.

ROC Department of Health. 2003. *Taiwan Diqu Minguo Bashiqi Nian Zhi Jiushi Nian Rengong Xiezhu Shengzhi Jishu Shixing Jieguo Fenxi* [Annual report of practices of Assisted Reproductive Technology in Taiwan, 1998–2001]. Taipei: ROC Department of Health.

———. 2005a. *Minguo Jiushiyi Nian Taiwan Diqu Rengong Xiezhu Shengzhi Shixing Jieguo Baogao* [Annual Report of Practices of Assisted Reproductive Technology in Taiwan, 2002]. Taipei: ROC Department of Health.

———. 2005b. *Minguo Jiushier Nian Taiwan Diqu Rengong Xiezhu Shengzhi Shixing Jieguo Baogao* [Annual Report of Practices of Assisted Reproductive Technology in Taiwan, 2003]. Taipei: ROC Department of Health.

———. 2009. *Minguo Jiushiliu Nian Taiwan Diqu Rengong Shengzhi Shixing Jieguo Fenxi Baogao* [Annual Report of Practices of Assisted Reproductive Technology in Taiwan, 2007]. Taipei: ROC Department of Health.

ROC Ministry of Health and Welfare. 2020. *Yilinqi Nian Rengong Shengzhi Shixing Jieguo Fenxi Baogao* [The assisted reproductive technology summary 2018 national report of Taiwan]. Taipei: ROC Ministry of Health and Welfare.

———. 2021a. *Yilinjiu Nian Rengong Shengzhi Shixing Jieguo Fenxi Baogao* [The assisted reproductive technology summary 2019 national report of Taiwan]. Taipei: ROC Ministry of Health and Welfare.

———. 2021b. *Yilinba Nian Chusheng Tongbao Tongji Nianbao* [2019 statistics of the birth reporting system]. Taipei: ROC Ministry of Health and Welfare.

Rosenwaks, Zev, Hung Ching Liu, Howard W. Jones, Linda Tseng, and Martin L. Stone. 1981. "In Vitro Inhibition of Endometrial Cancer Growth by a Neonatal Rat Testicular Secretory Product." *Journal of Clinical Endocrinology and Metabolism* 52(4): 817–19.

Rothman, Barbara Katz. 1989. *Recreating Motherhood: Ideology and Technology in a Patriarchal Society.* New York: W. W. Norton & Company.

Sackett, David L., William M. C. Rosenberg, J. A. Muir Gray, R. Brian Haynes, W. Scott Richardson. 1996. "Evidence Based Medicine: What It Is and What It Isn't." *British Medical Journal* 312: 71.

Saito, Hidekazu, Seung Chik Jwa, Akira Kuwahara, Kazuki Saito, Tomonori Ishikawa, Osamu Ishihara, Koji Kugu, Rintaro Sawa, Kouji Banno, and Minoru Irahara. 2017. "Assisted Reproductive Technology in Japan: A Summary Report for 2015 by the Ethics Committee of the Japan Society of Obstetrics and Gynecology." *Reproductive Medicine and Biology* 17(1): 20–8.

Saldeen, Pia, and Per Sundstrom. 2005. "Would Legislation Imposing Single Embryo Transfer Be a Feasible Way to Reduce the Rate of Multiple Pregnancy after IVF Treatment?" *Human Reproduction* 20(1): 4–8.

Sandall, J., H. Soltani, S. Gates, A. Shennan, and D. Devane. 2016. "Midwife-Led Continuity Models versus Other Models of Care for Childbearing Women." *Cochrane Database of Systematic Review* 4. doi: 10.1002/14651858. CD006178.pub2.

Schenker, Joseph G. 1993. "Medically Assisted Conception: The State of the Art in Clinical Practice." In *Tough Choices: In Vitro Fertilization and the Reproductive Technologies,* edited by Patricia Stephenson and Marsden G. Wagner, 25–36. Philadelphia, PA: Temple University Press.

Schenker, Joseph G., and Yossef Ezra. 1994. "Complications of Assisted Reproductive Techniques." *Fertility and Sterility* 61(3): 411–22.

Schenker, Joseph G., Shaul Yarkoni, and Menachem Granat. 1981. "Multiple Pregnancies Following Induction of Ovulation." *Fertility and Sterility* 35(2): 105–23.

Seeber, Beata E. 2012. "What Serial hCG Can Tell You, and Cannot Tell You, about an Early Pregnancy." *Fertility and Sterility* 98(5): 1074–77.

Semba, Yukari. 2005. "Tokutei Funin-chiryōhi Josei-Jigyō no Genjyō to kadai" [The current situation and issues of subsidy programs for infertility treatment]. *F-GENS Journal* 4: 85–92.

Senat, Marie-Victoire, Pierre-Yves Ancel, Marie-Helene Bouvier-Colle, and Gerard Breart. 1998. "How Does Multiple Pregnancy Affect Maternal Mortality and Morbidity?" *Clinical Obstetrics and Gynecology* 41(1): 79–83.

Seppala, Markku. 1985. "The World Collaborative Report on In Vitro Fertilization and Embryo Replacement: Current State of the Art in January 1984." *Annals of the New York Academy of Sciences* 442(1): 558–63. https://nyaspubs.onlinelibrary.wiley.com/toc/17496632/1985/442/1.

"Seventh Septuplet Dies." 1987. *Associated Press News*, 1 September. Retrieved 18 June 2021 from https://apnews.com/article/ab2b8fb38562 e3badaa3e5f0f496de28.

Shalev, Josef, Yair Frenkel, Mordechai Goldenberg, Eliezer Shalev, Shlomo Lipitz, Gad Barkai, Laslo Nebel, and Shlomo Mashiach. 1989. "Selective Reduction in Multiple Gestations: Pregnancy Outcome after Transvaginal and Transabdominal Needle-Guided Procedures." *Fertility and Sterility* 52(3): 416–20.

Shih, Ching-Ju. 2006. "Guoren Shengyu Taidu Diaocha Sanshiersui Xianghun Sanshiwusui Xiangsheng" [Survey on reproductive behaviors: Prefer to marry at 32, and birth at 35]. *United Daily News*, 27 August: A6.

Shih, L.-W. 2018. "Moral Bearing: The Paradox of Choice, Anxiety and Responsibility in Taiwan." In *Selective Reproduction in the 21st Century*, ed. A. Wahlberg and T. Gammeltoft, 97–122. Cham: Palgrave Macmillan.

Shih, Yen-Fei. 1998. "Duobaotai Zaochan Jilü Gao" [Higher chance of preterm babies for multiple pregnancy]. *China Times*, 28 May: 18.

Sobotka, Tomáš. 2010. "Shifting Parenthood to Advanced Reproductive Ages: Trends, Causes and Consequences." In *A Young Generation under Pressure: The Financial Situation and the "Rush Hour" of the Cohorts 1970–1985 in a Generational Comparison*, edited by Joerg Chet Tremmel, 129–54. Heidelberg: Springer.

Soong, Yung-Kuei. 1988. "Yu Yu Xiongzhang Liangzhe De Jian Da Yige Kunhuo De Muqin" [Have both fish and bear's paw: Answering "the confused mother"]. *Min-Sheng Daily*, 23 February: 14.

Sosa, Claudio G., Fernando Althabe, Jose M. Belizan, and Eduardo Bergel. 2015. "Bed Rest in Singleton Pregnancies for Preventive Preterm Birth." *Cochrane Database of Systematic Review* issue 3, art. no.: CD003581.

Speirs, A., A. Lopata, M. J. Gronow, G. N. Kellow, and W. I. H. Johnston. 1983. "Analysis of the Benefits and Risks of Multiple Embryo Transfer." *Fertility and Sterility* 39(4): 468–71.

Stanley, Fiona J., and Sandra M. Webb. 1993. "The Effectiveness of In Vitro Fertilization: An Epidemiological Perspective." In *Touch Choices: In Vitro Fertilization and the Reproductive Technologies*, edited by Patricia Stephenson and Marsden G. Wagner, 62–72. Philadelphia: Temple University Press.

Steinberg, Deborah Lynn. 1990. "The Depersonalisation of Women through the Administration of '*In Vitro* Fertilization.'" In *The New Reproductive*

Technologies, edited by Maureen McNeil, Ian Varcoe, and Steven Yearley, 74–122. New York: St. Martin's Press.

Stephenson, Patricia. 1993. "Ovulation Induction during Treatment of Infertility: An Assessment of the Risks." In *Touch Choices: In Vitro Fertilization and the Reproductive Technologies*, edited by Patricia Stephenson and Marsden G. Wagner, 97–121. Philadelphia: Temple University Press.

Stephenson, Patricia, and Marsden G. Wagner, eds. 1993. *Touch Choices: In Vitro Fertilization and the Reproductive Technologies*. Philadelphia: Temple University Press.

Steptoe, P. C., and R. G. Edwards. 1970. "Laparoscopic Recovery of Pre-ovulatory Human Oocytes after Priming of Ovaries with Gonadotrophins." *The Lancet* 295(7649): 683–89.

———. 1976. "Reimplantation of a Human Embryo with Subsequent Tubal Pregnancy." *The Lancet* 307(7965): 880–82.

Steptoe, P. C., R. G. Edwards, and J. M. Purdy. 1971. "Human Blastocysts Grown in Culture." *Nature* 229(5280): 132–33. doi:10.1038/229132a0.

Stern, Judy E., Marcelle I. Cedars, Tarun Jain, Nancy A. Klein, C. Martin Beaird, David A. Grainger, and William E. Gibbons. 2007. "Assisted Reproductive Technology Practice Patterns and the Impacts of Embryo Transfer Guidelines in the United States." *Fertility and Sterility* 88(2): 275–82.

Stilgoe, Jack, Richard Owen, and Phil Macnaghten. 2013. "Developing a Framework for Responsible Innovation." *Research Policy* 42: 1568–80.

Stone, J., K. Eddleman, L. Lynch, and R. L. Berkowitz. 2002. "A Single Center Experience with 1000 Consecutive Cases of Multifetal Pregnancy Reduction." *American Journal of Obstetrics and Gynecology* 187: 1163–67.

Su, Shu-Chen. 2006. "Tan Rengong Shengzhi Fa" [On the assisted repro-duction act]. *Taipei Bar Journal* 318: 30–35.

Sullivan, Walter. 1981. "'Test-Tube' Baby Born in the US, Joining Successes around the World." *New York Times*, 29 December: section C, page 1.

Sung, Jin-shiu. 1996. "Taiwan Chuantong Antai Ji Taishen De Guannian [The fetal sedative and the perception of '*Tai Shen*' in traditional Taiwan]." *Taiwan Historical Research* 3(2): 143–93.

———. 2000. "Renshen Antai Ji Renshen Yuzhouguan Xingbie Yu Wenhua De Guandian" [The concept of pregnancy, fetal sedative, and the tradi-tional cosmology: A perspective from gender and culture]. *Taiwan His-torical Research* 3(2): 117–62.

Suzuki, Masakuni. 1983. *Taigai-jusei: Seikou made no Documento* [Docu-mentation of the success of IVF to date]. Tokyo: Kyoritsu Publisher.

———. 2014. "In Vitro Fertilization in Japan—Early Days of In Vitro Fertilization and Embryo Transfer and Future Prospects for Assisted Reproductive Technology." *Proceedings of the Japan Academy Series B* 90: 184–201.

Svensson, Per-Gunnar, and Patricia Stephenson. 1993. "Equity and Resource Distribution in Infertility Care." In *Touch Choices: In Vitro Fertilization and the Reproductive Technologies*, edited by Patricia Stephenson and Marsden G. Wagner, 161–66. Philadelphia: Temple University Press.

Tai, Hsueh-Yung. 1988. "Duobaotai De Weiji Shouyun Guran Hao Kongzhi Geng Zhongyao" [Crisis of multiplets: Control is more important than pregnancy]." *China Times*, 10 February: 12.

Taiwan LGBT Family Rights Advocacy. 2010. *Dang Women Tong Zai Yi Jia Gei Xiang Sheng Xiaohai De Nü Tongzhi* [When we build a family: A childbearing guide for lesbians]. Taipei: Fembooks Publishing.

"Taiwan to Raise Subsidies to Boost Flagging Birthrate." 2021. *Taipei Times*, 28 April. Retrieved 12 December 2021 from https://www.taipeitimes .com/News/taiwan/archives/2021/04/28/2003756487.

Takeshima, Kazumi, Seung Chik Jwa, Hidekazu Saito, Aritoshi Nakaza, Akira Kuwahara, Osamu Ishihara, and Tetsuro Sakumoto. 2016. "Impact of Single Embryo Transfer Policy on Perinatal Outcomes in Fresh and Frozen Cycles—Analysis of Japanese Assisted Reproductive Technology Registry between 2007 and 2012." *Fertility and Sterility* 105(2): 337–46.

Tanaka, Akashi. 2015. "Nihon ni okeru Taigai-jusei no Donyu-katei no Rekishi Bunseki: Fukakujitsu-sei ka no Ishikettei to Sekinin" [The historical analysis of introducing IVF in Japan: Decision-making and responsibility under uncertainty]. *Tetsugaku, Kagakushi Ronso* [Annals of philosophy and history of science] 17: 83–102.

Templeton, Allan, and Joan K. Morris. 1998. "Reducing the Risk of Multiple Birth by Transfer of Two Embryos after In Vitro Fertilization." *New England Journal of Medicine* 339(9): 573–77.

Thompson, Charis. 2005. *Making Parents: The Ontological Choreography of Reproductive Technologies.* Cambridge, MA: MIT Press.

———. 2016. "IVF Global Histories, USA: Between a Rock and a Marketplace." *Reproductive BioMedicine and Society Online* 2: 128–35.

Thurin, Ann, Jon Hausken, Torbjörn Hillensjö, Barbara Jablonowska, Anja Pinborg, Annika Strandell, and Christina Bergh. 2004. "Elective Single-Embryo Transfer versus Double-Embryo Transfer in In Vitro Fertilization." *New England Journal of Medicine* 351: 2392–402.

Timmermans, Stefan, and Marc Berg. 2003. *The Gold Standard: The Challenge of Evidence-Based Medicine and Standardization in Health Care.* Philadelphia: Temple University Press.

Timmermans, Stefan, and Steven Epstein. 2010. "A World of Standards but Not a Standard World: Toward a Sociology of Standards and Standardization." *Annual Review of Sociology* 36: 69–89.

Timor-Tritsch, Ilan E., Asher Bashiri, Ana Monteagudo, Andrei Rebarber, and Alan A. Arslan. 2004. "Two Hundred Ninety Consecutive Cases of Multifetal Pregnancy Reduction: Comparison of the Transabdominal versus the Transvaginal Approach." *American Journal of Obstetrics and Gynecology* 191: 2085–89.

Timor-Tritsch, I. E., and A. Monteagudo. 2006. "Diagnosis of Chorionicity and Amnionicity." In *Multiple Pregnancy: Epidemiology, Gestation & Perinatal Outcomes*, 2nd ed., edited by Isaac Blickstein and Louis G. Keith, 291–307. Abingdon: Informa.

Timor-Tritsch, Ilan E., David B. Peisner, Ana Monteagudo, Jodi P. Lerner, and Shubhra Sharma. 1993. "Multifetal Pregnancy Reduction by Transvaginal Puncture: Evaluation of the Technique Used in 134 Cases." *American Journal of Obstetrics and Gynecology* 168: 799–804.

Tsai, Chia-Chang. 1999. "Danyi Peitai Zhiru Bushi Meng" [Single embryo transfer is not a dream]." *United Daily News*, 28 July: 34.

Tsai, Duu-Jian. 2002. *Taiwan waike yiliao fazhan shi* [The history of surgery in Taiwan]. Taipei: Tang-Shang.

Tsai, Horng-Der. 1999. "Meiguo Babaotai De Lianxiang Zhiru Duoshao Peitai Cai Suan Taiduo" [The connotation of octuplets in the US: How many embryos implanted are counted as too many]. *United Daily News*, 18 January: 34.

———. 2007. "Shuangbaotai Renshen Rengong Shouyun Bu Guli" [Assisted conception does not encourage twin pregnancy]. *United Daily News*, 26 May: E2.

Tseng, Fan-Tzu. 2017. "From Medicalization to Riskisation: Governing Early Childhood Development." *Sociology of Health & Illness* 39(1): 112–26.

Tseng, Yen-Jung. 2013. "Nü Tongzhi Jiating Qinzhi Shizuo" [Lesbian family and parenting practices]." Master's thesis, National Taiwan University, Taipei.

TSRM (Taiwan Society for Reproductive Medicine). 2012. "Taiwan Shengzhi Yi xuehui Peitai Zhiru Shu Zhiyin 2012" [TSRM guideline of recommended limits of the number of embryos to transfer]. *Taiwan Society for Reproductive Medicine*. Retrieved 17 December 2021 from http://www.tsrm.org.tw/news/content.asp?id=15.

Tsuge, Azumi. 1999. *Bunka to shiteno Seishoku-gijutsu: Funin-chiryo ni tazusawaru Ishi no Katari* [Reproductive technology as culture: Narratives of doctors involved in infertility treatment]. Kyoto: Shōraisha.

———. 2012. *Seishoku-gijutsu: Funin-chiryo to Saisei-iryo wa Shakai ni Nani wo motarasuka* [Reproductive technology: What infertility treatment and regenerative medicine bring to society]. Tokyo: Misuzu shobō.

———. 2016. "Josei no Kenko Seisaku no 20 nen: Reproductive Health/ Rights kara Shusshou Sokushin Seisaku made" [An overview of two decades of women's health policies in Japan: From the introduction of "reproductive health and rights" to policies addressing the declining birthrate]. *Kokusai Gender Gakkai-shi* [Journal for international society for gender studies] 14: 32–52.

Tsui, Kuan-Hao. 2021. "Shiguan Yinger Buzhu Fangan Qiangjiu Shengyulu Zhengfu Jichu Sanying Celüe" [Subsidy plans for IVF babies: Raising fertility rate! Triple-win strategy from the government]. Retrieved 12 December 2021 from https://www.youtube.com/watch?v=CWgsZP9nn3o&list=TLGGzkkNqycFREMxNDA5MjAyMQ.

Tzeng, Chii-Ruey. 2019. *Chen Chu Yitiao Shenglu Taiwan Shiguan Yinger Zhi Fu Zeng Qirui Yishi Ling Yu Yibai De Shengming Zhexue* [Make open a road of life: Taiwan's father of test-tube baby Tzeng Chii-Ruey's life philosophy between zero and one hundred]. Taipei: Business Weekly.

UK Department of Health and Social Care. 2021. "The Surrogacy Pathway: Surrogacy and the Legal Process for Intended Parents and Surrogates in England and Wales." Retrieved 8 December 2021 from https://www .gov.uk/government/publications/having-a-child-through-surrogacy/ the-surrogacy-pathway-surrogacy-and-the-legal-process-for-intended-parents-and-surrogates-in-england-and-wales.

Umstad, M. P., and P. A. L. Lancaster. 2005. "Multiple Birth in Australia." In *Multiple Pregnancy: Epidemiology, Gestation and Perinatal Outcomes*, 2nd ed., edited by Isaac Blickstein and Louis G. Keith, 26–32. Abingdon: Informa.

Urquhart, C., R. Currell, F. Harlow, and L. Callow. 2017. "Home Uterine Monitoring for Detecting Preterm Labour (Review)." *Cochrane Database of Systematic Review* 2, art. no.: CD006172.

Van Blerkom, Jonathan. 2009. "An Overview of Determinants of Oocyte and Embryo Developmental Competence: Specificity, Accuracy and Appplicability in Clinical IVF." In *Single Embryo Transfer*, edited by Jan Gerris, G. David Adamson, Petra De Sutter, and Catherine Racowsky, 17–50. Cambridge: Cambridge University Press.

Van Landuyt, Lisbet, G. Verheyen, H. Tournaye, M. Camus, P. Devroey, and A. Van Steirteghem. 2006. "New Belgian Embryo Transfer Policy Leads to Sharp Decrease in Multiple Pregnancy Rate." *Reproductive BioMedicine Online* 13(6): 765–71.

Vilska, S., A. Titinen, C. Hyden-Granskog, and O. Hovatta. 1999. "Elective Transfer of One Embryo Results in an Acceptable Pregnancy Rate and Eliminates the Risk of Multiple Birth." *Human Reproduction* 14: 2392–95.

Waggoner, Miranda R. 2017. *The Zero Trimester: Pre-pregnancy Care and the Politics of Reproductive Risk*. Oakland: University of California Press.

Wagner, M. G., and P. A. St. Clair. 1989. "Are In-Vitro Fertilisation and Embryo Transfer of Benefit to All?" *The Lancet* 330(8647): 1027–30.

Wagner, Marsden G., and Patricia Stephenson. 1993. "Infertility and In Vitro Fertilization: Is the Tail Wagging the Dog?" In *Touch Choices: In Vitro Fertilization and the Reproductive Technologies*, edited by Patricia Stephenson and Marsden G. Wagner, 1–22. Philadelphia, PA: Temple University Press.

Wahlberg, Ayo. 2016. "The Birth and Routinization of IVF in China." *Reproductive Biomedicine & Society Online* 2: 97–107.

———. 2019. *Good Quality: The Routinization of Sperm Banking in China*. Berkeley: University of California Press.

Wainwright, Steven P., Clare Williams, Mike Michael, Bobbie Farsides, and Alan Cribb. 2006. "Ethical Boundary-Work in the Embryonic Stem Cell Laboratory." *Sociology of Health and Illness* 28(6): 732–48.

Waldby, Catherine, and Robert Michell. 2006. *Tissue Economies: Blood Organs, and Cell Lines in Late Capitalism*. Durham, NC: Duke University Press.

Wang, Chi-Ching. 2000. "Chenggonglu Yizai Shuaxin Zhiliao Buyun Changgeng You Yitao" [The success rate creates a new record again: Infertility treatment is great in Chang-Cheng Hospital]." *United Daily News*, 27 September: 19.

Wang, Fu-chang. 2018. "Studies on Taiwan's Ethnic Relations." *International Journal of Taiwan Studies* 1: 64–89.

Wang, Hui-Lan, and Yu-Mei Yu Chao. 2006. "Lived Experiences of Taiwanese Women with Multifetal Pregnancies Who Receive Fetal Reduction." *Journal of Nursing Research* 14(2): 143–54.

Wang, Yueping Alex, Georgina M. Chambers, Mbathio Dieng, and Elizabeth A. Sullivan. 2009. *Assisted Reproductive Technology in Australia and New Zealand 2007.* Australian Institute of Health and Welfare, National Perinatal Statistics Unit.

Wang, Yueping Alex, Georgina M. Chambers, and Elizabeth A. Sullivan. 2010. *Assisted Reproductive Technology in Australia and New Zealand 2008.* Australian Institute of Health and Welfare.

Wang, Yueping Alex, Jishan Dean, Tim Badgery-Parker, and Elizabeth A. Sullivan. 2008. *Assisted Reproductive Technology in Australia and New Zealand 2006.* Australian Institute of Health and Welfare, National Perinatal Statistics Unit.

Wang, Yueping Alex, Jishan H. Dean, Narelle Grayson, and Elizabeth A. Sullivan. 2006. *Assisted Reproductive Technology in Australia and New Zealand 2004.* Australian Institute of Health and Welfare, National Perinatal Statistics Unit.

Wang, Yueping Alex, Jishan Dean, and Elizabeth A. Sullivan. 2007. *Assisted Reproductive Technology in Australia and New Zealand 2005.* Australian Institute of Health and Welfare, National Perinatal Statistics Unit.

Wang, Yueping Alex, Alan Macaldowie, Irene Hayward, Georgina M. Chambers, and Elizabeth A. Sullivan. 2011. *Assisted Reproductive Technology in Australia and New Zealand 2009.* Australian Institute of Health and Welfare.

Waters, Anne-Marie, Jishan H. Dean, and Elizabeth A. Sullivan. 2006. *Assisted Reproductive Technology in Australia and New Zealand 2003.* Australian Institute of Health and Welfare, National Perinatal Statistics Unit.

Wapner, Ronald J., George H. Davis, Anthony Johnson, Vivian J. Weinblatt, Richard L. Fischer, Laird G. Jackson, Frank A. Chervenak, and Laurence B. McCullough. 1990. "Selective Reduction of Multifetal Pregnancies." *The Lancet* 335(8681): 90–93.

Wei, Hsin-Hsin. 1999. "Rengong Shengzhi Buyun Fuqi Pan Jianbao Jifu Chenggong Qiuzi Chang De Huafei Baiwanyuan Jianbaoju Biaoshi Tiaogao Baofei Caineng Fudan" [Infertile couples hope for NHI to cover the assisted reproduction: Successful treatment costs millions of dollars / NHI Bureau not affordable unless raising premium]. *United Daily News,* 9 March: 6.

Wei, Li-Wen. 2005a. "Liangqiansibai Shiguan Yinger Made in Taibei Rongzong" [2,400 test-tube babies made in Taipei Veterans Hospital]. *United Daily News* 16 April: 4.

———. 2005b. "Duo Sheng Duo Fuqi Ciji Pailuan Bacheng Sanbaotai" [More births, more blessings? 80 percent of triplets caused by egg stimulation drug]. *United Evening News,* 28 August: 3.

Wennerholm, Ulla-Britt. 2009. "The Risks Associated with Multiple Pregnancies." In *Single Embryo Transfer*, edited by Jan Gerris, G. David Adamson, Petra De Sutter, and Catherine Racowsky, 3–16. Cambridge: University of Cambridge Press.

Whittaker, Andrea. 2015. *Thai In Vitro: Gender, Culture and Assisted Reproduction*. New York: Berghahn Books.

Wikler, Daniel, and Norma J. Wikler. 1991. "Turkey-Baster Babies: The Demedicalization of Artificial Insemination." *Milbank Quarterly* 69(1): 5–40.

Winner, Langdon. 1986. *The Whale and the Reactor: A Search for Limits in an Age of High Technology*. Chicago: University of Chicago Press.

Winston, Robert, and Raul Margara. 1987. "Effectiveness of Treatment for Infertility." *British Medical Journal* 295: 608–9.

Wolkowitz, Carol. 2006. *Bodies at Work*. London: Sage.

Wood, Carl, B. Downing, A. Trounson, and P. Rogers. 1984. "Clinical Implications of Developments in In Vitro Fertilization." *British Medical Journal* 289: 978–80.

Wood, Carl, Rex McMaster, George Rennie, Alan Trounson, and Jon Leeton. 1985. "Factors Influencing Pregnancy Rates Following In Vitro Fertilization and Embryo Transfer." *Fertility and Sterility* 43(2): 245–50.

Wood, Carl, and A. Westmore. 1984. *Test-Tube Conception*. London: George Allen & Unwin.

World Health Organization. 2012. *Born Too Soon: The Global Action Report on Preterm Birth*. Geneva: World Health Organization (WHO).

Wu, Chia-Ling. 2002a. "Taiwan De Xin Shengzhi Keji Yu Xingbie Zhengzhi, 1950–2000" [The new reproductive technologies and gender politics in Taiwan, 1950–2000]. *Taiwan: A Radical Quarterly in Social Studies* 45(1): 1–67.

———. 2002b. "Sho Wuming De Xingbie Xingbiehua De Wuming Cong Taiwan Buyun Nannü Chu jing Fenxi Wuming De Xingbie Zhengzhi" [Stigmatized gender and gendered stigma: The "infertile" men and women in Taiwan]. *Taiwanese Journal of Sociology* 29(1): 127–79.

———. 2012. "IVF Policy and Global/Local Politics: The Making of Multiple-Embryo Transfer Regulation in Taiwan." *Social Science & Medicine* 75(4): 725–32.

———. 2017a. "From Single Motherhood to Queer Reproduction: Access Politics of Assisted Conception in Taiwan." In *Gender and Health in East Asia*, edited by Angela Leung and Izumi Nakayama, 92–114. Hong Kong: Hong Kong University Press.

———. 2017b. "The Childbirth Reform Movement in Taiwan, 1995–2016." *Gender and Culture in Asia* 1: 99–112.

Wu, Chia-Ling, Jung-Ok Ha, and Azumi Tsuge. 2020. "Data Reporting as Care Infrastructure: Assembling ART Registries in Japan, Taiwan, and South Korea." *East Asian Science, Technology and Society* 14(1): 35–59.

Wu, Chia-Ling, Huang Yu-Ling, Ha Jung-ok, Chen Wei-Hong, and Huang Yu-Hsiang. 2020. "Gongping Jinyong Yufang Fengxian Huo Zengzhang

Renkou Zhuyun Keji Gongfei Buzhu De Ri Han Tai Bijiao" [Equal access, risk prevention, or pronatalism? Public financing on in vitro fertilization in Japan, South Korea, and Taiwan]. *Taiwan Democracy Quarterly* 17(4): 49–104.

Wyns, C., C. Bergh, C. Calhaz-Jorge, C. De Geyter, M. S. Kupka, T. Motrenko, . . . and V. Goossens. 2020. "ART in Europe, 2016: Results Generated from European Registries by ESHRE." *Human Reproduction Open* 2020(3): hoaa032.

Yamaguchi, Hiroyuki, Koizumi Yoshiyuki, Kagawa Chiaki, and Matsubara Yoko. 2005. "Tokushima Daigaku Rinri Iinkai Setsuritsu Keii no Chosa Interview: Mori Takahide" [Investigation and interview of Mori Takahide on the establishment of the ethics committee of Tokushima University]. Retrieved 10 June 2019 from http://www.ritsumei.ac.jp/acd/gr/gsce/2005/0219.htm.

Yanaihara, Takumi. 1998. *Funin-chiryo no Arikata ni kansuru Kenkyu: Kousei-sho Shinshin Shogai Kenkyu; Heisei 9 nen Kenkyu Houkoku-sho* [Research on the ideal practices of infertility treatment: 1997 report for the Ministry of Health and Welfare]. Tokyo: Ministry of Health and Welfare.

Yang, Hui-Chun. 2000. "Zaochan Siwanglu Gao Tuzeng Jiating Wenti Yu Shehui Chengben Zuoren Chenggong Duobaotai Jian Wei Shuangbaotai" [Premature births have a high mortality rate, and increase family troubles and social caste: Multiple pregnancy should be reduced to twin fetuses for successful infertility treatment]. *Min-Sheng Daily*, 11 October: D7.

———. 2002. "Rengong Shengzhi Duotai Fengxian Gao" [Assisted reproduction: Multiple birth had high risk]. *Min-Sheng Daily*, 4 March: A7.

Yeshua, Arilelle, Joseph A. Lee, Georgia Witkin, and Alan B. Copperman. 2015. "Female Couples Undergoing IVF with Partner Eggs (Co-IVF) Pathways to Parenthood." *LBGT Health* 2(2): 135–39.

Yu, Ching-Ju. 2015. "Taiwan Duobaotai Renshen Funü Yu Jieshou Jiantaishu Zhi Juece Licheng" [Decision-making process of Taiwanese women with multifetal pregnancies who receive fetal reduction]. Master's thesis, Graduate Institute of Molecular Medicine, National Taiwan University, Taipei.

Yuan, Tzu-Lun. 1995. "Jieshou Buyunzheng Funu Si Fen Zhi Yi Chan Duobaotai" [One-fourth of women with infertility treatment gave birth to multiplets]. *Min-Sheng Daily*, 4 August: 21.

Yui, Hideki. 2016. "Taigai-jusei no Risho Ouyou to Nihon Jusei-chakusho Gakkai no Seiritsu" [The clinical application of IVF and the establishment of the Japan Society of Fertilization and Implantation]. *Kagakushi kenkyu* [History of science studies] 278: 118–32.

Zegers-Hochschild, F., J. A. Crosby, C. Musri, M. D. C. B. de Souza, A. G. Martinez, A. A. Silva, . . . and N. Posada. 2020. "Assisted Reproductive Technology in Latin America: The Latin American Registry, 2017." *Reproductive Biomedicine Online* 41(1): 44–54.

INDEX

abduction, 12, 59, 64–68, 83, 120, 123

abortion: access to resources of, 115; fetal personhood in debates on, 171n7; legalization of, 78, 101; moral struggle over, 1, 46; spontaneous, 39, 55n10; suction, 43, 44, 56n15

ACOG. *See* American College of Obstetricians and Gynecologists

Adamson, David, 7

AI. *See* artificial intelligence

Almeling, Rene, 14

American College of Obstetricians and Gynecologists (ACOG), 157, 160, 169, 170n4

American Society for Reproductive Medicine (ASRM): annual meetings of, 90, 114; on fetal reduction, 47; NET guidelines from, 50–53, 71, 111–14, 120; on PGT-A, 67

amniocentesis, 43–44, 55n12, 99–100, 138, 149, 154

aneuploidies, 66–67. *See also* preimplantation genetic testing for aneuploidies

an-tai (keeping fetuses safe/calm): anticipatory labor and, 185; bed rest during, 172–74, 181, 183–84; leave from paid jobs during, 183–84; maternal body work during, 173, 174, 177–83; medical interventions during, 172, 173, 180–81; policy recommendations, 185–86

anticipatory governance: in Belgian Project, 74; components of, 13; definition of, 9–10; ensemblization and, 121; global variation in, 11, 51, 106–7; local/global dynamics in, 126–27; methodology for study of, 18–19; of NET, 12, 15–16, 52; responsible, 192–95; sociotechnical imaginaries and, 105–6

anticipatory labor: *an-tai* and, 185; definition of, 13, 21, 190; fetal reduction and, 155, 169, 191; maternal body work and, 14, 21, 191; maternal-fetal conflicts and, 13–14; methodology for study of, 19; in sociocultural contexts, 15, 192

anticipatory medicalization/ de-medicalization, 8, 40

anticipatory regimes: components of, 8; dimensions of, 9–15; power dynamics within, 188–90; in social studies literature, 9. *See also*

anticipatory governance;
anticipatory labor
anticipatory work: abduction and,
12, 59, 64–68, 83, 120, 123;
for eSET implementation,
59–68, 74, 76, 82–85; framing
of, 12, 84–85; hope work and,
12–13, 59–64, 68, 83, 123;
optimization of ARTs and, 130;
simplification and, 12, 16, 59,
67–68, 83
artificial insemination: egg
stimulation drugs and, 26,
55n10; interuterine, 5, 134–36,
146, 151n7; self-insemination,
145, 151n6, 151n10. *See also*
donor insemination
artificial intelligence (AI), 66
ARTs. *See* assisted reproductive
technologies
ASRM. *See* American Society for
Reproductive Medicine
Assisted Reproduction Act of 2007
(Taiwan), 16, 21, 115–20, 126,
129, 144, 190
assisted reproductive technologies
(ARTs): cross-border use of,
144–47; division of labor
in, 62, 80, 100, 144; global
comparison of eligibility
criteria for, 150n5; governance
of, 11, 37, 100–104, 106; as
hope technology, 9, 13, 59,
188; informed consent for,
111, 135; lesbian and gay
access to, 144–48, 151n6, 190;
methodology for study of,
18–19; in opposition to state
policy, 91; social studies of, 7,
9, 11. *See also* optimization of
ARTs; *specific technologies*
Australia: benefit and risk model
in, 41–42; competition for IVF
success in, 91; development of
IVF in, 27–29, 31, 32; multiple
pregnancy in, 33–36, 187, 190;
single embryo transfer in, 68;

success rate reporting for IVF
in, 63, 64

bed rest: during *an-tai*, 172–74,
181, 183–84; challenges related
to, 21, 181, 183–84; multiple
pregnancy and, 172, 176,
179, 181; for preterm birth
prevention, 172, 176, 181, 191
Belgium: Belgian Project, 72–75,
84, 193; NET guidelines in,
6–7, 72–73, 108, 116; public
financing for IVF in, 72–75, 84;
single embryo transfer in, 7,
68, 72–75, 83–84, 119, 124
Berg, Marc, 49
BFS. *See* British Fertility Society
Birenbaum-Carmeli, Daphna, 7
brain drain, 90, 107n2
Braude, Peter, 13
British Fertility Society (BFS), 49,
113
Brown, Leslie, 26–27, 39
Brown, Louise, 5, 20, 23, 27, 58
burden of care, 5, 36–37, 175–76,
189, 194

Canada: cross-border use of
ARTs in, 146, 147; multiple
pregnancy in, 61; NET
guidelines in, 108, 117
care burden. *See* burden of care
cerebral palsy (CP), 2–3, 5, 78, 154
Chang, Min Chueh, 90–91
Chang, Sheng-Ping, 88, 94, 105, 115
Chang, Shirley L., 107n2
Chang-Gung Hospital (Taiwan), 90,
92, 95–98
Chen, Min-Jer, 195
Chen, Shee-Uan, 117, 129–30
Chinese medicine. *See* traditional
Chinese medicine
chorionic villus sampling (CVS),
55n12, 162
Clarke, Adele, 12, 59, 64, 67
clinical pregnancy rate, 29, 54n5,
60, 68

clomiphene, 31–32, 55n10
Cohen, Jean, 68
Co-IVF (shared-motherhood IVF), 147
compulsory motherhood, 141–44, 151n6
compulsory single-embryo transfer (cSET), 58–59, 127
Conrad, Peter, 40
consent. *See* informed consent
Corea, Gena, 39
corporeal adjustment, 174, 177, 179–81
CP. *See* cerebral palsy
cp value (cost-performance ratio), 130, 148
cross-border use of ARTs, 144–47
cryopreservation, 44, 65–66, 69, 95, 100–102, 120
cSET. *See* compulsory single-embryo transfer
CVS. *See* chorionic villus sampling

delayed parenthood, 15, 17, 131, 135–39, 190
Denmark: ART governance in, 11; multiple pregnancy in, 61
DET. *See* double embryo transfer
donor insemination (DI): accreditation for institutions practicing, 122; HFEA report on birth rates with, 60; legal concerns regarding, 101; in queer reproduction, 144, 146, 151n6
double embryo transfer (DET): accreditation system and, 122; elective (eDET), 49; embryo selection for, 49; JSOG Project and, 76; multiple pregnancy and, 57–58, 67; single embryo transfer compared to, 65, 68, 72; subsidies for, 123–24; in surrogacy process, 187
dragon-phoenix twins, 130, 147

EBM. *See* evidence-based medicine

ectopic pregnancy, 55n10, 132, 163
eDET. *See* elective double-embryo transfer
Edwards, Robert, 23–25, 27, 29, 31, 35
egg banks, 122
egg freezing, 9, 65, 140
egg stimulation drugs: artificial insemination and, 26, 55n10; benefit and risk model for, 42; cSET and, 58; IUI with, 5, 136; JSOG Project and, 48, 79; multiple embryo transfer and, 31; multiple pregnancy and, 4, 17, 33–35, 78–79, 96, 98; in reproductive trajectories, 136
elective double-embryo transfer (eDET), 49
elective single-embryo transfer (eSET): anticipatory work for implementation of, 59–68, 74, 76, 82–85; assessment of, 64–67, 83, 121–22; Belgian Project and, 72–75; benefit and risk model for, 58–59; definition of, 58; disconnected patchworks of, 121–25, 194; emergence of, 20, 53, 58; feasibility of, 65–66, 69, 83; guidelines for, 67–68; individual exemplar experiments with, 121; in queer reproduction, 148; resistance to, 68–69; subsidies for, 69–71
embryo selection: for double embryo transfer, 49; genetic screening/testing and, 66, 120, 161; quality of, 102, 112, 120; as risk management strategy, 100; score system for, 121; sex selection prohibitions, 115; for single embryo transfer, 3, 65–67, 69–70, 81, 83
emotion work, 174, 177, 181–83
ensemblization, 121, 124–25
eSET. *See* elective single-embryo transfer

European Society of Human
   Reproduction and Embryology
   (ESHRE): conferences held
   by, 114; on embryo selection,
   66; on fetal reduction, 46–47;
   on IVF success rate reporting,
   61–62; journal published by,
   57; on multiple pregnancy
   recognition, 80
Evans, Mark I., 44–46
Evers, Johannes L. H., 62
evidence-based medicine (EBM):
   fetal reduction and, 164; as
   global governance mechanism,
   189; on home monitoring
   of pregnancy, 179; NET
   guidelines and, 49, 51; on
   preterm birth prevention, 176,
   185, 191; reproductive politics
   and, 16; single embryo transfer
   and, 11, 65, 68

false hope, 12, 20, 59–62
feminism: on anticipatory labor, 14;
   on compulsory motherhood,
   143, 151n6; on fetal reduction,
   38, 115; health movements
   and, 21, 52, 188–89; IVF as
   critiqued by, 38–40, 193; JSOG
   Project and, 79, 87n7; on
   medicalization of infertility, 38,
   143; on multiple pregnancy,
   16, 20, 39, 118; on NET
   regulation, 115–18; on social
   causes of infertility, 40
Feminist International Network
   for Resistance to Reproductive
   and Genetic Engineering
   (FINRRAGE), 38, 79, 87n7,
   115, 118
Ferber, Sarah, 90
Fertility Clinic Success Rate and
   Certification Act of 1992 (US),
   63
fertility drugs: multiple pregnancy
   and, 1, 4, 15, 55n10, 133,
   150, 158–59, 166; in queer

reproduction, 147; in
   reproductive trajectories, 133,
   135. *See also specific names and
   types of drugs*
Fertility Information Network
   (FINE), 81
fertility rate, 17, 81, 123, 131, 137,
   194–95
fetal personhood, 167–68, 171n7
fetal reduction: anticipatory labor
   and, 155, 169, 191; benefit
   and risk model for, 45–46,
   97–98, 160; decision-making
   process for, 153–55, 162–70,
   191; doctors with contrasting
   opinions on, 162, 164–65,
   168–69; emergence of, 20,
   43–45, 52, 155, 157; feminist
   views of, 38, 115; framing of,
   106; global rates of, 46–47,
   158; husbands as allies in,
   166–67; intensity of direction
   guides for, 162–68; as last
   resort, 47; maternal-fetal
   conflicts and, 13–14, 162,
   167–68; methods of, 43–45,
   56n16, 98–99; miscarriage
   risk and, 13, 18, 45–46, 98,
   159–60, 170n5; mobilization
   of science and emotion in,
   165–66; moral struggle over, 1,
   13, 46, 99, 100; as safety net,
   47, 98; selection of fetuses for,
   160–61; skill-based autonomy
   and, 168–69; social concerns
   regarding, 78–79; technological
   assessment of, 98–100, 159–62,
   169–70
feto-centrism, 170, 185, 191
FINE. *See* Fertility Information
   Network
Finland: NET guidelines in, 103;
   single embryo transfer in, 68
FINRRAGE. *See* Feminist
   International Network for
   Resistance to Reproductive and
   Genetic Engineering

Fox, Bonnie, 180
framing: of anticipatory work, 12, 84–85; of fetal reduction, 106; of IVF, 10, 24, 52–53, 89, 100; of multiple pregnancy, 15–16, 21; power dynamics and, 11, 189
France: fetal reduction in, 44; insurance coverage for IVF in, 117; multiple pregnancy in, 35–37; NET guidelines in, 48–49
Franklin, Sarah, 9, 14, 28, 127, 135
Frydman, Rene, 91

gamete intrafallopian transfer (GIFT), 48, 95, 97
Gatrell, Caroline, 14, 181
gays. *See* lesbian and gay community
Gender Equality in Employment Act of 2010 (Taiwan), 184
Genetic Health Act of 1984 (Taiwan), 99
genetic screening, 120, 122
genetic testing: age guidelines for, 138; amniocentesis and, 99; for embryo quality, 12; fetal reduction and, 43, 45, 55n13. *See also* preimplantation genetic testing for aneuploidies
Germany: ART governance in, 11; NET guidelines in, 6, 48, 102–3
GIFT. *See* gamete intrafallopian transfer
governance. *See* anticipatory governance
Grimes, David A., 185–86
Guston, David H., 10

hCG. *See* human chorionic gonadotrophin
HFEA. *See* Human Fertilisation and Embryology Authority
HFE Act. *See* Human Fertilisation and Embryology Act of 1990
higher-order multiple pregnancy: egg stimulation drugs and, 33–34, 79; nonuplets, 33, 98; octuplets, 4, 33, 43, 45, 98; quintuplets, 4–5, 33–34, 44–45, 110; septuplets, 33, 37–38, 45, 98, 110; sextuplets, 33–34, 45. *See also* fetal reduction; quadruplets; triplets
hMG. *See* human menopausal gonadotrophin
home uterine monitoring, 176, 178
homosexuals. *See* lesbian and gay community
hope work, 12–13, 59–64, 68, 83, 123
Huang, Shu-Ying, 115–18, 129, 184, 189–90
human chorionic gonadotrophin (hCG), 26, 31, 33, 156, 163
Human Fertilisation and Embryology (HFE) Act of 1990 (UK), 48, 101–2, 107n5
Human Fertilisation and Embryology Authority (HFEA), 49, 60–61, 69–70, 102, 123
human menopausal gonadotrophin (hMG), 26, 33, 55n10

ICMART. *See* International Committee for Monitoring Assisted Reproductive Technologies
ICSI. *See* intracytoplasmic sperm injection
IFFS. *See* International Federation of Fertility Societies
Ince, Susan, 39
infertility: age and, 137–38; anticipatory, 9, 138; medicalization of, 38, 143; PCOS as cause of, 141; social causes of, 40, 189. *See also* assisted reproductive technologies
informed consent, 111, 135, 169
Inhorn, Marcia, 7
insemination. *See* artificial insemination

insurance coverage, 70–71, 81, 113–14, 117. *See also* National Health Insurance

International Committee for Monitoring Assisted Reproductive Technologies (ICMART): alliance with JSOG Project, 82; data collection and reporting by, 15; as global governance mechanism, 189; on IVF success rate reporting, 60–61; on NET by selected countries, 103; on single embryo transfer, 11; on twin rates, 4–5

International Federation of Fertility Societies (IFFS): conferences held by, 114; on eligibility criteria for ARTs, 150n5; as global governance mechanism, 189; on insurance coverage for IVF, 117; on NET guidelines, 48, 108, 111–13; on PGT-A, 66–67; on resistance to eSET, 68; surveys on IVF conducted by, 15

International Working Group for Registers on Assisted Reproduction. *See* International Committee for Monitoring Assisted Reproductive Technologies

interuterine insemination (IUI), 5, 134–36, 146, 151n7

intracytoplasmic sperm injection (ICSI), 5–6, 57, 73

in vitro fertilization (IVF): accreditation for institutions practicing, 122; adverse outcomes of, 36, 60, 95, 110; anticipatory practices of, 20, 23–30, 38, 52; benefit and risk model for, 41–43; Co-IVF (shared-motherhood IVF), 147; cost redistribution for, 70–71, 74–75, 82; feminist critiques of, 38–40, 193; framing of, 10, 24, 52–53, 89, 100; gatherings of children born by, 2, 104–5; global governance mechanisms for, 189; hesitancy in utilization of, 134–35, 190; insurance coverage for, 70–71, 81, 113–14, 117; as nationalist glory, 12, 20, 88–93, 100, 105–6; natural cycle method of, 20, 26–28, 31–32, 43, 52, 58; professional conflicts among experts, 10–11; promissory capital in, 9, 70–71, 74, 84, 125; queer reproduction and, 144–47; redefining success of, 59–64, 83; scientific breakthroughs in, 20, 23–28; self-regulation model for, 77, 102, 106, 126; social concerns regarding, 76–80, 92–93; sociotechnical imaginaries of, 11–12, 20, 84–85, 92, 100; success rate of, 16, 20, 28–30, 52; on US healthcare priority list, 86n5. *See also* multiple pregnancy; number of embryos transferred; public financing for IVF

Ishihara, Osamu, 82, 189

Israel: ART governance in, 11; fetal reduction in, 44; insurance coverage for IVF in, 117; IVF as nationalist glory in, 89

IUI. *See* interuterine insemination

IVF. *See* in vitro fertilization

JAOGMP. *See* Japan Association of Obstetrics and Gynecology for Maternal Protection

Japan: abortion legalization in, 78; ART governance in, 106; competition for IVF success in, 91; cross-border use of ARTs in, 146; fetal reduction in, 44, 78–79; multiple pregnancy in, 5, 17, 34, 61, 76–81, 127; NET

guidelines in, 6, 48, 76–77, 79, 108; public financing for IVF in, 81, 123; single embryo transfer in, 3, 75–76, 81–85, 106, 119, 124; social concerns of IVF in, 76–80, 92–93
Japan Association of Obstetrics and Gynecology for Maternal Protection (JAOGMP), 78
Japan Society of Obstetrics and Gynecology (JSOG): alliance with ICMART, 82; on egg stimulation drugs, 48, 79; feminist involvement with, 79, 87n7; interprofessional conflict and, 80–83; on multiple pregnancy, 48, 77–81; NET guidelines from, 48, 76–77, 79, 113; registry data from, 77, 79–82, 193; on single embryo transfer, 75–76, 81–82, 106
Jasanoff, Sheila, 11, 51, 76
Johnston, Ian, 27–29
Jones, Georgeanna, 90
Jones, Howard, 31, 68, 90
JSOG. *See* Japan Society of Obstetrics and Gynecology

Kim, Sang-Hyun, 11, 76
Ko, Tsang-Ming, 170n5
Kuan, Bi-Ling, 124

Lai, Hui-Chen, 111
Lai, Ying-Ming, 112
Lee, Kuo-Kuang, 2–3, 12, 110–11, 121
Lee, Maw-Sheng, 100, 104–5, 121
Lee, Tzu-Yao, 102
lesbian and gay community: ART access for, 144–48, 151n6, 190; marriages of convenience in, 145, 151n7; same-sex marriage in, 142, 147–48, 154; surrogacy options for, 148
LH. *See* luteinizing hormone
Liu, Chih-Hong, 137
Liu, Helen Hung Ching, 90

low birthweight: complications of, 5; multiple pregnancy and, 33, 35–36, 61, 95–96, 105, 110, 127; on US healthcare priority list, 86n5
Lu, Tien-Lin, 129–30
luteinizing hormone (LH), 26, 32
Lyerly, Anne Drapkin, 185–86

MacKay Memorial Hospital (Taiwan), 110–11, 121
Mackie, Vera, 90
Marks, Nicola J., 90
marriage: average age of first marriage, 132, 136; of convenience, 145, 151n7; late marriage trends, 15, 21, 131, 136–37, 190; same-sex, 142, 147–48, 154; social norm of motherhood within, 40, 132; voluntary childlessness within, 142
Martin, Lauren Jade, 136, 143
maternal body work: during *an-tai*, 173–74, 177–83; anticipatory labor and, 14, 21, 191; corporeal adjustment, 174, 177, 179–81; emotion work, 174, 177, 181–83; self-palpation for prediction, 174, 177–79
maternal-fetal conflicts, 13–14, 162, 167–68, 182
maternal mortality, 5, 36, 46, 160, 167, 182–83, 189, 191
McCall, Christina A., 185–86
medicalization of infertility, 38, 143
Men Having Babies (MHB), 148
MET. *See* multiple embryo transfer
Meyers, Diana Tietjens, 168
MHB. *See* Men Having Babies
midwives, 157, 176, 178v79, 186
miscarriages: aneuploidies and, 66; emotional reactions to, 134; fetal reduction and, 13, 18, 45–46, 98, 159–60, 170n5;

JSOG Project and, 77–78; multiple pregnancy and, 35; post-IVF pregnancy, 30

motherhood: compulsory, 141–44, 151n6; shared-motherhood IVF (Co-IVF), 147; as social norm within marriage, 40, 132

Mukerji, Subhas, 54n3

multifetal pregnancy reduction. *See* fetal reduction

multiple embryo transfer (MET): accreditation system for reduction of, 122; benefit and risk model for, 41–42, 97–98; criticisms of, 96–97; emergence of, 30–32; global comparisons, 16, 125; as hope work, 59; multiple pregnancy with, 2–6, 20, 24, 33–37, 52, 95–98, 139–40, 150; in optimization of ARTs, 130, 133, 190; in queer reproduction, 146–48; success rate of, 2, 9, 31–32, 42. *See also* double embryo transfer

multiple pregnancy: *an-tai* and, 172–74, 177–86; bed rest and, 172, 176, 179, 181; Belgian Project reduction of, 74–75; benefit and risk model for, 41–42, 97; complications of, 2–3, 5, 13, 35–38, 95–97; detection of, 156–57; double embryo transfer and, 57–58, 67; egg stimulation drugs and, 4, 17, 33–35, 78–79, 96, 98; feminist views of, 16, 20, 39, 118; fertility drugs and, 1, 4, 15, 55n10, 133, 150, 158–59, 166; framing of, 15–16, 21; ICSI and, 5–6, 57; JSOG Project and, 48, 77–81; low birthweight and, 33, 35–36, 61, 95–96, 105, 110, 127; maternal mortality and, 5, 36, 160, 182–83; miscarriage rate with, 35; multiple embryo transfer and, 2–6, 20, 24,

33–37, 52, 95–98, 139–40, 150; preterm births and, 18, 33, 35, 96, 109–11, 172–76, 184, 191; quantitative assessment of, 14; queer reproduction and, 144–48. *See also* fetal reduction; higher-order multiple pregnancy; twins

National Health Insurance (NHI), 110, 114, 165, 174

nationalist glory, IVF as, 12, 20, 88–93, 100, 105–6

National Taiwan University (NTU) Hospital, 90–92, 98–99, 102, 110

natural cycle method of IVF, 20, 26–28, 31–32, 43, 52, 58

Neiterman, Elena, 180

NET. *See* number of embryos transferred

Netsu, Yahiro, 44, 56n17, 78–79

NHI. *See* National Health Insurance

nonuplets, 33, 98. *See also* multiple pregnancy

NTU Hospital. *See* National Taiwan University Hospital

number of embryos transferred (NET): age guidelines for, 48–51, 56n18, 112–13, 120, 122, 139; anticipatory governance of, 12, 15–16, 52; ASRM guidelines on, 50–53, 71, 111–14; Belgian Project and, 72–73; benefit and risk model for, 41–43, 47, 64; feminist calls for regulation of, 115–18; global comparisons, 82, 103–4, 108, 116; international guidelines on, 6–7, 20–21, 48–53, 101–4, 111–17; JSOG Project and, 76–77, 79; local considerations for, 116–17; optimization of ARTs and, 129–30, 185; pregnancy success rate and, 32, 41–42, 116–19; public financing for IVF and, 71–73; self-regulation model for, 102; seminars and continuing education on, 111; TSRM guidelines on, 112–14. *See also* multiple embryo transfer; single embryo transfer

octuplets, 4, 33, 43, 45, 98. *See also* multiple pregnancy
OHSS. *See* ovarian hyperstimulation syndrome
Ombelet, Willem, 72
optimization of ARTs: anticipatory work and, 130; cp value and, 130, 148; healthcare costs and, 74; multiple embryo transfer in, 130, 133, 190; NET guidelines and, 129–30, 185; in queer reproduction, 147; reproductive trajectories and, 21, 131–41, 149
ovarian hyperstimulation syndrome (OHSS), 38, 44, 46, 55n10, 189, 194
ovary stimulation drugs. *See* egg stimulation drugs

patient selection, for single embryo transfer, 3, 66–67, 70
PBFT. *See* Premature Baby Foundation of Taiwan
PCOS. *See* polycystic ovary syndrome
Pennings, Guido, 60
PGS. *See* preimplantation genetic screening
PGT-A. *See* preimplantation genetic testing for aneuploidies
polycystic ovary syndrome (PCOS), 141
population control policies, 91
preimplantation genetic screening (PGS), 120
preimplantation genetic testing for aneuploidies (PGT-A), 66–67, 140–41, 146, 148, 161

Premature Baby Foundation of Taiwan (PBFT), 107, 109–11, 121
prenatal care, 78, 156, 164–65
preterm births: complications of, 3, 5, 33, 110, 163, 175–76; epidemiological data on, 105, 174–75; healthcare costs for, 73–74, 148; medical definition of, 172, 174; multiple pregnancy and, 18, 33, 35, 96, 109–11, 172–76, 184, 191; prevention strategies, 1–2, 21, 172–73, 176, 181, 185–86, 191
productive labor, 174, 183–84
promissory capital, 9, 70–71, 74, 84, 125
pronatalism, 11, 71, 81, 123–24, 193–95
public financing for IVF: in Belgian Project, 72–75, 84, 193; family financial burdens lessened by, 37; NET guidelines and, 71–73; single embryo transfer and, 67–71, 123–24, 194. *See also* subsidies

quadruplets: egg stimulation drugs and, 33; fetal reduction for, 45, 78, 98, 142, 166–67; global rates of, 4, 17, 35, 57, 158; low birthweight among, 95–96; preterm births among, 96. *See also* multiple pregnancy
queer reproduction, 144–48, 151n6. *See also* lesbian and gay community
quintuplets, 4–5, 33–34, 44, 45, 110. *See also* multiple pregnancy

Raymond, Janice G., 38, 40, 41
Reed, Candice Elizabeth Reed, 28
regulatory agency, 16, 67, 100–104
reproductive labor, 7, 14, 144, 174, 183–84

responsible anticipatory governance, 192–95
ROC Infertility Foundation, 104
Rothman, Barbara Katz, 14

same-sex marriage, 142, 147–48, 154
SART. *See* Society for Assisted Reproductive Technology
Schenker, Joseph G., 42
self-insemination, 145, 151n6, 151n10
self-palpation for prediction, 174, 177–79
self-regulation, 77, 102, 106, 126
septuplets, 33, 37–38, 45, 98, 110. *See also* multiple pregnancy
SET. *See* single embryo transfer
sextuplets, 33–34, 45. *See also* multiple pregnancy
sexual minorities. *See* lesbian and gay community
shared-motherhood IVF (Co-IVF), 147
simplification, 12, 16, 59, 67–68, 83
single embryo transfer (SET): age-specific guidelines on, 120; Belgian Project and, 72–75, 84, 193; compulsory, 58–59, 127; double embryo transfer compared to, 65, 68, 72; embryo selection for, 3, 65–67, 69–70, 81, 83; evidence-based medicine and, 11, 65, 68; feasibility of, 68, 111, 117; global comparisons, 83–84, 116, 124–28, 130; international guidelines for, 3, 7, 11, 67–68; JSOG Project and, 75–76, 81–85, 106; natural cycle method for, 20, 26–28, 31–32, 43, 52, 58; patient selection for, 3, 66–67, 70; in queer reproduction, 148; subsidies for, 7, 69–71, 81–82, 123–24, 194–95; success rate of, 41, 68. *See*

also elective single-embryo transfer
singletons: cerebral palsy rate for, 3, 154; global rates of, 61; in IVF success rate reporting, 62–63, 83; preterm births among, 174; queer reproduction and, 144, 148; stillbirth risk for, 95
skill-based autonomy, 168–69
social parenthood, 143
Society for Assisted Reproductive Technology (SART): eSET as defined by, 58; on IVF success rate reporting, 63; NET guidelines from, 50–51
sociotechnical imaginaries: anticipatory governance and, 105–6; definition of, 11, 76; of IVF, 11–12, 20, 84–85, 92, 100; medical achievement in, 89; power dynamics within, 189
sociotechnical networks, 18, 27, 191
Soong, Yung-Kuei, 97–98
South Korea: multiple pregnancy in, 34–35, 61, 190; NET guidelines in, 16, 103; opposition of ARTs to state policy in, 91; public financing for IVF in, 123
sperm banks, 18, 122, 147
spontaneous abortion, 39, 55n10
Stephenson, Patricia, 40, 55n10
Steptoe, Patrick, 23–24, 26–28, 31, 91
stillbirths, 39, 60–61, 81, 95
Su, Fa-Chao, 144
subsidies: age limits for, 138, 141, 194; for double embryo transfer, 123–24; for single embryo transfer, 7, 69–71, 81–82, 123–24, 194–95
suction abortion, 43–44, 56n15
Suleman, Nadya, 4
surrogacy: commercial, 127, 177; cross-border use of, 145; feminist opposition to, 115;

legalization of, 101, 115, 134–35; for same-sex parents, 148

Suzuki, Masakuni, 92, 93

Sweden: ART governance in, 11; multiple pregnancy in, 61, 67–68; NET guidelines in, 103, 108; public financing for IVF in, 67–68; single embryo transfer in, 67–68, 83–84, 119

Taipei Veterans General Hospital, 88, 91–95, 98, 105, 115

Taiwan: accreditation for IVF institutions in, 122; ART governance in, 100–104, 106; benefit and risk model in, 97; brain drain in, 90, 107n2; competition for IVF success in, 91–92; delayed parenthood in, 15, 17, 131, 135–39, 190; ethnic tensions in, 91–92, 107n4; fertility rate in, 17, 131, 137, 194–95; fetal reduction in, 97–100, 106, 157–59; framing of multiple pregnancy in, 15, 21; gatherings of IVF children in, 2, 104–5; international political isolation overcome by, 89–90; IVF as nationalist glory in, 20, 88–93, 100, 105–6; multiple pregnancy in, 5, 17, 61, 94–100, 127–28, 139–40, 158–59, 187, 190; National Health Insurance in, 110, 114, 165, 174; NET guidelines in, 16, 21, 101–4, 108, 112–20, 129–30, 139; population control policy in, 91; prenatal care in, 164–65; preterm births in, 17–18, 96, 175; public financing for IVF in, 123–24, 128n3, 194; public support for IVF in, 93; queer reproduction in, 144–48; registry building in, 122–23, 192; single embryo transfer in, 84, 120–28, 130,

194–95; US influence on IVF in, 90–91, 112–15, 189; voluntary childlessness in, 138, 141–44, 166

Taiwanese Society for Reproductive Medicine (TSRM): annual meetings of, 2–3, 121; establishment of, 101; NET guidelines from, 112–14, 117, 119–20, 139; seminars and continuing education classes by, 111; on subsidy program for IVF, 194; survey of reproductive knowledge by, 137

Taiwan LGBT Family Rights Advocacy, 145, 151n8

Taiwan Women's Link (TWL), 115

Tea Tree Moms, 146–47

Testart, Jacques, 91

test-tube babies. *See* in vitro fertilization

Thailand: cross-border use of ARTs in, 144–46; multiple pregnancy as viewed in, 7

Thompson, Charis, 7, 70

Timmermans, Stefan, 49

tocolytic therapy, 173, 181

traditional Chinese medicine, 1, 132, 134–36, 149, 190

transabdominal reduction, 43–45, 56n16, 98–99

transcervical suction aspiration, 43–44, 56n16, 98

transvaginal reduction, 43–45, 98–99

triplets: in benefit and risk model, 42; cerebral palsy rate for, 3, 154; fetal reduction for, 45, 153–55, 157, 160, 163; global rates of, 4, 6, 35, 57, 61, 158–59; healthcare costs for, 37, 55n11; low birthweight among, 36, 61; preterm births among, 105, 163, 174; queer reproduction and, 145. *See also* multiple pregnancy

TSRM. *See* Taiwanese Society for
    Reproductive Medicine
Tsuge, Azumi, 79
Tsuo, Kuo-Inn, 110
twins: in benefit and risk model,
    41–42; cerebral palsy rate for,
    3, 154; dragon-phoenix, 130,
    147; egg stimulation drugs and,
    35; fetal reduction for, 43, 45,
    157; global rates of, 4–6, 17,
    57, 187; healthcare costs for,
    37, 55n11; low birthweight
    among, 35–36; maternal
    mortality and, 182–83; preterm
    births among, 33, 105, 173–74;
    queer reproduction and,
    146–48; stillbirth risk for, 95.
    See also multiple pregnancy
TWL. *See* Taiwan Women's Link

umbilical cord blood banks, 70
United Kingdom: ART governance
    in, 11, 37; development of
    IVF in, 20, 23–27, 29–32; fetal
    reduction in, 46, 158; multiple
    pregnancy in, 17, 33–37, 61,
    69–70, 127; NET guidelines
    in, 6, 20, 48–51, 102–3, 108;
    public financing for IVF in,
    37, 69–70; single embryo
    transfer in, 69–70; success
    rate reporting for IVF in, 64;
    surrogacy process in, 187

United States: ART governance in,
    11; competition for IVF success
    in, 91; cross-border use of
    ARTs in, 146; development of
    IVF in, 30–32; fetal reduction
    in, 44, 46; healthcare priority
    list in, 86n5; influence on IVF
    in Taiwan, 90–91, 112–15,
    189; multiple pregnancy in,
    61, 187; NET guidelines in,
    16, 20, 49–51, 56n18, 103,
    111–14; single embryo transfer
    in, 3, 68, 71, 84; success rate
    reporting for IVF in, 63–64

value systems, 155, 161–62, 169
voluntary childlessness, 40, 138,
    141–44, 166

Waggoner, Miranda, 40
Wagner, Marsden G., 38, 40
Wang, Chien-Shun, 144
Whittaker, Andrea, 7
Wood, Carl, 42
World Health Organization (WHO),
    38, 175
Wu, Hsiang-Da, 94

Yanaihara, Takumi, 79
Yu, Ching-Ju, 162, 164, 171n6

zygote intrafallopian transfer
    (ZIFT), 95